Health Psychology in Digital, Educational, and Creative Contexts

Agathi Argyriadi
American University, Dubai, UAE

Alexandros Argyriadis
https://orcid.org/0000-0001-5754-4787
Hellenic Mediterranean University, Greece

IGI Global
Scientific Publishing
Publishing Tomorrow's Research Today

Vice President of Editorial	Melissa Wagner
Director of Acquisitions	Mikaela Felty
Director of Book Development	Jocelynn Hessler
Production Manager	Mike Brehm
Cover Design	Jose Rosado

Published in the United States of America by
IGI Global Scientific Publishing
701 East Chocolate Avenue
Hershey, PA, 17033, USA
Tel: 717-533-8845 | Fax: 717-533-7115
Website: https://www.igi-global.com E-mail: cust@igi-global.com

Library of Congress Cataloging-in-Publication Data

LCCN: 2026032283 (CIP Data Pending)
ISBN13: 9798260030851
Isbn13Softcover: 9798260030868
EISBN13: 9798260030875
British Cataloguing in Publication Data
A Cataloguing in Publication record for this book is available from the British Library.

Table of Contents

Detailed Table of Contents

This chapter provides an exploration of psychological resilience, challenging traditional views of the concept as a fixed trait. Moving beyond narrow models, the discussion supports resilience as an interplay of biological, social, and psychological factors that build an individual's ability to recover and grow from their stressors. The chapter reviews strength-based perspectives, evaluating the role of attachment, developmental perspectives, and life tasks. This includes diverse populations, including racial, ethnic, gender, and sexual minorities, highlighting how systemic factors shape resilience and the crucial role of community support. The chapter also investigates resilience in acute and chronic health challenges, and collective resilience during large-scale crises, emphasising meaning-making. The chapter also reviews established resilience-building techniques such as CBT, ACT, digital health tools, mobile applications, and telehealth platforms to build resilience. Ultimately, the chapter urges a collaborative strategy to foster a more globally resilient society.

The concept of health has altered dramatically throughout time. It used to be primarily concerned with not becoming sick, a deficit-oriented viewpoint. It has now evolved into something that emphasises well-being and positive outcomes in life. This chapter examines the forefront of that transition. It explains how to build and implement personalised digital PPIs. These draw on the PERMA model of well-being and Self-Determination Theory. Digital technologies make them scalable and accessible while also being able to personalise things. The chapter proposes that humans should be at the centre of digital PPI design. It emphasises relational and ethical aspects right from the outset. The chapter contributes an integrative, ethically grounded framework for designing and implementing digital PPIs that preserve human empathy while advancing scalable well-being solutions.

Quick commerce delivery workers in Southeast Asia face significant health risks from long working hours, environmental exposure, and limited access to healthcare. This narrative review explores how telemedicine can address these challenges by analysing literature from South and Southeast Asia. Thematic analysis highlights three key areas: barriers to adoption (low digital literacy, poor internet connectivity, financial limitations, and mistrust), policy and platform gaps (fragmented regulations, weak accountability, and data security concerns), and climate-linked vulnerabilities (heat stress, pollution, and mental health strain). Findings suggest that telemedicine offers affordable consultations, mental health support, and flexible digital platforms that are well-suited to the unpredictable schedules of gig workers. However, broader adoption requires policy integration, literacy training, and inclusive initiatives. While evidence remains emergent, telemedicine shows strong potential as a scalable, preventive health solution for quick commerce workers in Southeast Asia.

Art therapy stands at the intersection of health psychology, education, and child development, offering unique ways to support resilience, meaning-making, and well-being in primary schools. Rooted in health psychology, it demonstrates how embodied creative expression promotes adaptive behavior and holistic wellness. Since children often lack the vocabulary to express complex emotions, art activities—drawing, painting, collage—enable symbolic communication and self-discovery. Research confirms benefits such as reduced anxiety, improved focus, and stronger relationships. Multisensory art-making enhances neural integration, memory, and regulation. Activities like "safe place" drawings, "strength shields," and group murals foster resilience, inclusion, and collaboration. While not a substitute for clinical therapy, arts-based interventions in classrooms provide preventative, accessible tools that promote emotional health and cultivate creativity, affirming children's innate capacity to flourish.

Health psychology examines links between psychological processes, health, and social context. Within this field, art functions as a mediator of resilience, identity, and behavioural change. Creative expression is an embodied practice through which people process experience and develop coping strategies. Engagement in visual arts, music, dance, or writing bridges cognition, emotion, and bodily awareness, turning illness into meaning (Stuckey & Nobel, 2010; Fuchs, 2018). Dance, for example, aligns movement and rhythm to reduce stress (Koch et al., 2014), while visual art externalises trauma (Kaimal & Ray, 2017). Such practices resonate with enactive approaches to cognition (Varela et al., 1991). Meaning-making is central in illness (Park, 2010); art provides symbolic language for suffering and agency (Puig et al., 2006). It fosters resilience, self-efficacy, and social connectedness (Forgeard & Elstein, 2014). Thus, art enriches health psychology as embodied creativity, offering holistic tools for wellbeing and behavioural change.

The intersection of art, neuroscience, and health psychology offers a transformative lens on primary education, showing how creative engagement fosters cognitive, emotional, and behavioural growth. Neuroscience highlights children's heightened neuroplasticity, making them highly responsive to artistic experiences that stimulate neural networks. Arts practices activate motor, sensory, emotional, and cognitive regions, strengthening executive functions and socio-emotional regulation. Health psychology frames art as a behavioural intervention that supports resilience, coping, and wellbeing. Evidence shows that creative expression reduces stress, enhances motivation through dopamine release, and fosters prosocial behaviour. Activities like drawing and storytelling help children symbolise experiences, building self-efficacy and meaning. Art thus bridges brushstrokes and brainwaves, integrating scientific insight with humanistic values to position creativity as a cornerstone of holistic learning and resilience in education.

Preface

The rapid pace of technological innovation, changing educational environments, and evolving models of work are reshaping the ways people experience health and psychological well-being. These developments have created new opportunities for promoting resilience and improving quality of life, but they have also introduced challenges that were scarcely imaginable only a generation ago. Health psychology now extends well beyond hospitals and clinics. It informs digital health, education, workplace practice, creative expression, and community development, offering valuable insights into how individuals adapt to an increasingly interconnected world.

This volume brings together contributions that reflect this expanding scope of the discipline. Although the chapters examine diverse topics, they are united by a shared conviction that psychological well-being is influenced by the environments people inhabit, the technologies they use, the relationships they develop, and the opportunities they have to create meaning in everyday life. Throughout the book, theory and practice are presented as complementary rather than separate pursuits, with each chapter illustrating how psychological knowledge can be translated into interventions that are relevant to contemporary society.

CHAPTER OVERVIEW

The opening chapters consider resilience as a lifelong process and explore the growing role of digital technologies in supporting mental health. Human-centred approaches to digital positive psychology demonstrate how technological innovation can be designed around individual needs rather than technological capability alone. The discussion of telemedicine further illustrates how digital health services have become an important means of improving access to care, particularly for populations facing geographical, economic, or social barriers.

Digital environments also influence the ways people learn, work, and connect with one another. The experiences of young people in Jammu and Kashmir, together with discussions of psychological safety within virtual teams and the well-being of faculty working in private higher education, reveal that psychological health is shaped by far more than individual characteristics. Organisational culture, social support, educational systems, and the quality of interpersonal relationships remain fundamental determinants of well-being, even when interactions increasingly occur through digital platforms.

Alongside these technological developments, the volume highlights the enduring value of creativity as a resource for psychological growth. The chapters devoted to art therapy, embodied creativity, and the relationship between neuroscience and artistic expression demonstrate that creative activity is not simply an educational enrichment but an important pathway through which children and adults explore emotions, construct meaning, and strengthen resilience. These contributions encourage readers to view creativity as an integral component of psychological health rather than as an activity existing on its margins.

The final chapters turn to mathematics education, examining innovative pedagogical approaches that seek to reduce anxiety while fostering confidence, curiosity, and engagement among young learners. The use of Dienes Blocks and Cuisenaire Rods illustrates how thoughtfully designed educational practices can influence emotional development as well as academic achievement. Such perspectives remind us that learning environments are also health-promoting environments, capable of shaping children's beliefs about themselves, their abilities, and their future.

One of the strengths of this collection lies in its interdisciplinary character. Psychology is placed in dialogue with education, digital innovation, neuroscience, organisational studies, public health, and the creative arts. Rather than treating these disciplines as separate domains, the contributors demonstrate how they enrich one another when addressing complex questions concerning human adaptation and well-being. This breadth reflects the direction in which health psychology itself continues to evolve.

The chapters gathered here are intended for researchers, educators, psychologists, health professionals, students, and practitioners interested in understanding how psychological principles can be applied across diverse contemporary settings. Whether the focus is digital intervention, educational innovation, workplace well-being, or creative practice, the underlying objective remains the same: to identify approaches that support healthier, more resilient individuals and communities.

The editors are deeply grateful to all contributing authors for the care and expertise reflected in their work. Their willingness to share ideas from different cultural, disciplinary, and professional perspectives has given this volume both its richness and its relevance. We also acknowledge the reviewers and editorial staff whose thoughtful feedback has strengthened the quality of the final manuscript.

We hope this book encourages readers to think broadly about the future of health psychology. As societies continue to change, the field will increasingly be called upon to respond to new forms of human experience shaped by technology, education, creativity, and global interconnectedness. The chapters that follow offer not definitive answers but thoughtful contributions to an ongoing conversation about how psychological science can help individuals and communities flourish in a rapidly changing world.

Dr. Agathi Argyriadi

Dr. Alexandros Argyriadis

Chapter 1
Psychological Resilience Across the Lifespan and in Diverse Communities

Shreya Giridhar Chenji
http://orcid.org/0009-0009-3342-7848
PES University, India

Shreya Ghosh
http://orcid.org/0009-0008-9309-3424
PES University, India

ABSTRACT

This chapter provides an exploration of psychological resilience, challenging traditional views of the concept as a fixed trait. Moving beyond narrow models, the discussion supports resilience as an interplay of biological, social, and psychological factors that build an individual's ability to recover and grow from their stressors. The chapter reviews strength-based perspectives, evaluating the role of attachment, developmental perspectives, and life tasks. This includes diverse populations, including racial, ethnic, gender, and sexual minorities, highlighting how systemic factors shape resilience and the crucial role of community support. The chapter also investigates resilience in acute and chronic health challenges, and collective resilience during large-scale crises, emphasising meaning-making. The chapter also reviews established resilience-building techniques such as CBT, ACT, digital health tools, mobile applications, and telehealth platforms to build resilience. Ultimately, the chapter urges a collaborative strategy to foster a more globally resilient society.

DOI: 10.4018/979-8-2600-3085-1.ch001

INTRODUCTION

Introduction to resilience

Adversity refers to tough situations that introduce difficulties in the lives of individuals. How these individuals react to the adversity dictates whether an individual will flourish and grow from the adversity or whether they will experience hopelessness or failure (Singh & Sharma, 2017). Positive psychology, as given by Seligman and Csikszentmihalyi (2014), endorses the shift in focus of psychology research and practice from fixing problems or unwanted challenges to enhancing favourable qualities. In the current era, individuals are often confronted by an overwhelming amount of challenges that influence various aspects of their lives. These stressors can range from global issues (such as a global pandemic) to personal pressures and workplace concerns. Positive psychology research aims to explain why certain individuals are able to tolerate and recover from the adversity and stressors that they experience (Fullerton et al., 2021). Our reactions to stress are influenced by biological factors, social factors, and psychological factors such as mindset (Southwick et al., 2014).

Defining Resilience

There is no common definition of resilience, even though the concept is used worldwide to explain reactions to adversity (Aburn et al., 2016). Instead, various models and definitions of resilience from various physiological and psychological perspectives explain the concept. These define resilience as a trait, a continuum, or a binary approach (Southwick et al., 2014). This makes it complex to understand resilience, especially when we examine resilience through various developmental stages and cultural contexts. However, similar themes that have been recognised when defining resilience are experiencing stressors or adversities, and the capacity to positively adapt to them (Fletcher & Sarkar., 2013).

Modern studies on psychological resilience generally include four main components: 1) pre-adversity, 2) adversity, 3) the resilient outcome, and 4) predictors of these outcomes (Bonanno et al., 2015). When defining resilience, it is crucial to clarify whether we are looking at it as a stable characteristic (a trait), an ongoing process, or a successful outcome (Southwick et al, 2014). Integrating resilience research into clinical practice, psychological intervention, and medicine is driving a paradigm shift. In studying the effects of trauma, this change represents a changed focus from traditional models, which are more deficit-focused, to a strength-based approach. This model does not solely focus on the treatment of existing conditions;

it also focuses on the prevention of illness and improving psychological competence (Southwick et al, 2014).

Biological Basis of Resilience

Resilience is an active process including various biological adaptations that benefit healthy functioning in the face of stressors. The central component in the biology of resilience is the hypothalamic-pituitary-adrenal axis or the HPA axis, which is the body's primary stress response system. Chronic stress can lead to dysregulation of the HPA axis (Russo et al., 2012). A higher ratio of ehydroepiandrosterone (which can counteract the effects of cortisol) to cortisol has been associated with better coping mechanisms and reduced stress-related symptoms (Russo et al., 2012; Ryan & Ryznar, 2022).

Twin studies suggest that resilience is partially heritable, since genes involved in the regulation of neurotransmitters like serotonin and dopamine, along with CRHR1 and FKBP5 (genes related to the HPA axis), have been identified as important in protecting against Major Depressive Disorder and PTSD (Russo et al., 2012; Ryan & Ryznar, 2022). Epigenetic modifications, such as DNA methylation of the FKBP5 gene was observed in Holocaust survivors (though the level of methylation was lower) and may act as a protective factor against adversity (Ryan & Ryznar, 2022).

The biological interplay of factors influencing resilience includes genetic predisposition, epigenetic modifications, regulation of the neuroendocrine system, and neural adaptations, and can help counteract stress-induced changes in the brain.

Critique of Narrow Models of Resilience

Early research, including simplistic or biomedical models, treated resilience as a stable personality trait that individuals either possessed or did not, often comparing it with characteristics such as hardiness, optimism, or an internal locus of control (Rutter, 2006). When viewing resilience as an interaction between genes and the environment rather than solely biological determinants, challenges to the biomedical view include viewing resilience as an interactive process, evaluating resilience from a lifespan perspective, determining which psychological processes constitute protective factors for adverse situations, variations in coping among different communities and cultures, and exposure to risk.

This chapter aims to provide a comprehensive exploration of psychological resilience by examining its expression and development across the human lifespan and within diverse populations. The initial focus will be on understanding how resilience manifests and can be nurtured through distinct developmental stages, from the foundational role of a secure attachment style to identity formation in adolescence, to generativity in adulthood. It will explore how specific adversities in each life phase (as well as protective factors) shape the ability of an individual to adapt and thrive. The chapter will then analyse the purpose of resilience as well as how it is expressed across various diverse populations. This includes moving beyond a universal model to consider how sociocultural context, economic conditions, careers, and group identities can influence resilience pathways. This analysis can help highlight that the very definition and development of resilience are shaped by an individual's environment and their lived experiences, rather than their resilience being a binary or a fixed trait. Ultimately, the chapter seeks to bridge theoretical knowledge with real-world application to offer insights into the creation of more tailored and culturally sensitive interventions. This chapter is theoretical in nature and utilises secondary data collection from peer-reviewed sources on the subjects of positive psychology, neurobiology, sociology, health psychology, and medical sciences.

RESILIENCE ACROSS THE LIFESPAN

Defining Resilience from a Developmental Perspective

To move beyond viewing resilience as a fixed trait and to conceptualise it as a dynamic process, resilience can be defined from modern perspectives using a developmental approach. From a developmental perspective, resilience can be defined as the capacity of a system to adapt successfully to challenges that threaten its function, survival, or future development (Masten & Barnes, 2018). This definition is scalable; it can be applied to individuals (here, children), but also their families, schools, or communities. Resilience from a developmental perspective is not a trait, i.e., it is not something a child has or possesses as a stable, static concept. Resilience is instead a process that unfolds through positive adaptation (Masten & Barnes, 2018); the capacity of the individual to adapt can be strengthened or weakened by their life experiences. Masten & Barnes (2018) outline three specific questions that have guided research in resilience. These questions are necessary to understand resilience from a developmental point of view. These questions include:

1. What are the challenges? This involves identifying and measuring specific adversities that threaten the system. This question is broad and applicable to various challenges, from personal challenges such as individual neglect to broader challenges like poverty or other socioeconomic challenges.
2. How is the person doing? This question adds to the definition of resilience by creating criteria for what constitutes adaptive successes. This, according to

Masten & Barnes, can be assessed through multiple categories, like achieving age-related developmental tasks and showcasing social competence.

3. What processes support success? The main goal of resilience research is to pinpoint the protective factors which can display why some individuals adapt successfully, whereas others are unable to. These factors, as constructed over decades of research, include caring and supportive relationships, effective parenting, and self-regulation abilities, and represent the adaptive systems that benefit resilience.

Early childhood is a sensitive period where stress can have lasting negative effects; this is also a key window of opportunity for interventions that can foster resilience (Masten & Barnes, 2018).

The Process of Developing Resilience Across the Lifespan

An assessment of the impact of various factors during the developmental trajectory of resilience throughout the lifespan can be structured through developmental frameworks. Foundational theories, such as Bowlby's (influenced by his Kleinian education, as per Bowlby, 1944; Bretherton & American Psychological Association, Inc., 1992) and Ainsworth's Attachment theory, provide a crucial lens for understanding how the quality of early caregiver relationships establishes an internal working model that can shape an individual's ability to adapt to future stressors. Adding to this, Erikson's theory of psychosocial development offers a stage-based model elucidating the age-specific psychosocial crises that individuals must navigate. Resolving these crises (Orenstein & Lewis, 2022), from the identity process in adolescence to how middle-aged adults resolve their generativity stage conflict, can contribute to the development of ego strengths. Integrating these perspectives can help researchers analyse resilience as a dynamic and cumulative process rather than a static one. This section will assess two key developmental frameworks: Bowlby and Ainsworth's attachment theory and Erikson's Psychosocial stages, and evaluate their effect on resilience across early childhood, middle childhood, adolescence, and adulthood in diverse populations.

Bowlby's and Ainsworth's attachment theory

Bowlby's and Ainsworth's attachment theory is a foundational framework in developmental psychology, positing that the emotional bond formed between an infant and primary caregiver is a necessity for lifelong emotional development (Bretherton & American Psychological Association, Inc., 1992). Bowlby was dissatisfied with the the explanations of a child's bond with their mother, since both the psychoanalytic view and the behaviorist view saw it as a learned dependency. Bowlby argued that attachment ensures survival of an infant through proximity to a protective caregiver (Bretherton & American Psychological Association, Inc., 1992). From his early clinical work such as his 1944 study on *Forty-Four Juvenile Thieves,* Bowlby observed a link between maternal deprivation and maladjustment later in life (Bowlby, 1944). Bowlby's other enduring theory (Internal Working Model) argued that through mental representations of the self, infants construct a mental representation of their relationship. This model becomes a prototype for all future relationships, guiding their expectations, emotions, and behavior through life (Cassidy et al., 2013).

Later on, Mary Ainsworth provided empirical testing of these ideas. Ainsworth created the Strange Situation procedure to assess the quality of an infant's attachment to their caregiver. The procedure consisted of eight episodes of brief separation and reunion of an infant with their caregiver over a span of 20 minutes in an unfamiliar playroom (Bretherton & American Psychological Association, Inc., 1992). The researchers then observed how the infant uses caregivers as a secure base when distressed. Ainsworth and her colleagues identified three types of attachment based on this experiment in 1978, which were secure, insecure-ambivalent, and insecure-avoidant.

Ainsworth found a link between attachment style and the quality of maternal care (Bretherton & American Psychological Association, 1992). Later, a fourth category (Disorganised attachment) was identified by Ainsworth's student (Bretherton & American Psychological Association, Inc., 1992).

Since then, various studies have linked the importance of secure attachment to the emotional expression and coping of individuals in the following stages of life.

Infancy, Early, and Middle Childhood

Children develop their models of emotional expression and regulation from their interactions with their caregivers (Ainsworth et al., 1985; Bowlby, 1944). A 2023 study by Tabacknick et al. investigated the association between secure attachment in infancy and the child's emotional expression in middle childhood within a high-risk sample of families. The sample (N=78) included children who are at risk of maltreatment since they are known to have a higher likelihood of insecure attachment (avoidant, resistant, and disorganised attachments). In middle childhood, the children's positive and negative affect (along with the appropriateness of their emotional expression) was coded from video recordings of the two discussion tasks utilised by the study. The study included a longitudinal perspective, linking attachment to observed emotional functioning in middle childhood. Secure attachment was associated with greater emotional flexibility and significantly more appropriate ability to downregulate distress as compared to the insecure peers.

In 2023, Quintana et al. conducted an examination of the perceived security in childhood attachment and the influence of this on adult self-concept. The study suggested that this is mediated by resilience and self-esteem. Self-concept refers to an individual's perception of their own characteristics, abilities, and values (Quintana et al., 2023). This relationship between secure attachment, resilience, and self-concept emphasises that trust in a caregiver's availability and sensitivity can foster a coherent self-concept in adulthood (Bowlby, 1944; Ainsworth et al., 1985). Resilience plays a role that is mediating in nature, which means that secure attachment builds a foundation for resilience. Post this, resilience reinforces a positive self-perception (Quintana et al., 2023). The study also investigated positive self-evaluation as a mediator for developing a positive self-concept. The study utilised a quantitative approach (cross-sectional design) with 383 adults. Data was collected using the following scales: The CaMir-R Questionnaire (to measure perceived security in childhood attachment), the AF-5 Self-Concept Scale (to assess five dimensions of self-concept, the Connor and Davidson Resilience Scale (to measure global resilience), and the Rosenberg Self-Esteem Scale (to evaluate positive self-esteem). The sequential mediation model was tested using the PROCESS Macro model. The study found that there were significant positive correlations between all four key variables (perceived security of attachment, resilience, positive self-esteem, and self-concept). The study found that the sequential mediation effect showed that perceived security positively influences resilience, which in turn enhances positive self-esteem, which leads to a higher positive self-concept. This provided strong evidence that the influence of childhood attachment was significantly explained by the development of resilience and positive self-esteem.

Erikson's Theory of Psychosocial Development

Erikson's 1950 theory of psychosocial development is a foundational framework for understanding human growth across the entire lifespan. Each stage is characterised by a specific psychosocial conflict that must be resolved. This theory was revolutionary for being one of the first theories to extend developmental theory beyond childhood and adolescence, emphasising that development does not stop at adolescence or early adulthood, but continues across the lifespan in an interplay of various factors (biological, psychological, and social) (Sokol, 2009). Erikson's (1950s) theory outlines the following developmental tasks, of which successful resolution results in the development of a corresponding virtue or stress, whereas failure leads to a maladaptive outcome. The outcome of each stage, as posited by Erikson in the 1950s, influences the resolution of subsequent stages. The two stages evaluated here, from their significance in resilience studies, are identity vs role confusion in adolescence and generativity vs stagnation in middle adulthood.

Adolescence

A 2023 study (Bogaerts et al) investigated the developmental pathways of identity formation in a sample of Flemish adolescents (N=2,123). The study focused on adaptive and disturbed dimensions of identity. It aimed to evaluate how various developmental trajectories are associated with key indicators of psychological functioning, such as self-esteem, resilience, symptoms of depression, and features of Borderline Personality Disorder. The study evaluated three dimensions of identity in the adolescents, including consolidated identity (a coherent sense of self), disturbed identity (confusion, instability), and a lack of identity (inner feelings of emptiness). The researchers used longitudinal data to identify distinct patterns of how these changed over time in different subgroups of adolescents. The analysis displayed four developmental trajectory groups. The first group was identified as the adaptive identity group. This group, consisting of nearly 70% of the sample, displayed a stable sense of consolidated identity. This included a low level of identity disturbance as well. The adolescents in this group consistently displayed high resilience as well as high self-esteem and low negative symptoms (depressive symptoms with Borderline Personality disorder features). The second group was the Diffused Identity group, showing the opposite pattern. This group made up approximately 12% of the sample and had a consistently low sense of consolidated identity, a high level of disturbed identity, and a lack of identity. They reported low levels of resilience and self-esteem, and high negative symptoms. The third group, the identity progression group, included approximately 8% of the population. These adolescents showed improvement over time, with an increase in their consolidated identity and a decrease in their disturbed identity. This shift in their identity included an improvement in their psychological functioning. The fourth and last group, Identity regression, included approximately 10% of the sample. These adolescents began the study with a healthy identity but experienced a decline. The findings emphasise that the process of identity formation is deeply connected to adaptive psychological functioning. A stable identity is a key factor in adaptive psychological processes such as resilience, whereas emerging identity problems could represent a significant risk factor for psychopathology.

A longitudinal study conducted by Shrima et al. in 2024 aimed to understand two developmental trajectories: identity formation and resilience. The study sought to understand how these two processes occurred over time and interacted with each other. The study was based on the five-dimensional dual cycle model (including the dimensions of commitment making, exploration in breadth, and ruminative exploration) developed by Luyckx et al., and evaluated resilience in a non-Western and under-resourced setting. The study followed 546 adolescents over a 12-month period, utilising the Dimensions of Identity Development Scale and a subscale of the Resilience Questionnaire for Middle Adolescents in Township Schools to measure the constructs. The findings highlighted the effects of context on adolescent development. Firstly, stable identity trajectories. The authors suggested that the lack of resources and opportunities in the community may have limited the adolescents' ability to explore different identity alternatives. However, resilience showed significant fluctuation. There was a notable decrease in resilience, coinciding with the timings of the COVID-19 lockdown. This furthers the idea that resilience is contingent on contextual stressors or not a stable trait. The results underscore the need for support systems that benefit resilience and healthy identity exploration in vulnerable youth.

Adulthood

A 2023 study by Ong et al. examined the relationship between generativity and social asymmetry (the discrepancy between the objective level of loneliness and the subjective feeling of loneliness of an individual. Individuals, according to Ong et al., can be either socially vulnerable (experience more loneliness as compared to their level of isolation) or socially resilient. The study, conducted in 2 waves (2008 and 2012) of the Midlife Japan Survey, included 645 adults aged 30-79. These adults were situated in the metropolitan area of Tokyo. The study concluded that generativity was linked to social resilience. However, a change in the level of generativity of the adults was not a predictive factor of social asymmetry in the second wave. The authors suggest that this may be due to the fact that Generativity is a relatively stable aspect. They also suggested that a four-year interval was an insufficient time gap to capture a change that was meaningful to the individuals.

A 2014 study by Landes et al. investigated the impact of childhood adversity on well-being later in life with a focus on the role of midlife generativity as a potential indicator for resilience. Childhood adversity was described as harsh parenting (familial adversity) or poverty (socioeconomic adversity). The capacity to positively develop and create meaning in their lives is an important facet of Generativity vs Stagnation (Landes et al., 2014). The study measures two primary outcomes: physical health status and psychological well-being. The study utilised a sample of 636 white men from the 73-year longitudinal study of Adult Development. The study revealed that the men who experienced childhood adversity from both cohorts were less likely to achieve generativity. Generativity in the rest of the sample reduced the psychological impact of the adversity they experienced, showing a higher level of resilience.

In 2025, Jung et al. provided an in-depth evaluation of the factors that could predict generativity among LGBTQ individuals in late life. The study's findings revealed that a number of psychological factors were associated with higher levels of generativity. These included resilience, social support, and community engagement. Within the group, resilience was a stronger predictor of generativity, elaborating on how posttraumatic growth was potentially possible. The research also noted that certain factors held different levels of importance for different age groups in the given sample. For the younger participants of the study, resilience as well as the size of their social network were revealed to be stronger predictors of their capacity for generativity and meaning making.

In 2020, Windle et al. aimed to understand how resilience develops in older adults who are managing multiple health problems (co-morbidity). The model within which the qualitative research is framed is ecopsychosocial. This means that the resilience of these individuals, as theorised by the authors, arises from an interplay of various factors such as personal, social, and environmental. This paper describes adversity as the presence of two or more chronic health conditions, something that is a fairly common challenge in later life. The study employed semi-structured interviews with its 20 participants (aged 65 and above). The findings revealed four primary life experiences that shaped the participants' resilience. The life experiences were childhood experiences (involving material hardship as well as family responsibility), work and employment (this was a formative source of their identity and contributed greatly to their capacity for meaning making), adverse experiences (bereavement and significant illness specifically), and caring experiences (providing and receiving care). Three mechanisms for resilience identified were character and self-identity, a positive outlook and an active life, and strong connections with family and community.

From the above studies, we can conclude that resilience is not a static trait, but a process that unfolds over a lifetime. Resilience is also not an isolated concept, since it is clear that it affects and is affected by the context, the role of other individuals, and significant life events.

RESILIENCE IN DIVERSE COMMUNITIES

Racial and Ethnic Minorities and Systemic Factors

For racial and ethnic minorities, resilience cannot be evaluated without considering systemic and institutional factors that contribute to chronic stress. Race is a social construct that groups individuals based on physical characteristics. It has historically been used to establish dominance over another group (Chang et al., 2007). Racism is an ideology that considers White individuals to be superior in comparison to other races, including both behavioural and institutional practices in its oppression (Chang et al., 2007). Ethnicity, also attributed at birth, refers to a group of individuals who share characteristics including a common culture, historical memories, and generally a symbolic link to a homeland (Berreman, 1972). Racial and ethnic minorities experience increased amounts of self-blame and poor mental health due to racism. A strong sense of ethnic identity can offer some protective factors against this self-blame. Individual factors are limited in their ability to protect against systemic discrimination (Barrita & Wong-Padoongpatt, 2023). Additionally, among diverse ethnic communities, meaning-making often includes a non-eurocentric model of spiritual beliefs, stronger community support and reliance, and collective ways of coping with adversity (Theron & Theron, 2014). This section will elaborate on the interaction between individual protective factors and systemic oppression.

Research on the effects of systemic oppression also aims to shift the focus of the field from solely deficit-based models to strength-based and trauma-informed perspectives, synthesising protective factors against adversity. This assesses factors that disproportionally affect racial minorities' youth. At an individual level, positive self-concept and effective coping skills during adversity (resilience) were identified as protective factors. At the family level, strengths included strong family bonds, supportive parents, and transmission of cultural values. At the community level, resources for resilience included cultural connectedness, ethnic and racial identities, spirituality, and supportive relationships with their peers. Yoon et al. provide an interconnected system to support the well-being of youth who are part of minority groups, with resilience being one of the main factors due to the amount of adversity faced.

Critical questions surrounding the impact of racial microaggressions are regarding the extent to which protective factors are effective (Yoon et al., 2025). Barrita & Wong-Padoongpatt (2023) explored whether resilience and connection to ethnic identity can moderate the negative psychological effects of oppression. When People of Colour experience racial microaggressions, they sometimes internalise the blame for the actions of their microaggressors. Resilience and connection to ethnic identity can offer protective effects, but do not completely mitigate the psychological distress. Individual-level factors need to be understood within the larger sociopolitical context.

In 2021, Wilcox et al. studied ecological factors that mediate the resilience of adolescents in rural Eastern North Carolina. The study utilised five groups (with a total sample of 49) of African American and Latinx adolescents aged 12-16. The study found that the most significant factors decreasing resilience were related to two factors: social justice and power and control. The most significant risk factors identified were racism and discrimination. Adversities faced by the African American adolescents included racial profiling and police brutality. The study also identified four tensions that *enhanced* resilience: cultural adherence, identity, cohesion, and access to material resources. Findings in another factor, relationships, highlighted that the role of the family on resilience was dual in nature; supportive relationships with mothers and grandmothers improved coping abilities for challenges related to suicidal ideation, whereas individuals with parents who engaged in substance abuse or were absent experienced higher levels of adversity due to their relationships rather than being protected by them (Wilcox et al., 2021). The study calls for interventions that empower ethnic minority youth and address the systemic inequities they face. Fleming & Ledogar (2008) also evaluate the role of community support in the development of resilience. This can lead to protective factors for the entire community. For example, there was a strong correlation between a First Nations community's efforts to preserve its cultural heritage and lower the rates of suicide (Chalnder & Lalonde, 1998).

There were three models that explained how positive factors can mitigate the effects of adversity. The first is a compensatory model, where a positive factor directly counteracts the effects of a risk factor (Andersson & Ledogar, 2008; Fleming & Ledogar, 2008). The protective model explains that positive factors can either improve the effect of other positive factors or reduce the effect of risks, but they cannot completely mitigate the risk (Fleming & Ledogar, 2008). The Challenge model suggests that exposure to a moderate level of adversity can build coping skills (Fleming & Ledogar, 2008).

Estrada-Moreno et al. in 2025 assessed the role of resilience as a resource for immigrants. The study sought to identify what factors promote well-being and successful adaptation in the immigrant population, who generally experience increased amounts of racial and ethnic discrimination. Immigrants endure large amounts of psychological negative symptoms during the different phases of their immigration process, which greatly affects their psychological and physical health (Anisman et al., 2024). During migration, refugees and migrants often encounter a set of challenges and then experience acculturative stress once settled in the destination country (Anisman et al., 2024). There is a strong positive relationship between resilience and successful social integration (Estrada-Moreno et al., 2025). More resilient immigrants were more likely to report higher satisfaction with life. They were also more likely to engage with social events within their new community, displaying successful integration.

GENDER AND SEXUAL MINORITIES AND RESILIENCE: SYSTEMIC FACTORS

Gender (typically used to assign individuals to male or female categories) is a construct influenced by biological, psychosocial, and cultural elements (Mayer et al., 2008). Sexual orientation refers to individuals who identify with a particular sexual minority group (Johnson et al., 2008). Gender and Sexual Minorities are populations that are statistically misrepresented and have decreased health outcomes due to discrimination (Mayer et al., 2008).

A central focus in resilience studies in Gender and Sexual Minorities research is shifting from a deficit-based model to a strengths-based health promotion approach. This refers to the focus on HIV (Human immunodeficiency virus) infection rates, rates of sexually transmitted diseases, obesity and depression (Colpitts & Gahagan, 2016). This reinforces negative stereotypes and can have negative health outcomes for these individuals (Colpitts & Gahagan, 2016; Morales et al., 2017). Most models used to measure resilience (such as the compensatory, protective, and challenge models) did not apply to LGBTQ populations since the focus in these models is often individual-level, whereas LGBTQ health disparities are often created because of systemic adversity. To address these disparities, resilience studies need to be from an intersectional lens (Colpitts & Galahan, 2016).

The persistent stress experienced by LGBTQ individuals can be explained as a direct result of their marginalised social position, which subjects them to injustice, discrimination, violence, and stigmatisation (Meyer, 1995; Meyer, 2003; Meyer, 2013; Meyer, 2015). 'Minority stress' (Meyer, 1995) describes stress as originating from minority status, which is particularly relevant in schools, where students who are bullied or harassed by peers are likely to suffer higher stress levels (Ferbežar et al., 2025). Additionally, school environments are generally where Gender and sexual minorities experience their first signs of discrimination (Stańczykiewicz & Senczyszyn, 2024), leading to negative outcomes at various levels, from increased likelihood of not attending school. Resilience theories for LGBTQ individuals suggest that adverse experiences do not necessarily always lead to negative outcomes, but that LGBTQ individuals can cultivate resilience and flourish (Meyer, 2015).

In 2025, Ferbežar et al. used qualitative narrative interviews to explore resilience among 27 students who were part of Gender and Sexual Minorities. The study aimed to identify key stressors as well as protective factors. Individual factors included personal knowledge, positive characteristics, and optimism. However, community-based factors, such as social support from friends, affirming school staff, and family, were noted as significantly more protective. By addressing these aspects of their students' experiences, educational institutions can support their LGBTQ students more effectively (Ferbežar et al., 2025). In 2022, the Trevor Project conducted a study on nearly forty thousand LGBTQ youth from ages 13-24. The study found that external factors associated with higher resilience were affirming families and schools, a strong sense of community, and supportive social networks. The study also found that the older youth in the sample (ages 18 to 24) had significantly higher resilience than younger adolescents, which suggests that resilience can be developed over time.

Resilience is a factor that predicts generativity in older adults (Jung et al., 2025). The findings highlight the potential for posttraumatic growth, where experiences of adversity turn into a capacity to be resilience. Resilience was seen as a powerful predictor of this generative capacity compared to other factors, especially for the younger participants (of a sample greater than 2000) in the late-life sample (who ranged in age from 50 to over 100), suggesting that the ability to adapt and grow from challenges is important for developing a generative outlook.

Individual characteristics that act as protective factors can be beneficial to Gender and Sexual minorities. It is also clear that the role of community-based support in coping with adversity is far more significant. A better understanding of resilience in this population requires a shift away from individualistic models.

Resilience in Health Challenges and Large-Scale Crises

Resilience in Health Challenges

Resilience in health challenges represents how individuals adapt to acute and chronic health challenges, which require long-term management (Gheshlagh et al., 2016). For acute stress, resilience includes the ability to manage essential functions a crisis (Emami et al., 2024). In this context, resilience does not always mean the ability to bounce back after the stressor. The focus for individuals experiencing chronic illness is more about finding ways to make meaning despite the ongoing challenges (Eggenberger et al., 2011). This section explores resilience in health challenges, community-based resilience in emergencies, and the importance of developing context-specific strategies that build on the strengths of the community.

The entire family dynamic and roles can change as lives adapt to an individual's chronic illness (Eggenberger et al., 2011). For example, cancer survivors often express psychological distress from their disease and from the adverse side effects of their cancer therapies. They also struggle with carrying on with regular life (Mosher & DuHamel, 2006). Similarly, the growing prevalence of co-morbid health problems in aging populations is a challenge to maintaining their well-being. A life course perspective for elderly adults includes a framework where resilience is developed throughout a lifetime of adverse experiences, including their early life, work experience, bereavement, and illness (Windle et al., 2020).

From a health psychology perspective, creating resilience involves a dynamic process that aims to reduce these negative effects. Better health outcomes, such as decreased levels of distress as well as better physical condition, were recorded in patients who had a higher positive outlook (Segerstrom et al., 2018). Meaning-making processes can provide a sense of control over the lives of individuals who experience chronic illness. These interventions, including meaning-making components, can reduce the level of psychological distress being experienced (Ghosh & Deb, 2017). During health crises like COVID-19, individuals with chronic illnesses experience less distress if they are more resilient. This is generally due to the fact that increased resilience is linked to less avoidant coping strategies (Elliott et al., 2023).

Schetter & Dolbier (2011) suggest a definition of resilience that is more accurate for chronic illness, since usual definitions of resilience are based on acute stressors. Resilience from the context of chronic illness can be explained as a process wherein an individual is able to cope with continuous adversity while also carrying on with regular functioning in various aspects of life (Schetter & Dolbier, 2011). The paper reviews three major research focuses in the study of resilience: developmental psychopathology for children experiencing adversity, adjustment to life-threatening medical conditions, and responses to acute adversity for adults, to create a categorisation of resources. These include six sections of characteristics that can build resilience in the face of chronic stress: 1) Personality traits such as optimism and hardiness, 2) Self and Ego Related resources such as self-esteem, mastery, secure attachment, and belief in one's capabilities, 3) Social networks and observed support, 4) Spirituality, world views, and culturally-relevant beliefs, 5) Cognitive and Behavioural coping skills, problem-focused coping ability, and cognitive reappraisal, 6) Resources such as socioeconomic status, health, intelligence, and previous history of adversity.

Positive outcomes from resilience are also relevant for health crises and critical illnesses. In a 2024 study, Matheiu et al. assessed resilience in survivors of critical illnesses, who generally experience Post Traumatic Stress Disorder symptoms. and decrease health-related quality of life. Patients with a higher level of resilience, specifically the individuals' perception of their diseases and increased social support, showed a higher quality of life and displayed a smaller prevalence of Post Traumatic Stress Disorder symptoms. From these, it is clear that social support based resilience practices as well as individual resilience practices can be beneficial for an individual.

Collective Resilience in Times of Crisis

Recent literature on resilience has expanded from a focus on individual traits to collective and community-based capacities instead (Fan & Lyu, 2021). 'Community resilience', abbreviated as *CR*, has emerged as an interdisciplinary topic, referring to the ability of a social unit to proactively prepare for, adapt to, and recover from adversities (Brown & Kulig, 1996). While there is no singular definition for community resilience, the themes that were visible in various definitions were local knowledge, support from the social network of the community, support from interpersonal relationships, health, the leadership of the community, how prepared the community was for adversity, and either a positive or negative outlook (Patel et al., 2017).

Even within Community Resilience research, the focus has evolved over the past 20 years (Fan & Lyu, 2021). Earlier frameworks focused on disaster response, whereas studies from 2015-16 onwards have shifted to the importance of social capital, the capacity of the community, and the importance of these in navigating adversities that are both on a personal level and major crises such as natural disasters (Fan & Lyu, 2021). This section explores community-based resilience in emergencies and the importance of developing context-specific strategies that build on the strengths of the community.

To identify the core components of community resilience in health emergencies, van Kessel et al. (2025) conducted a scoping review on 38 articles investigating community resilience in response to various health crises. The main focus was on making the core characteristics more clearly defined so that they could be explained. From this, there were 21 clear components of community resilience that were categorised into Abilities and Resources. Abilities included 10 observable capabilities that a resilient community displayed. The most frequently identified abilities were adaptation, connection, transformation, and self-organisation. The other abilities were the capacity to anticipate, prepare, prevent, absorb, include, and cope with the health emergencies that caused adversity. The main resources out of the eleven identified were grouped under social resources. Under this category, they included social networks, social capital, social cohesion amongst the community, and support within the community. The other essential resources were physical infrastructure, economic conditions, environment, the leadership and governance of the community, available human capital, capacity for emergency management, and socioeconomic resources present. Encouraging a sense of shared identity between the community and the responders to the crisis can be done through sharing useful and applicable information to build trust (van Kessel et al., 2025).

During mass emergencies, a shared sense of identity leads to a shared sense of fate among the affected. This often leads to collaboration between survivors of disasters and emergencies (Cocking, 2013). Survivors often act as what is now referred to as 'zero responders' and provide mutual aid to each other (Cocking, 2013). This collective resilience displayed is a predictable function of psychological processes (such as social psychological processes) (Drury et al., 2019). Based on CR in emergencies, Drury et al. (2019) offer 12 actionable recommendations for emergency responders. Key aspects of this include: educating responders about group psychology, planning to work with existing group norms instead of against them, building relationships with at-risk communities during the phase of preparation for an emergency, prioritising informative communication to build trust and reinforce shared identity, and avoiding undermining the shared sense of identity.

In supporting the community resilience processes during disasters and emergencies, emergency management practices can be significantly improved.

The Link between Spirituality and Resilience Levels

Spirituality can be defined as experiencing a meaningful connection to either ourselves, other individuals, or a higher power, as expressed through our life narratives and behaviours (Schulz, 2002). Across various populations and contexts, studies consistently display that spiritual beliefs and practices can serve an important role in navigating adversity. This section will explore the evidence linking spirituality to resilience, examining the mechanisms through which spiritual engagement increases an individual's capacity to withstand stress and thrive in significant life challenges.

Howard et al. (2023) examined spirituality, resilience, and well-being among a sample of 529 adults who were previously in alternative care settings, recognising that care leavers are at a higher risk of Adverse Life experiences. Spirituality was identified as various categories, such as a relationship with a higher power, a sense of purpose, and spiritual practices. Six themes of spirituality were identified, and resilience was associated with four out of them. These were related to God, community support, higher purpose, and spiritual teachings.

Reyes-Perez et al. (2025) looked into the interrelationships between spirituality, resilience, and happiness among higher education students in Northern Peru. The study utilises developmental and religious coping theory to see whether religious belief can moderate negative outcomes of adversity, and used 459 university students as its sample. The findings revealed significant direct effects wherein spirituality benefitted resilience, and demonstrated a positive effect on happiness. This, according to the study, was independent of the specific religious orientation of the students.

Manning et al. (2019) explored the interplay between spirituality and resilience in older adults who had experienced adversity earlier in their lives, using interviews on a sample of 46 individuals who identified spirituality to be a key resource in managing their hardships. The study identified five key areas wherein participants utilised their spiritual resilience. These are, reliance on relationships (with their faith community as well as a divine entity), power of belief (trust that things would work out as they intended them to), spiritual coping (for meaning-making out of adversity), commitment to spiritual values and practices, (to manage stress), and openness to spiritual growth and transformation (adversity was reframed as an opportunity for growth and expansion). Spiritual resilience is thus an active and cumulative process (Manning et al., 2019).

In short, research consistently shows that spirituality and resilience are strongly connected. Spirituality gives people the tools to cope with hardship through personal belief systems and belief in a higher power. The sense of hope it provides can help bounce back from stress at a much quicker rate. Ultimately, having a spiritual belief system can be a key factor in maintaining well-being throughout life

Resilience in Occupations

Resilience across different workplaces is a focus for health psychology since it emphasises the challenges faced by various professional groups. It aims to suggest interventions specific to these settings to promote well-being. Health professionals and first responders see trauma and emotional exhaustion very often and are at risk for a lower sense of purpose, burnout, and compassion fatigue (Jeanmonod et al., 2024; Deriglazov et al., 2025). Teaching resilience within health occupations should emphasise building reflection. This encourages practical application that can complement workplace culture shifts and then decrease burnout and compassion fatigue (McAllister & McKinnon, 2009).

Singh & Sharma's 2017 study on Indian IT Sector employees' capacity to face adversity and suggested that interventions targeted to boost the 'Adversity Quotient' of the individual can act as a protective factor against the high-pressure demands of the industry.

Along similar lines to workplace performance, for students, research shows a strong relationship between academic resilience and motivation. This highlights that resilience is also related to the drive to succeed (Yang & Wang, 2022).

Where the stress comes from may be specific to the individual, due to differing life experiences. However, these shared principles of adapting to stress and coping with stress can be applied across the globe. Interventions for resilience that are relevant to the patient or person can improve resilience in individuals, providing protective factors in workplace settings. This, combined with systems supporting the well-being of their employees, can better psychological well-being (Jeanmonod et al., 2024).

APPLICATIONS AND INTERVENTIONS

There is a visible modern shift in health psychology from earlier models of resilience, which see it as a fixed personality trait, to a process. Effective interventions to support this shift should be tailored to the group or individual it aims to support.

A meta-analysis by Joyce et al. (2018) reviewed over a hundred papers on resilience interventions and found the following interventions to have the strongest positive effect on enhancing individual resilience. CBT-based approaches for identifying and reframing maladaptive thought patterns related to stressors lead to increased adaptive coping strategies and a greater sense of personal agency. Mindfulness-based interventions focus on the emotional and attentional aspects of resilience. This includes practices such as meditation and body scan exercises, and can benefit emotional regulation and reduce physiological reactions to stress. Combining these techniques, according to Joyce et al. (2018), can teach and strengthen resilience.

Resilience interventions in the modern day include applications, digital health tools, mobile apps, and telehealth platforms. These interventions aim to make resilience support more scalable and accessible. A 2023 trial of smartphone CBT (accessed by an app called *Resilience Training*) by Furuwaka et al. showed a reduction in depressive symptoms for all participants. These technologies offer context-sensitive support that can adapt to a user's needs. A scoping literature review (Voth et al., 2022), found that the 22 mental health apps that they reviewed were beneficial in assisting the military members, public safety officers, and veterans, with a focus on mindfulness, CBT, ACT, and education about psychological resilience.

A modern approach must recognise that individual capacity cannot be separated from the surrounding environment. This means that a collaborative strategy, as explained in previous sections, is crucial for improved psychological outcomes. In the current era, this looks like individual support, technological advancements, and systemic change to build a more resilient society.

CONCLUSION

This chapter details that resilience is not a static trait but a dynamic process that takes place over the lifetime of an individual and is deeply connected to the context of the individual or group. This context refers to early attachment relationships, developmental tasks and is strongly influenced by family and community. From a forward-looking perspective in health psychology, the field is moving away from solely deficit-based models to focus on growth and enhancement. This includes strength-based approaches to prevent illness and improve quality of life, culturally relevant interventions that leverage community support, technological inventions to improve scale and accessibility, and building collective resilience to address challenges that affect entire communities in times of need. Ultimately, there is a clear need for researchers, clinicians, and policy makers to move beyond narrow models of resilience to address systemic barriers so that the burden of overcoming adversity does not rest on the individual. By building supportive systems and addressing structural inequalities, individuals can be enabled to not only bounce back from adversity but also to make meaning in their lives and thrive.

REFERENCES

Aburn, G., Gott, M., & Hoare, K. (2016). What is resilience? An integrative review of the empirical literature. *Journal of Advanced Nursing*, *72*(5), 980–1000. DOI: 10.1111/jan.12888 PMID: 26748456

Ainsworth, M. D. (1985). Patterns of infant-mother attachments: Antecedents and effects on development. *Bulletin of the New York Academy of Medicine*, *61*(9), 771. PMID: 3864510

Andersson, N., & Ledogar, R. J. (2008). The CIET Aboriginal Youth Resilience Studies: 14 Years of Capacity Building and Methods Development in Canada. *Pimatisiwin*, *6*(2), 65–88. PMID: 20862230

Anisman, H., Doubad, D., Asokumar, A., & Matheson, K. (2024). Psychosocial and neurobiological aspects of the worldwide refugee crisis: From vulnerability to resilience. *Neuroscience and Biobehavioral Reviews*, *165*, 105859. DOI: 10.1016/j.neubiorev.2024.105859 PMID: 39159733

Barrita, A. M., & Wong-Padoongpatt, G. (2023). Ethnic identity and resilience: A moderated mediation analysis of protective factors for self-blame and racial microaggressions. *Frontiers in Psychology*, *14*, 1198375. DOI: 10.3389/fpsyg.2023.1198375 PMID: 37457064

Berreman, G. D. (1972). Race, caste, and other invidious distinctions in social stratification. *Race*, *13*(4), 385–414. DOI: 10.1177/030639687201300401

Bogaerts, A., Claes, L., Raymaekers, K., Buelens, T., Bastiaens, T., & Luyckx, K. (2023). Trajectories of adaptive and disturbed identity dimensions in adolescence: Developmental associations with self-esteem, resilience, symptoms of depression, and borderline personality disorder features. *Frontiers in Psychiatry*, *14*, 1125812. DOI: 10.3389/fpsyt.2023.1125812 PMID: 37168080

Bonanno, G. A., Romero, S. A., & Klein, S. I. (2015). The temporal elements of psychological resilience: An integrative framework for the study of individuals, families, and communities. *Psychological Inquiry*, *26*(2), 139–169. DOI: 10.1080/1047840X.2015.992677

Bowlby, J. (1944). Forty-four juvenile thieves: Their characters and home-life. *The International Journal of Psycho-Analysis*, *25*, 19.

Bretherton, I. & American Psychological Association, Inc. (1992). The Origins of Attachment Theory: John Bowlby and Mary Ainsworth. In Developmental Psychology (Vol. 28, Issue 5, pp. 759–775). American Psychological Association, Inc. https://psychology.psy.sunysb.edu/attachment/online/inge_origins%20DP1992.pdf

Brown, D. D., & Kulig, J. C. (1996). The concepts of resiliency: Theoretical lessons from community research.

Cassidy, J., Jones, J. D., & Shaver, P. R. (2013). Contributions of attachment theory and research: A framework for future research, translation, and policy. *Development and Psychopathology*, *25*(4pt2), 1415–1434. DOI: 10.1017/S0954579413000692 PMID: 24342848

Chang, R., Barrita, A. M., & Wong-Padoongpatt, G. (2007). Race (racism). *The Blackwell Encyclopedia of Sociology*, 1-3.

Cocking, C. (2013). The role of "zero-responders" during 7/7: Implications for the emergency services. *International Journal of Emergency Services*, *2*(2), 79–93. DOI: 10.1108/IJES-08-2012-0035

Colpitts, E., & Gahagan, J. (2016). The utility of resilience as a conceptual framework for understanding and measuring LGBTQ health. *International Journal for Equity in Health*, *15*(1), 60. DOI: 10.1186/s12939-016-0349-1 PMID: 27048319

Deriglazov, D., Halamová, J., & Kernová, L. (2025). Burnout, Compassion Fatigue, and Compassion Satisfaction Interventions via Mobile Applications: A Systematic Review and a Meta-Analysis. *Worldviews on Evidence-Based Nursing*, *22*(3), e70033. DOI: 10.1111/wvn.70033 PMID: 40361274

Drury, J., Carter, H., Cocking, C., Ntontis, E., Tekin Guven, S., & Amlôt, R. (2019). Facilitating Collective Psychosocial Resilience in the Public in Emergencies: Twelve Recommendations Based on the Social Identity Approach. *Frontiers in Public Health*, *7*, 429165. DOI: 10.3389/fpubh.2019.00141 PMID: 31214561

Eggenberger, S. K., Meiers, S. J., Krumwiede, N., Bliesmer, M., & Earle, P. (2011). Reintegration within families in the context of chronic illness: A family health promoting process. *Journal of Nursing and Healthcare of Chronic Illness*, *3*(3), 283–292. DOI: 10.1111/j.1752-9824.2011.01101.x

Elliott, T. R., Perrin, P. B., Powers, M. B., Duffeck, D., & Warren, A. M. (2023). Resilience and distress among individuals with chronic health conditions during the initial wave of the COVID-19 pandemic. *Journal of Affective Disorders Reports*, *15*, 100710. DOI: 10.1016/j.jadr.2023.100710

Emami, S. G., Lorenzoni, V., & Turchetti, G. (2024). Towards Resilient Healthcare Systems: A Framework for Crisis Management. *International Journal of Environmental Research and Public Health, 21*(3), 286. DOI: 10.3390/ijerph21030286 PMID: 38541286

Estrada-Moreno, I. S., Palma-Garcia, M. D. L. O., Gomez Jacinto, L., & Hombrados-Mendieta, M. I. (2025). Resilience in immigrants: A facilitating resource for their social integration. *Journal of Ethnic & Cultural Diversity in Social Work*, •••, 1–16.

Fan, Y., & Lyu, X. (2021). Exploring Two Decades of Research in Community Resilience: A Content Analysis Across the International Literature. *Psychology Research and Behavior Management, 14*, 1643–1654. DOI: 10.2147/PRBM.S329829 PMID: 34675704

Ferbežar, N., Kopinič, A., & Gavriloski Tretjak, M. (2025). Elements of minority stress and resilience in LGBTQ+ students' experience of education. *Journal of Homosexuality, 72*(3), 520–543. DOI: 10.1080/00918369.2024.2326473 PMID: 38470515

Fleming, J., & Ledogar, R. J. (2008). Resilience, an Evolving Concept: A Review of Literature Relevant to Aboriginal Research. *Pimatisiwin, 6*(2), 7–23. PMID: 20963184

Fletcher, D., & Sarkar, M. (2013). Psychological resilience. *European Psychologist, 18*(1), 12–23. DOI: 10.1027/1016-9040/a000124

Fullerton, D. J., Zhang, L. M., & Kleitman, S. (2021). An integrative process model of resilience in an academic context: Resilience resources, coping strategies, and positive adaptation. *PLoS One, 16*(2), e0246000. DOI: 10.1371/journal.pone.0246000 PMID: 33529232

Ghanei Gheshlagh, R., Sayehmiri, K., Ebadi, A., Dalvandi, A., Dalvand, S., & Nourozi Tabrizi, K. (2016). Resilience of Patients With Chronic Physical Diseases: A Systematic Review and Meta-Analysis. *Iranian Red Crescent Medical Journal, 18*(7), e38562. DOI: 10.5812/ircmj.38562 PMID: 27703800

Ghosh, A., & Deb, A. (2017). Positive psychology interventions for chronic physical illnesses: A systematic review. *Psychological Studies, 62*(4), 354–362. DOI: 10.1007/s12646-017-0421-y

Howard, A. H., Roberts, M., Mitchell, T., & Wilke, N. G. (2023). The Relationship Between Spirituality and Resilience and Well-being: A Study of 529 Care Leavers from 11 Nations. *Adversity and Resilience Science, 4*(2), 177–190. DOI: 10.1007/s42844-023-00088-y PMID: 36816809

Jeanmonod, D., Irick, J., Munday, A. R., Awosika, A. O., & Jeanmonod, R. (2024). Compassion Fatigue in Emergency Medicine: Current Perspectives. *Open Access Emergency Medicine : OAEM*, *16*, 167–181. DOI: 10.2147/OAEM.S418935 PMID: 39045605

Johnson, C. V., Mimiaga, M. J., & Bradford, J. (2008). Health care issues among lesbian, gay, bisexual, transgender and intersex (LGBTI) populations in the United States: Introduction. *Journal of Homosexuality*, *54*(3), 213–224. DOI: 10.1080/00918360801982025 PMID: 18825859

Joyce, S., Shand, F., Tighe, J., Laurent, S. J., Bryant, R. A., & Harvey, S. B. (2018). Road to resilience: A systematic review and meta-analysis of resilience training programmes and interventions. *BMJ Open*, *8*(6), e017858. DOI: 10.1136/bmjopen-2017-017858 PMID: 29903782

Jung, H. H., Emlet, C. A., Kim, H. J., & Fredriksen-Goldsen, K. (2025). Predictors of Generativity Among SGM Midlife and Older Adults. *The Gerontologist*, *65*(4), gnaf023. DOI: 10.1093/geront/gnaf023 PMID: 39878371

Landes, S. D., Ardelt, M., Vaillant, G. E., & Waldinger, R. J. (2014). Childhood adversity, midlife generativity, and later life well-being. *The Journals of Gerontology. Series B, Psychological Sciences and Social Sciences*, *69*(6), 942–952. DOI: 10.1093/geronb/gbu055 PMID: 24870028

Luyckx, K., Goossens, L., Soenens, B., Beyers, W., & Vansteenkiste, M. (2005). Identity statuses based on 4 rather than 2 identity dimensions: Extending and refining Marcia's paradigm. *Journal of Youth and Adolescence*, *34*(6), 605–618. DOI: 10.1007/s10964-005-8949-x

Manning, L., Ferris, M., Rosario, C. N., Prues, M., & Bouchard, L. (2019). Spiritual resilience: Understanding the protection and promotion of well-being in the later life. *Journal of Religion, Spirituality and Aging*, *31*(2), 168–186. DOI: 10.1080/15528030.2018.1532859 PMID: 33335455

Martín Quintana, J. C., Alemán Ramos, P. F., & Morales Almeida, P. (2023). The Influence of Perceived Security in Childhood on Adult Self-Concept: The Mediating Role of Resilience and Self-Esteem. *Healthcare (Basel)*, *11*(17), 2435. DOI: 10.3390/healthcare11172435 PMID: 37685469

Masten, A. S., & Barnes, A. J. (2018). Resilience in Children: Developmental Perspectives. *Children (Basel, Switzerland)*, *5*(7), 98. DOI: 10.3390/children5070098 PMID: 30018217

Mayer, K. H., Bradford, J. B., Makadon, H. J., Stall, R., Goldhammer, H., & Landers, S. (2008). Sexual and gender minority health: What we know and what needs to be done. *American Journal of Public Health, 98*(6), 989–995. DOI: 10.2105/AJPH.2007.127811 PMID: 18445789

McAllister, M., & McKinnon, J. (2009). The importance of teaching and learning resilience in the health disciplines: A critical review of the literature. *Nurse Education Today, 29*(4), 371–379. DOI: 10.1016/j.nedt.2008.10.011 PMID: 19056153

Meyer, I. H. (1995). Minority stress and mental health in gay men. *Journal of Health and Social Behavior, 36*(1), 38–56. DOI: 10.2307/2137286 PMID: 7738327

Meyer, I. H. (2003). Prejudice, social stress, and mental health in lesbian, gay, and bisexual populations: Conceptual issues and research evidence. *Psychological Bulletin, 129*(5), 674–697. DOI: 10.1037/0033-2909.129.5.674 PMID: 12956539

Meyer, I. H. (2013). Prejudice, social stress, and mental health in lesbian, gay, and bisexual populations: Conceptual issues and research evidence.

Meyer, I. H. (2015). Resilience in the study of minority stress and health of sexual and gender minorities. *Psychology of Sexual Orientation and Gender Diversity, 2*(3), 209–213. DOI: 10.1037/sgd0000132

Morales, M. J., King, M. D., Hiler, H., Coopwood, M. S., & Wayland, S. (2017). The greater St. Louis LGBT health and human services needs assessment: An examination of the silent and baby boom generations. In *Community-Based Research on LGBT Aging* (pp. 103–128). Routledge.

Mosher, C. E., & DuHamel, K. N. (2006). An examination of distress, physical symptoms, and health behaviors among cancer survivors. *Cancer, 107*(4), 831–838.

Ong, A. D., Graham, E. K., Jackson, K., Atherton, O. E., Luo, J., Willroth, E. C., Beck, E. D., Yoneda, T., Cintron, D. W., Mroczek, D. K., & Steptoe, A. (2024). Associations Between Generativity and Social Asymmetry Among Older Adults in Japan. *The Journals of Gerontology. Series B, Psychological Sciences and Social Sciences, 79*(2), gbad183. Advance online publication. DOI: 10.1093/geronb/gbad183 PMID: 38149998

Orenstein, G. A., & Lewis, L. (2022). Erikson's stages of psychosocial development. In *StatPearls* [Internet]. StatPearls Publishing.

Patel, S. S., Rogers, M. B., Amlôt, R., & Rubin, G. J. (2017). What Do We Mean by 'Community Resilience'? A Systematic Literature Review of How It Is Defined in the Literature. *PLoS currents, 9*, ecurrents.dis.db775aff25efc5ac4f0660ad9c9f7db2. DOI: 10.1371/currents.dis.db775aff25efc5ac4f0660ad9c9f7db2

Reyes-Perez, M. D., Carreño Saucedo, L., Sanchez-Levano, M. J., Cabanillas-Palomino, R., Monje-Yovera, P. F., Jaime-Rodríguez, J. P., Atoche-Silva, L. A., Alarcón-Bustíos, J. M., & Fernández-Altamirano, A. E. F. (2025). The Spirituality-Resilience-Happiness Triad: A High-Powered Model for Understanding University Student Well-Being. *European Journal of Investigation in Health, Psychology and Education*, *15*(8), 158. DOI: 10.3390/ejihpe15080158 PMID: 40863280

Russo, S. J., Murrough, J. W., Han, M. H., Charney, D. S., & Nestler, E. J. (2012). Neurobiology of resilience. *Nature Neuroscience*, *15*(11), 1475–1484. DOI: 10.1038/nn.3234 PMID: 23064380

Rutter, M. (2006). Implications of resilience concepts for scientific understanding. *Annals of the New York Academy of Sciences*, *1094*(1), 1–12. DOI: 10.1196/annals.1376.002 PMID: 17347337

Ryan, M., & Ryznar, R. (2022). The Molecular Basis of Resilience: A Narrative Review. *Frontiers in Psychiatry*, *13*, 856998. DOI: 10.3389/fpsyt.2022.856998 PMID: 35599764

Schetter, C. D., & Dolbier, C. (2011). Resilience in the Context of Chronic Stress and Health in Adults. *Social and Personality Psychology Compass*, *5*(9), 634–652. DOI: 10.1111/j.1751-9004.2011.00379.x PMID: 26161137

Schulz, E. K. (2002). *The meaning of spirituality in the lives and adaptation processes of individuals with disabilities*. Texas Woman's University.

Segerstrom, S. C., Carver, C. S., & Scheier, M. F. (2018). Optimism, psychosocial well-being, and adaptation to chronic illness. *Health Psychology Review*, *12*(2), 71–93.

Seligman, M. E., & Csikszentmihalyi, M. (2014). *Positive Psychology: An Introduction*. Springer.

Singh, S., & Sharma, T. (2017). Affect of adversity quotient on the occupational stress of IT managers in India. *Procedia Computer Science*, *122*, 86–93. DOI: 10.1016/j.procs.2017.11.345

Sokol, J. T. (2009). Identity development throughout the lifetime: An examination of Eriksonian theory. Graduate journal of counseling psychology, 1(2), 14.

Southwick, S. M., Bonanno, G. A., Masten, A. S., Panter-Brick, C., & Yehuda, R. (2014). Resilience definitions, theory, and challenges: interdisciplinary perspectives. European journal of psychotraumatology, 5, . DOI: 10.3402/ejpt.v5.25338

Stańczykiewicz, B., & Senczyszyn, A. (2024). Bullying of LGBTQ+ children and adolescents in schools: Understanding the phenomenon, consequences, and international standards with a focus on the polish context. *Frontiers in Psychiatry, 15*, 1493745. DOI: 10.3389/fpsyt.2024.1493745 PMID: 39524124

The Trevor Project. (2022, June). *Resilience and mental health among LGBTQ youth.*

Theron, L. C., & Theron, A. M. (2014). Meaning-making and resilience: Case studies of a multifaceted process. *Journal of Psychology in Africa, 24*(1), 24–32. DOI: 10.1080/14330237.2014.904099

van Kessel, G., Milanese, S., Dizon, J., de Vries, D. H., MacGregor, H., Abramowitz, S., Enria, L., Burtscher, D., Yeoh, E. K., Thomas, B. E., Kwang, R., de Almeida, J. R., & Gobat, N. (2025). Community resilience to health emergencies: A scoping review. *BMJ Global Health, 10*(4), e016963. DOI: 10.1136/bmjgh-2024-016963 PMID: 40221140

Voth, M., Chisholm, S., Sollid, H., Jones, C., Smith-MacDonald, L., & Brémault-Phillips, S. (2022). Efficacy, effectiveness, and quality of resilience-building mobile health apps for military, veteran, and public safety personnel populations: Scoping literature review and app evaluation. *JMIR mHealth and uHealth, 10*(1), e26453. DOI: 10.2196/26453 PMID: 35044307

Wilcox, L., Larson, K., & Bartlett, R. (2021). The role of resilience in ethnic minority adolescent navigation of ecological adversity. *Journal of Child & Adolescent Trauma, 14*(4), 507–515. DOI: 10.1007/s40653-020-00337-7 PMID: 33456643

Windle, G., Bennett, K. M., & MacLeod, C. (2020). The Influence of Life Experiences on the Development of Resilience in Older People With Co-morbid Health Problems. *Frontiers in Medicine, 7*, 502314. DOI: 10.3389/fmed.2020.502314 PMID: 33072779

Yang, S., & Wang, W. (2022). The Role of Academic Resilience, Motivational Intensity and Their Relationship in EFL Learners' Academic Achievement. *Frontiers in Psychology, 12*, 823537. DOI: 10.3389/fpsyg.2021.823537 PMID: 35153940

Yoon, S., Tomlinson, C. A., Lorenzo Benavides, J., Chang, Y., Stanek, C., Wang, X., Ishiekwene, M., Susana Mariscal, E., Duron, J. F., & Howell, K. H. (2025). Resilience and Strengths Among Minoritized Racial and Ethnic Groups of Children in the United States Exposed to Trauma, Violence, and Maltreatment: A Scoping Review. *Trauma, Violence & Abuse, 26*(2), 220–234. DOI: 10.1177/15248380241309382 PMID: 40022617

Chapter 2

Individualised Digital Positive Psychology Interventions: A Human-Centred Approach to Well-Being

Peri Anantha Lakshmi Sharvani
http://orcid.org/0009-0002-0755-3284
PES University, India

Shreya Ghosh
http://orcid.org/0009-0008-9309-3424
PES University, India

ABSTRACT

The concept of health has altered dramatically throughout time. It used to be primarily concerned with not becoming sick, a deficit-oriented viewpoint. It has now evolved into something that emphasises well-being and positive outcomes in life. This chapter examines the forefront of that transition. It explains how to build and implement personalised digital PPIs. These draw on the PERMA model of well-being and Self-Determination Theory. Digital technologies make them scalable and accessible while also being able to personalise things. The chapter proposes that humans should be at the centre of digital PPI design. It emphasises relational and ethical aspects right from the outset. The chapter contributes an integrative, ethically grounded framework for designing and implementing digital PPIs that preserve human empathy while advancing scalable well-being solutions.

DOI: 10.4018/979-8-2600-3085-1.ch002

INTRODUCTION: THE SHIFT TOWARDS POSITIVE HEALTH

The definition of health has changed, and it is no longer regarded as a disease free, but taking the dynamic form of wellbeing that includes social, psychological, and physical aspects. This development is congruent with the salutogenic approach that focuses on the determinants of health and health maintenance. Keyes (2002) claimed that a distinction exists between languishment and flourishing where mental health implies optimal functioning and lack of mental disease. The conceptualisation of mental health services and interventions has far-reaching implications in the shift of paradigm of a deficiency model to a model that actively promotes thriving. Positive psychology provides a paradigm of perceiving life, meaning and improvement beyond the lack of dysfunction. It is especially important that this way of redefining human potential is essential since the active development of wellbeing is not a priority in the conventional biomedical paradigm. Positive psychology accounts the existence of life, purpose and growth alongside the lack of dysfunction and thus forms a paradigm change in the estimation of human potential.

As theorised by Seligman and Csikszentmihalyi (2000), positive psychology represents a scientifically grounded research into strengths, virtues, and positive functioning of human beings. In this context, Positive Psychology Interventions (PPIs) are evidence-based, formulated practices which augment wellbeing, meaning, optimism and resilience (Sin & Lyubomirsky, 2009). The interventions include exercises of both the identification of strengths and the feeling of gratitude as well as altruistic behaviour and savouring. The meta-analysis of 39 trials (Bolier et al., 2013) revealed that the PPI's diminish depressive symptoms (mean = -0.23) and improve wellbeing (mean = -0.34) and the effects last up to six months after the intervention. Such findings imply that PPIs have the potential of significantly and sustainably enhancing psychological functioning beyond the effects of a palliative effect only.

To provide an example, when I was interning with a student during summer one day, I was involved in a counselling session with a student who had a low level of motivation and self-doubt following a failed exam. Instead of attending to his negative cognitions only, we also adopted a strengths-based PPI, which had the effect of aiding the client to recognize and apply his personal strengths, such as kindness, curiosity and tenacity to the everyday aspects of his life. After six weeks, the student said that he felt more self-confident and dedicated to his academic pursuits, saying that he had finally felt competent again and his self-rated wellbeing had increased.

Technological advances have enabled the digital delivery of PPIs, improving accessibility and scalability (Bakker et al., 2016). Firth et al. (2017) emphasized that smartphone-based interventions can reach populations traditionally underserved by mental health services, including those in rural areas, individuals with mobility limitations, and people who face stigma in seeking traditional therapy. However, this digitalisation raises ethical and relational questions concerning empathy, authenticity, and privacy (Torous et al., 2021; Miner et al., 2016). The promise of universal access through technology must be balanced against the risk of creating superficial, mechanistic interventions that fail to honour the complexity of human experience.

I've tried several gratitude apps myself and honestly, some of them feel more like completing a daily checklist than actual reflection. You tap "I'm grateful for my coffee" and move on without really thinking about it. But I've also seen digital tools work really well. A friend of mine has been dealing with social anxiety and she started using this app that had small exposure exercises or things like "make eye contact with a cashier for 3 seconds" or "ask one question in class." She'd practice these between her therapy sessions, and then talk about how it went with her therapist. The app didn't replace therapy but it gave her a way to practice between sessions which made a real difference.

Therefore, a human-centred and ethically mindful approach is essential to ensure that digital PPIs promote authentic flourishing rather than mechanised well-being (Schueller et al., 2017). Positive psychology is the science of what enables individuals, organizations and societies to develop and flourish to their fullest potential. It represents a paradigm shift from pathology to possibility, from deficit to strength from surviving to thriving.

THE EVOLUTION AND FOUNDATIONS OF POSITIVE PSYCHOLOGY

Positive psychology is the science of successful living. Its focus is on the empirical study of human resources, strengths and potential as well as well-being. The fields of research are wide-ranging they range from the effects of positive emotions on the psyche and physical body, to flow experiences and supportive social relationships, to questions of motivation, mindfulness, passion and the experience of meaning. This breadth reflects the recognition that human flourishing is multifaceted, requiring attention to emotional, cognitive, behavioral, relational and existential domains.

With this resource-oriented approach, positive psychology stands clearly in the tradition of humanistic psychology and philosophy of the 20th century. Abraham Maslow is therefore considered a pioneer of this young scientific discipline. Maslow's hierarchy of needs provided an early framework for understanding human motivation beyond mere deficit reduction, culminating in the concept of self-actualization as it is the realization of one's full potential.

"Humanistic philosophy offers a new conception of learning, of teaching and of education," Maslow stated. In a nutshell, this theory holds that the "self-actualiza-

tion" of a person the achievement of the maximum level that the human species or a particular individual may reach, is the ultimate aim of education and its objective the human goal, the humanistic goal, the goal from the perspective of humans. As stated in the paper, p. 168f, it is simply helping the person become the best version of himself. This concept, which was revolutionary at the time and is still revolutionary now sees psychology as a freeing science as opposed to a healing one.

Self-actualization and personality development are both themes found in positive psychology but without describing them exhaustively because the findings clearly point to the relevance of social relationships and self-transcendent areas of life and experience of meaning for human well-being (Seligman, 2011). Positive psychology also differs methodologically from humanistic psychology: While the latter is more likely to be understood as a philosophical discipline due to its theoretical orientation, positive psychology is an empirical science based on quantitative and qualitative methods of social research

The new perspective of psychological research toward positive psychology was initiated in particular by the American psychologist Martin Seligman. He began his presidency of the American Psychological Association (APA) in 1998 with a keynote speech on focusing psychological research on aspects of a successful life and coined the term Positive Psychology. Since then research in these areas has "exploded" internationally.

A corresponding European research network (ENPP) was established in 2000. This international proliferation demonstrates the universal appeal of studying what makes life worth living, transcending cultural and geographical boundaries.

Since the 2010s, the field of positive psychology study has grown more specialised. These days there are a number of distinct subdisciplines, such as Positive Education, Positive Health and Positive Neuroscience, each of which advances certain application areas and research methodologies. Positive education examines how character characteristics, optimism and engagement may enhance student's academic achievement and overall well-being by incorporating the concepts of positive psychology into educational environments.

Positive Health integrates well-being promotion with medical care because health is more than just the absence of illness and pleasant neuroscience investigates the neurological foundations of flourishing by charting how pleasant experiences modify the structure and function of the brain.

ELEMENTS OF A SUCCESSFUL LIFE: THE PERMA MODEL

Seligman (2011) summarized the factors that empirically contribute to subjective well-being in the so-called PERMA scheme. Each of the five elements of this scheme by definition that fulfils the following three criteria:

(1) It contributes to human well-being
(2) A sufficiently large number of people strive for it for its own sake
(3) It is defined independently of the other elements and can also be measured independently of them.

This operationalization allows researchers to study well-being components systematically while respecting their distinct contributions. The abbreviation PERMA stands for positive emotions, engagement, relationship, meaning and accomplishment. Each element represents a pillar of psychological flourishing and together they constitute a comprehensive framework for understanding human well-being.

Positive Emotions

Barbara Fredrickson's Broaden-and-Build theory is based on a number of findings regarding the resource-building effects of positive emotions Positive emotions like hope, gratitude, enthusiasm, love and curiosity don't just feel good they also foster an open, exploratory mindset (the Broaden effect) and support the long-term development of psychological resources and skills (the Build effect). For instance, in the context of resilience, hope is linked to action tendencies towards resource building and planning, whereas interest is linked to a propensity to learn and explore which eventually results in the creation of new knowledge.

This theory has profound implications for intervention design. If positive emotions don't just feel good but actually build psychological, social and physical resources, then cultivating them becomes a strategic investment in future well-being. One experiencing gratitude doesn't just provide momentary pleasure it strengthens social bonds, increases prosocial behavior and enhances sleep quality.

Engagement

Engagement entails being fully involved in something that puts your competencies to the right use. The concept of flow states that in this state, the time passes unnoticed, one is less self-conscious and able to act and pay attention simultaneously. On their own, these moments are good and the life is made more satisfying. The digital tools can assist individuals to seek flow-creating activities that set the appropriate environment to remain active.

Relationships

In most cultures and circumstances, good relationships can be regarded as the most potent element that makes people happy. Research is always conducted that demonstrating the ability of social bond protection against mental disease, enhances physical health, and has been associated with increased longevity. Programs that contribute to a healthier relationship through promoting positive reactions, expressing gratitude, or using compassionate forms of communication have tangible positive effects on well-being. In the digital realm this begs the question of the way in which technology can assist us to connect in a real way rather than superficial encounters.

Meaning

PPI's make life meaningful when you feel that you are part of something bigger than yourself. This meaning grounds us, regardless of whether it is through a spiritual practice, serving others, making art or working on a cause. Viktor Frankl through his experience in logotherapy revealed that meaning can make people go even when they are in great distress. Digital programs can assist individuals to derive meaning by making sense of values, doing legacy projects, and connecting them to a purpose.

Accomplishment

Attempting to achieve and pursue goals is a source of well-being by its own without the other elements of PERMA. It is human nature to become more adept at things, learn and fulfil our goals. Achievement can be facilitated using apps to set objectives, monitor development and celebrate the achievements. Nevertheless, this area should be carefully balanced: too difficult goals will result in frustration, whereas too easy will be demotivating.

THEORETICAL FOUNDATIONS OF INDIVIDUALISED PPIs

Self-Determination and Autonomy

Self-Determination Theory (SDT) suggests that we are at our best when we get to decide on what we want to do, have something we enjoy about what we are doing and feel loved by our people who are dear to us. The reason why individualised PPIs are so cool is that people get to choose the activities to do which will be aligned with their values and what is going on with their life. One child may be more invigorated by gratitude lists and another will be more peaceful through mindfulness or compassion training. Such corresponding observation adheres to the differences of personality, culture, circumstances of life of people and their development level.

SDT simply asserts that we are all programmed to require specific psychological items that their presence support our development and remain happy. Autonomy concerns the capacity to make decisions that are genuine to yourself and not merely doing what other people indicate. Competence refers to having the sense that you are doing well in whatever you are doing and being able to master it. Relatedness implies real relations with caring people. Programs that provide people with what they require in these three bring about real inspirations and transformations. Studies concerning the person activity fit model reveal that interventions that suit a person properly in terms of their alignment with his or her real self-perform much better.

Sheldon and Lyubomsky discovered that individuals who pursued self-concordant goals or goals that align with their values, received more well-being compared to those goals that were imposed upon them. It puts the one size fits all philosophy out of the field and demands personalisation at all levels. This personalisation as a result of autonomy is a big thing since it promotes intrinsic motivation, and that is how being happy is attached.

Nonetheless, the question remains, to what extent is an excessive choice? Excesses of choice may become paralysis and fewer may seem like an exclusion. It takes good conversation, and not an algorithm, to find that sweet spot. The paradox of choice informs us that excess choice can always work against us leading to decision-fatigue and regret, therefore good personalisation must lead you with few meaningful choices within a clear system.

The Biopsychosocial Model

Engel is the founder of the Biopsychosocial Model which postulates the coming together of the brain, the body and the social life to create health.

Personalised PPI accesses emotional resilience, physical health and relationships simultaneously. It is an integrated way of thinking and making the realization that we are not brains but complete bodies existing in social worlds. A program that concentrates only on one of those components is normally inadequate.

Research supports that higher well-being correlates with improved immune response, lower inflammation and greater longevity (Steptoe et al., 2015; Diener & Chan, 2011). Independent of negative affect, positive affect predicts lower morbidity and death according to research evaluated by Pressman and Cohen (2005). These results imply that therapies for well-being have real physiological advantages in addition to psychological ones. The mechanisms are complex, involving neuroendocrine pathways, inflammatory processes and health behaviors.

Ryff et al. (2004) demonstrated that psychological well-being is associated with lower cardiovascular risk, better neuroendocrine regulation, and reduced inflammatory markers. This physiological embedding of well-being underscores the importance of interventions that target multiple systems simultaneously (Ryff, 2014). The interventions that promote social connection reduce cortisol levels. Gratitude practices improve sleep quality. Purpose in life predicts healthier aging trajectories. These connections between psychological and biological processes validate the integrated approach of the biopsychosocial model.

The biopsychosocial model isn't just a framework it's a reminder that humans are irreducibly complex. Any intervention that ignores biological rhythms, social contexts or psychological nuances is bound to fall flat. Digital tools that reduce well-being to a single metric which is a daily mood score, step count or meditation streak that miss this complexity. Effective PPIs must therefore integrate multiple dimensions, recognizing their dynamic interactions.

Human-Centred Design in Positive Psychology

Human-Centred Design (HCD) focuses on empathy, co-creation and feedback (Norman, 2013; Brown, 2008). When HCD is used on PPIs, interventions become culturally relevant, accessible and context-sensitive (Hollis et al., 2017). HCD does not impose a single model on all and instead, it takes a stance by matching scientific evidence with human experience, closing the gap between the theory and the real world. This process starts with a profound insight into users, their requirements, situations and problems, prior to any intervention design being used. HCD has a number of principles it should begin with the empathy of users and should brainstorm on a number of possible solutions, should prototype by quickly and cheaply, should test with actual users and should iterate on the basis of feedback.

This is a collaborative process in nature, which puts them in the position where they impart their knowledge, frustrations and innovations, to influence the intervention on a given stage. End-users have been demonstrated to make interventions more acceptable and effective in participatory design techniques, in which end-users participate in the development process (Mohr et al., 2017). According to Yardley et al. (2015), recently, the approaches based on persons that involve the synthesis of evidence and qualitative knowledge of the target users to develop evidence-based interventions that are both theoretically correct and practically feasible. This dual emphasis on empirical validity and user experience distinguishes successful interventions from those that are scientifically rigorous but practically unusable.

HCD isn't optional rather it's the difference between theoretical elegance and real-world impact. It requires humility from researchers and designers, acknowledging that expertise about interventions doesn't equate to expertise about user's lives. The most sophisticated evidence base means nothing if the intervention sits unused on someone's phone. By centering human experience HCD ensures that scientific innovation translates into meaningful benefit.

Digitalisation of Positive Psychology Interventions

The integration of technology into Positive Psychology has revolutionised well-being promotion. Digital platforms, mobile applications and online therapy modules offer scalability and convenience (Parks et al., 2012; Seligman et al., 2005). Digital PPIs can personalise user experiences through adaptive algorithms and real-time feedback (Schueller et al., 2017; Krebs et al., 2010). This technological transformation has democratized access to evidence-based interventions that potentially reach millions who would never engage with traditional therapeutic services.

The advantages of digital delivery are substantial. Digital interventions are available 24/7, eliminating barriers of geography, scheduling and cost. They can be delivered at scale without proportional increases in resources. They offer anonymity that reduces stigma. They can incorporate multimedia elements video, audio, interactive exercises etc that enhance engagement. They generate rich data that can inform personalization and continuous improvement. For populations facing access barriers like in rural communities, individuals with disabilities those in underserved regions digital PPIs represent unprecedented opportunity.

Smartphone-based mental health therapies had moderate impact sizes ($d = 0.38$) for depressed symptoms, according to a 2019 meta-analysis by Firth et al. While encouraging, that is not a miracle. Although these technologies are effective, they are not miracle cures.

In a similar vein, Bakker et al. (2016) examined the data regarding mental health apps and came to the conclusion that although many of them exhibit promise, thorough evaluation is still uneven. Apps are becoming more and more popular than science creating a market where verified and unvalidated tools compete. But problems still exist. One important factor influencing psychological change is the therapeutic alliance, which may be weakened by a lack of human connection (Watts et al., 2020; Horvath et al., 2011). The therapeutic relationship, which is defined by warmth, empathy and genuine understanding, has been repeatedly demonstrated to predict therapy success across modalities. Can this be replicated by algorithms? At least not entirely, given the knowledge available today.

Also there are still unresolved ethical issues with digital literacy, accessibility and data protection (Nebeker et al., 2019; Luxton et al., 2011). Many questions like

"Who is the owner of the information produced by apps for mental health? In what ways is it kept, examined and possibly made profitable? When a user's data indicates crisis- level distress, what happens?" all of these arise. Technology companies frequently neglect to sufficiently address the legal, ethical and clinical aspects of these issues. Regulations are unable to keep up with the rapid commercialisation of mental health technology which has led to a Wild West of privacy issues and possible abuse.

Think about this situation where an elderly person with little technological expertise downloads a well- regarded app for wellbeing. After a few minutes, they become frustrated and delete it after becoming lost in nested menus and perplexed by terms like "CBT modules" and "affect regulation." The app wasn't poorly designed; it just wasn't designed for them. According to research by Choi and Dinitto (2013) perceived complexity and lack of relevance are two major obstacles to older adults' adoption of technology. Access to devices is only one aspect of the digital divide and also other factors include usability, literacy and cultural relevance.

The digital PPI ecosystem can be conceptualised as a triadic model of interaction and of balancing the personalisation, technology and ethics. For sustainability, all three must remain in equilibrium while technology must amplify not replace human empathy (Mohr et al., 2013). Interventions lose their human nature when they are treated as an end in themselves and not a means to an end. As soon as efficiency is used as the key indicator, we start losing depth in favor of reach. This is the difficulty in balancing it and increasing interventions to serve the needs of the population. Lattie et al. (2019) showed that digital interventions that are supported by human beings are more effective than the fully automated interventions, and the effect sizes are almost two times more than usual self-guided interventions.

The implication of this finding is that we cannot and will not replace humans with technology, but we can and will employ both with a strategic approach. The hybrid models capitalize on the competencies of both strategies. Technology brings about uniformity, accessibility and data-informed personalization. The human beings offer compassion, sensitive judgment and morality. Technology handles routine monitoring and skill-building. Humans address complex decision-making and crisis intervention. By thoughtfully integrating both we can achieve greater reach without sacrificing relational depth.

At a policy level, individualised digital PPIs can inform the development of inclusive national well-being strategies, integrating psychological support into education and workplace systems. By embedding ethical digital design in institutional practices, policymakers can advance equitable mental health promotion at scale

ETHICAL AND RELATIONAL CONSIDERATIONS

The basis of the psychological interventions is the ethical integrity. The principles of beneficence, non-maleficence, autonomy, and justice should be followed during the creation of digital personalised psychological interventions (PPIs) (Beauchamp and Childress, 2019; Mittelstadt et al., 2016). Beneficence binds interventions to vigorously facilitate user well-being. Non-maleficence demands that they should not cause harm, which is a complicated issue when the interventions are on a large scale and we have minimal control over them. The principle of autonomy gives users the freedom to make informed decisions about involvement and data use. Justice requires fair accessibility and a safeguard against the increase of the existing inequalities.

Participants have to be assured of privacy, informed consent, and the issue of transparency in terms of data use, which will help them maintain trust (Nebeker et al., 2019). The real-life application of these ethical mandates creates a lot of complexity. Genuinely informed consent is a facet of the issue in that a big percentage of the users will scroll past the terms of service without using the content. The idea that data collection is required to make it more personal and the privacy issues which are the basis of trust imposes a constant strain. They are not some forms of abstract dilemmas, but rather everyday operational problems. The severity of the problem has been proven by empirical evidence: Obar and OeldorfHirsch (2020) established that 74% of users did not read the privacy policies, which, in its turn, makes the concept of informed consent questionable.

The standard consent model a lengthy legal document filled with technical jargon—fails its purported purpose. Users don't read these documents, let alone understand them. Yet legally, their checkbox constitutes consent. This fiction serves institutional protection more than ethical practice. Genuine informed consent requires comprehensible information, meaningful choice, and ongoing opportunity to revise decisions. Digital interventions must innovate beyond checkbox compliance toward authentic transparency.

I once worked with a team developing a mood-tracking app. Our algorithm detected patterns suggesting suicidal ideation in a user's data. Ethically, we were obligated to intervene. But legally, our terms of service didn't grant us permission to contact users directly. We had designed a system that could identify crisis but couldn't respond to it. That's the gap between theoretical ethics and operational reality. Bauer et al. (2017) discuss similar dilemmas in their framework for ethical mobile health research, emphasizing the need for clear crisis protocols.

This case illustrates a fundamental tension in digital mental health: the duty to protect versus the duty to respect privacy. When does data-driven risk detection justify intervention? How do we build systems that can respond to crisis without becoming surveillance tools? These questions have no easy answers, but they demand thoughtful consideration before interventions reach users, not after crises emerge.

Moreover, digital inequality may pose problems to individuals who lack a proper connection or literacy (Bhardwaj et al., 2021; Veinot et al., 2018). In India where I am studying, the disparity is enormous. A rural Maharashtra farmer might entirely be served by a PPI, but high-speed internet is required, along with English literacy, and you are essentially banned. Ramsetty and Adams (2020) demonstrated how COVID-19 increased digital health inequities, particularly among rural and low-income populations.

The pandemic made it quite evident that the claim of telehealth as a method of universal access fails in the communities that do not have the necessary infrastructure, equipment, or digital skills. Diversity is not a buzzword but an ethical and design challenge (Graham et al., 2011). It implies consideration of technology (ensuring compatibility with low-bandwidth and low-tech devices), language (more than one, right literacy rate), price (free or affordable) and culture (suited to other worldviews and practices). The hybrid models of intervention, involving a combination of digital technologies with human assistance, offer a moderate solution, preserving the emotional purity but at the same time applying the precision of technologies (Mohr et al., 2017).

As an example, a community health worker can organize a group on a digital PPI platform to overcome the technology divide and remain culturally and linguistically inclusive. Patel et al. (2010) endorse task-sharing models of global mental health where the community resources are combined with digital tools. These models disseminate mental health promotion among specialists to trained lay people making a massive reach without compromising quality. In India, it would imply ASHA workers (Accredited Social Health Activists) conducting digital PPIs in the villages, translating texts into the local languages, and modifying exercises to the cultural contexts. Hybrid intervention models combining digital tools with human facilitation offer a balanced approach, ensuring emotional authenticity while retaining technological precision (Mohr et al., 2017). For instance, a community health worker could facilitate a group using a digital PPI platform, bridging the technology gap while maintaining cultural and linguistic relevance. Patel et al. (2010) advocate for task-sharing models in global mental health that leverage community resources alongside digital tools. Such models distribute mental health promotion beyond specialized professionals to trained lay workers, dramatically expanding reach while maintaining quality.

In the Indian context, this might involve ASHA workers (Accredited Social Health Activists) facilitating digital PPIs in village settings, translating content into local languages, and contextualizing exercises within cultural frameworks. Technology provides structure and evidence-based content; local facilitators provide cultural translation and relational support. This integration respects both scientific validity and cultural wisdom, creating interventions that are globally informed but locally rooted.

ETHICAL IMPLEMENTATION REFLECTIVE FRAMEWORK

The present reflective framework is the basis of designing and implementing ethically justified and individualized positive psychology interventions (PPIs). It consists of the five elements that are interconnected and include Assessment, Co-Design, Personalisation, Ethical Oversight and Evaluation which are detailed below.

Figure 1. Ethical Implementation Reflective Framework

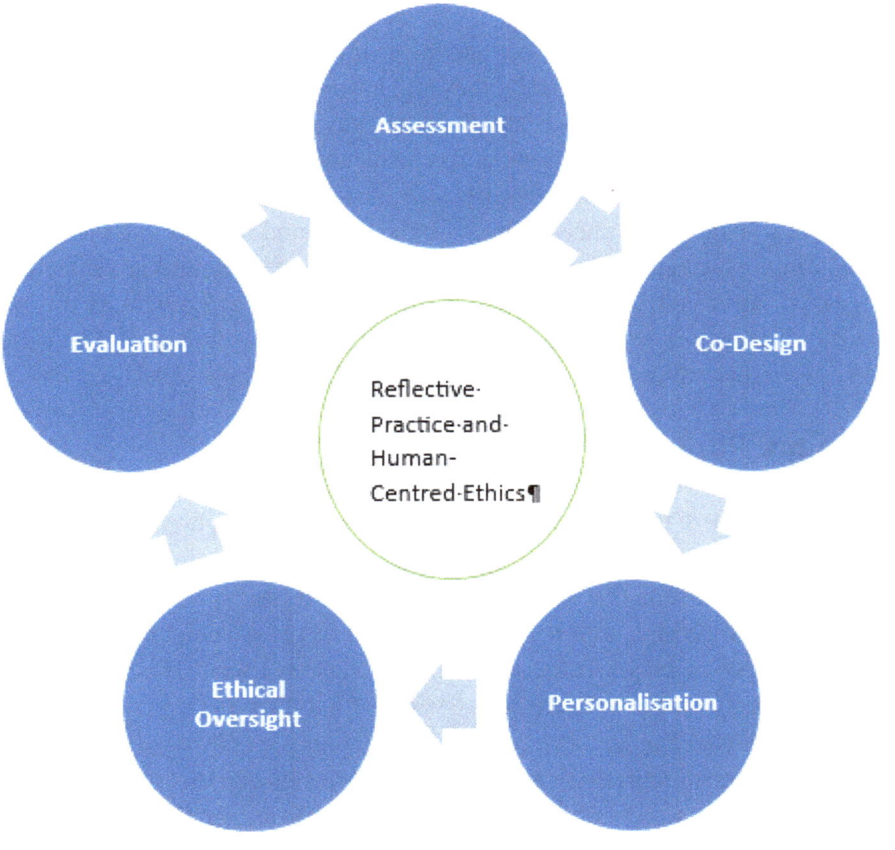

This model depicts the cyclical and reflective process that guides the development and delivery of tailored digital Positive Psychology Interventions (PPIs). Each component such as Assessment, Co-Design, Personalisation, Ethical Oversight and Evaluation, interacts dynamically to guarantee that digital tools are ethical, context-sensitive and human-centered.

Evaluation: Determine User Requirements, Objectives and Contextual Strengths

At the operational level, the establishment of effective interventions requires a strict investigation of the real needs of patrons instead of assumptions. The empirical data provided by Horne et al. (2015) show that a subtle understanding of the real needs of patients is the key to maintaining the engagement and improving the results; therefore, user-defined needs should be considered a priority rather than researcher-prescribed desiderata.

The evaluation procedure goes beyond the primitive surveys in exploring the real world of the participants, the capacity they still have, their culture and their personal limits. The relevant interrogatives are: What resources are already available? What are the obstacles being faced? What is the influence of antecedent experiences in expectations? Cooperation is a necessity both parties are realized as domain experts in their own life and researchers bring with them methodological knowledge.

Wellbeing is evaluated with quantitative measures, values and goals are elucidated in qualitative interview, daily fluctuations in ecological momentary measures and cultural relevance are added with community stakeholder input. The general objective is an overall understanding that guides all decisions of design.

Co-Design: Participatory Design With Users.

The importance of bona fide participation of users is highlighted in the literature. Sanders and Stappers (2008) argue that co-design cannot be done without in the creation of interventions that work in practice. In one study, the researchers held monthly design meetings with the end-users, one of the participants called Aisha proposed the use of prayer-time reminders to Muslim users. This feature being rooted in her daily routine of keeping up with the habit formation and the practice of religion enhanced engagement among the religious users by 45 percent and was well integrated into the current rituals. Effective co-design does not only end at initial consultation. During the developmental process, the participants criticize the prototypes, suggest features, find the problems and test the solutions. Researchers should surrender themselves and the user expertise should question the expert assumptions.

The outcome is a utilitarian intervention that is seen to co-own. Milieus have to be built to enable the free articulation of participants to facilitate actual collaboration. The time and knowledge should be compensated, and researchers need to communicate clearly with the limitations that do not allow applying the specific recommendations. Co-design can produce innovations when carried out in the right manner and might not be realized in processes where researchers are in charge.

Personalisation: Change Feedback, Content and Pacing

Krebs et al. (2010) have also proven that customized interventions are more effective in retention and result in better outcomes than generic interventions. As an example, to prevent dropout an intervention can also control the intensity based on the current level of stress of the user, where more mild exercises can be provided during times of distress. The adaptive personalization recognizes that wellbeing work takes place in the contexts of the real world that are complicated. Personalization exists on several levels and various choice of exercises, time-related delivery, level of difficulty, the source of modality (text, audio, video, interactive) and feedback nature.

The best personalization combines what users have stated they like with behavioral cues, based on empirical evidence of similar user cohorts. However, personalization needs to be fine-tuned. Extreme customization can seem invasive, like the system is spying in your face or lack of customization can make the content sterile and useless. The ideal balance is one that includes transparency about the algorithmic processes, user agency over settings that are vital and so on and iterative tuning based on the ongoing feedback. The users are supposed to understand the reasoning behind certain content and have the right to change it.

Ethical Oversight: Be Transparent, Consent and Fair Access.

According to Grady (2015), we require actual, useful consent material and not dull legality. Rather than a 30 minutes tedious form, a plain-no frills form of about three minutes reading would be preferable. It must provide explicit information regarding the use of data, present straightforward flow charts, provide specific examples and indicate how to acquire new consent in case of modifications in features. Ethical checks are not supposed to be made only once a time the IRBs or ethics committees should intervene whenever there is a drastic change. We should have actual bad event and user complaints reporting systems, and independent audits of algorithm bias.

Responsibility is maintained through direct connections that allow users to pose questions and obtain answers very quickly. Other programs provide user advisor boards, which convene quarterly to discuss the engagement statistics, grievance, and ethics. These boards may consist of past users, community leaders, ethicists, and physicians to provide an external view, with a higher degree of accountability and consistent ethical course.

Evaluation: Continued Mixed Methods Evaluation.

According to Creswell and Plano Clark (2017), it is more appropriate to employ more than one method than a single method as it provides more information. It is both examining numbers (such as the number of people who continue using it or their wellness scores) and actual stories (such as someone said this exercise felt forced). Patterns of numbers are explained by stories.

Success should not be measured on who gets the help, when or why. We run analyses on users, make comparisons across different groups and cause and effect to avoid making a guess that is too broad. Other areas are also checked by a complete check-list, such as user satisfaction, the level of control, its compatibility with their culture and the bad side effects. We do not simply tally, we can observe the level of engagement of people immediately and in the long run to determine whether it becomes permanent. This cycle maintains the programs as flexible, caring and respectful towards the dignity and health of people. Although there are rules, it is success that we have to be cautious with the manner we utilize them.

CHALLENGES AND LIMITATIONS IN DIGITAL PPI IMPLEMENTATION

Despite the promise of digital PPIs, significant challenges persist that must be acknowledged and addressed. The field's rapid growth has sometimes outpaced careful consideration of limitations, creating unrealistic expectations and potential harm when interventions fail to deliver on inflated promises.

The Engagement Problem

One of the most persistent challenges in digital mental health is user engagement. While millions download well-being apps, the vast majority abandon them within days. Research indicates that retention rates for mental health applications remain critically low, with fewer than 15% of users maintaining engagement beyond one month (Parks et al., 2012). This attrition crisis reflects fundamental gaps between user needs and intervention design, highlighting the paradoxical nature of digital accessibility. The ease of access that makes digital tools appealing simultaneously reduces commitment, as users face no scheduled appointments, financial investments or social accountability structures that characterize traditional therapeutic settings. As Parks and colleagues (2012) observed, the elimination of traditional barriers ironically undermines sustained engagement, as users can abandon interventions without consequence. Digital well-being tools compete for attention within saturated digital ecosystems, where engagement demands exceed available time and cognitive resources. The challenge lies in creating intrinsic commitment mechanisms without reintroducing the barriers that digital interventions aimed to eliminate.

I remember reading this paper (Parks et al., 2012) that nailed it. They talked about this paradox: that an app being super easy to get is also its biggest weakness. Because if there's no commitment and no appointment you paid for, no therapist waiting for you, it feels weightless. You can bail. It's like how paying for a gym membership hurts if you don't go, but that free yoga video on YouTube? You'll skip it without a second thought. All those "barriers" in traditional therapy, like the cost and the scheduled time, they actually force you to show up. So the real trick for these digital tools is to figure out how to create that sense of commitment without it just becoming an expensive, inconvenient thing they were trying to replace in the first place. It's a seriously tough puzzle.

The Measurement Challenge

Digital PPIs produce enormous amounts of data, but abundance does not equal actionable insight. The area is confronted with considerable challenges regarding what to measure, how to measure it, and what the measures mean. Self-report is still the gold standard for subjective well-being, but repeated questioning every day causes burden that decreases response quality and raises attrition. Passive sensing (utilizing phone sensors to monitor behavior) provides invisible collection of data but enhances privacy concerns and yields data of questionable validity.

The classic well-being scales were crafted for research environments where administration was well controlled. Their equivalence when presented in the context of apps, filled out on phones while riding public transportation, and with high frequency is not adequately established. The measurement context affects responses in ways we're only just coming to appreciate. Does a sunny morning well-being survey generate the same information as one filled out at a stressful evening commute? Most likely not, but we equate these measurements as if they are the same.

Diener and Chan (2011) highlighted the fact that well-being is multidimensional, involving emotional, cognitive, psychological, and social aspects. No one measure captures all these dimensions, but digital interventions tend to collapse well-being into a single daily rating. Reducing well-being in this way may be expedient but it's also limiting, risking the omission of valuable elements of users' experiences.

The problem is how to create measurement solutions that are both comprehensive and user-friendly.

The Generalizability Gap

Nearly all studies on digital PPIs have been done with WEIRD populations i.e. the Western, Educated, Industrialized, Rich and Democratic populations. However, these populations are a small minority of humanity. How much what is found generalizes to other cultural settings is unknown. Gratitude interventions built and tested in the United States might not generalize well to collectivist cultures in which gratitude is experienced and expressed differently. Mindfulness practices separated from their Buddhist context can lose critical components that made them effective.

Cultural adaptation means a lot more than simple translation. It calls for a real grasp of how people think about well-being in their own way. You have to consider what practices fit smoothly with local customs. Values that get top priority matter too. Everyday life situations play a big role as well. An approach to treat depression made for wealthy Americans who have steady homes and easy access to doctors ends up looking quite different. That is compared to what someone in poverty needs. Those folks might deal with violence and big systemic barriers too. Still, many digital positive psychology interventions get rolled out worldwide. They often skip much adaptation at all. The idea seems to be that they work the same everywhere.

Bhardwaj and colleagues in 2021 pointed out the importance of building digital mental health tools around local cultures in India. They noted how Western ideas of self-care can clash with group-oriented values there. Take interventions that push focusing on yourself and chasing personal joy. Those might come off as self-centred in places where family obligations and group peace come first. To make cultural adaptation work well, you need to bring in people from the community right from the start. Do not just translate what already exists.

The Efficacy-Effectiveness Gap.

Things that succeed in tight lab settings do not always hold up the same in everyday life. That difference shows up clearly in studies on talk therapy. It looks just as true for digital positive psychology interventions. People in research get carefully picked and screened. They feel motivated and get plenty of help. Someone keeps an eye on them too. Real users out in the world miss all that. They try the tools under far from perfect setups. Technical help from experts stays out of reach. Attention from researchers vanishes as well. Everyday folks run into cut-off sessions. Glitches pop up often. Life pulls them in other directions. No one holds them accountable from outside.

Bolier and team back in 2013 saw that these interventions deliver solid results in controlled trials. Doubts linger though about if those gains stick around in normal everyday use. Studies on how they work when people actually grab them on their own stay pretty rare. That compares to the flood of lab-based efficacy work. The mismatch leaves questions about true real-life punch. Something with great trial numbers might deliver real help at large scale. Or it might not, especially without much backup.

On top of that, journals tend to publish only the wins. Flops get buried and ignored. The body of work ends up painting too rosy a view of how well these things perform. Reviews that pull together studies can only draw from what sees the light of day. That leaves out key pieces of the puzzle. The whole area would benefit from more open talk about failures. Share the hurdles in rolling things out too. Only then can we get a straight sense of what digital positive psychology interventions truly offer. And where they fall short.

Integration With Clinical Practice

This paper focuses mainly on tools for everyday folks, but those digital well-being options, or PPIs, could fit into real clinical settings too. We have to watch out closely when blending them in. It is not straightforward to suggest an app for happiness to a person dealing with depression.

These tools act more like a supporting element, not the core treatment. Consider PPIs, such as keeping a gratitude journal or spotting personal strengths, as helpful extras during recovery. They support the process without taking centre stage. The main focus stays on therapy or medication when required. There is a serious risk in promoting these apps as complete mental health solutions. A person facing deep struggles might rely on the app alone and delay proper care, which only worsens the situation. Studies support this view. One from Sin and Lyubomirsky in 2009 showed that PPIs ease depressive symptoms somewhat, but the impact remains limited and suits lighter cases best. In severe situations, they work only as supplements.

This goes beyond ideas on paper. Friends of mine in therapy have used mindfulness apps between visits to reinforce their efforts. It helps maintain progress and provides topics for discussion next time. Still, it never substitutes the thorough sessions with a professional.

One key point stands out here that the apps cannot launch without proper safeguards in place. They require built-in protections. Directing someone in suicidal thoughts or a sharp crisis toward positive exercises proves not only useless, but harmful too. Developers must include checks for such risks and direct users straight to expert assistance right away. Building that feature well in an app presents a huge hurdle that remains unsolved for now.

Many users will not accurately report symptoms that might disqualify them from an intervention they want to use. Others may not recognize the severity of their condition. Digital screening lacks the clinical judgment that face-to-face assessment provides. These limitations necessitate conservative approaches: when in doubt, refer. Better to over-refer than to have someone in crisis using an insufficient intervention.

Torous et al. (2021) emphasize the need for clear crisis protocols in digital mental health interventions. These protocols should include immediate access to crisis resources, clear communication about limitations of the intervention, and where possible, connection to human support. The earlier example of detecting suicidal ideation in user data illustrates the complexity: identifying risk without capacity to respond is ethically untenable. Systems must be designed to detect and respond to crisis, not merely collect concerning data.

Training and Integration for Providers

Digital PPIs can really fit into clinical work only if mental health providers get proper training on how to use them, along with their evidence and any limits they have. A lot of clinicians just do not know much about the tools out there. They also feel unsure about which ones to suggest to patients. Training programs for professionals ought to cover digital health literacy. That way, future clinicians learn to check out apps carefully. They can match the right tools to what clients actually need. Plus, they figure out how to blend digital options with regular therapy approaches.

Technical side of things counts a lot too. When digital PPIs run on their own, away from patient records, they do not add much real value. Providers end up blind to what clients try on their own. Clients have to juggle separate systems that do not connect at all. In the end, no one gets a full view of the overall care plan. Interoperability could help here. It lets digital tools talk directly to clinical systems. That might improve how everything works together. Still, it brings up big issues around privacy. Technical hurdles come with it as well.

Mohr and his colleagues in 2017 pushed for stronger links between research and real-world practice in digital mental health. They pointed out that most apps get built without any say from clinicians. At the same time, clinicians barely know about tools backed by solid evidence. Closing that divide means using team-based development. Researchers, clinicians, users and developers all join in right from the start.

FUTURE DIRECTIONS AND INNOVATIONS

The area of digital PPIs keeps changing fast. New technologies and methods come along that open up better ways to support well-being for many people.

Artificial Intelligence and Machine Learning

AI and machine learning have gotten pretty advanced. They help with personalization that feels more tailored over time. For instance, algorithms look at user data to spot patterns. Those patterns show which interventions work best for specific people. They also predict the right time to deliver those interventions for the biggest effect. Plus, they flag when someone might drop off or disengage. Natural language processing adds another layer. It lets conversational agents give responses that seem empathetic. They offer guidance that adjusts as needed.

Still, using AI brings up some big ethical issues. If algorithms learn from biased data, they just keep that bias going. Black-box systems in machine learning make choices that people struggle to understand or question. There's this sense that algorithms are neutral, but really, they hide the values built into how they're designed, and as AI gets even smarter, calls for strong ethical checks grow louder.

Mittelstadt and others from 2016 laid out a solid way to think about ethics in algorithms. It covers things like fairness, who takes responsibility, and how transparent everything is. These points hit hard in mental health areas. Errors from algorithms there can lead to real damage. So the field needs to build AI tools with care. That means keeping humans in the loop for oversight. It also requires clear ways to hold people accountable.

Virtual and Augmented Reality

Virtual reality and augmented reality technologies provide immersive experiences. They might help improve positive psychology interventions in meaningful ways. You can think about feeling nature's healing power through VR scenes of the outdoors or picture practising gratitude in fully wrapped moments that feel real. Even building compassion comes alive with perspective-taking in these setups. Such tools turn interventions into something more hands-on. They go beyond just mental workouts. Instead, they create experiences that involve the whole body.

Early studies on VR for mental health look promising. This holds true especially for treatments based on exposure. Work in positive psychology stays limited so far. Still, it feels intriguing. VR could mimic activities that lead to flow states. AR might add layers of information that boost meaning right into everyday surroundings. Ideas like this call for more investigation. Yet access to VR and AR stays restricted for many people. The gear costs a lot. It demands a good level of tech know how. Plus, some folks end up feeling unwell from it. Things like motion sickness or cyber sickness can hit hard. Even feelings of disconnection pose risks. Like any new tech these bring excitement. But people need to balance that with a clear look at the downsides. Fairness matters too in terms of who gets to use it and who gets left out.

Social and Collaborative Features

Early digital tools targeted single users mostly. Newer methods see the value in social ties for better well-being. Forums for peer support help a lot, and share goal-setting sessions. Practices like group gratitude or team challenges build in more involvement. They boost results through a sense of accountability from others. Connection plays a big role there.

Still social elements need smart handling. Online groups can turn negative without strong oversight. Seeing others' advances might hurt more than help sometimes. It can spark unhelpful comparisons. Privacy issues grow when people share personal details in groups. The benefits of social features must be balanced against these risks.

Parks et al. (2012) discuss how digital platforms can facilitate positive interpersonal processes, but warn against assuming that online connection substitutes for face-to-face relationships. The most effective approaches may combine digital social features with opportunities for in-person connection, as in hybrid models where app users also attend occasional group meetings.

Preventive and Developmental Applications

Most mental health intervention occurs after problems emerge. Digital PPIs offer potential for prevention and proactive well-being promotion. School-based programs could build resilience before students face major stressors. Workplace interventions could prevent burnout rather than responding after it occurs. Developmental interventions could support well-being across the lifespan, with age-appropriate content from childhood through late life.

Seligman et al. (2005) demonstrated that PPIs can be effective as universal preventive interventions, not just treatments for existing problems. This preventive potential represents a paradigm shift from reactive to proactive mental health care. However, implementing prevention requires different models: population-wide reach rather than clinical referral, sustained engagement over months or years rather than time-limited treatment, and addressing well-being before crisis rather than symptom relief.

The challenge is maintaining engagement when distress is absent. People seek help when suffering, not when functioning adequately. Preventive interventions must therefore provide immediate value that not just future protection to sustain participation. Framing PPIs as performance enhancement rather than illness prevention might increase uptake: not "prevent future depression" but "thrive in your daily life."

CONCLUSION

Individualized and digital PPIs represent a big shift in how we promote health. They blend technology with personal touches and strong ethics. This approach goes past the old mechanical ways of care. It heads toward something more whole and focused on people. Parks and Biswas-Diener talked about this in 2013. The change brings a lot of hope. It also brings real challenges that need constant focus.

After spending years in this area, I really think the future of digital well-being tools does not come down to fancier algorithms or nicer looking screens. The key thing is to keep in mind that every bit of data comes from a real person. That person has dreams and tough times. They have cultural backgrounds and lives that no numbers can fully capture. Tech can do a lot. Still, it stays just a tool and not the full answer. True well-being promotion comes down to human efforts. We need to figure out what people care about most. We support their development. We respect their worth as individuals.

Health psychology's path forward does not involve swapping out human links for computer programs. Instead, it means mixing sharp science with real kindness. Riva and others pointed this out in 2012. I have watched what happens when we strike that balance well. One example is a teenager dealing with depression. She gained some hope from a digital tool backed by peers. It let her connect with folks who got her pain in ways regular talks could not match. Another case involved a worn-out health worker. She turned to short PPIs in her breaks. This helped her keep going during the pandemic. She found bits of thanks and purpose even in heavy pressure. Then there was a dad mourning a loss. He worked through it with a mix of app activities and person-to-person help. Over time, he started putting his life back together after a huge heartbreak.

Stories like these show me the point of all this effort. They also keep me grounded. They point out how much we still have to learn. Specific parts of these tools make them work well. We wonder how to fit them right to each person. The mix of human help and digital parts needs the best setup. Equity has to come with growth in new ideas. No clear fixes exist for these issues just yet. The area is still new and acting too sure would not make sense.

Ethics have to lead any new steps. People require solid proof in practice along with caring support where tech by itself falls short. Human ties stay one of a kind and fairness counts a great deal. Tools must get built together with all kinds of groups, not just handed to them.

Positive Psychology can hold to its main goal by rooting digital advances in ethics and understanding. That goal goes beyond easing pain. It aims to help people thrive in all sorts of settings. Seligman laid this out in 2011. Huppert and so added to it in 2013. This idea drove the start of the field. It needs to keep shaping how it grows. Tech keeps getting better. This makes it easier to chase what we can count over what truly counts. We might favour big scale over fine details. Quick and easy could beat out what feels right for people. Staying alert against these pulls takes steady effort.

Technology fits into well-being tools without question. It sits right in the middle of how millions handle mental health and personal growth. The real issue comes down to how we shape it. We need the smarts, attention, and human touch that this area calls for. Human worth and respect for different cultures must stay at the centre. Fairness should run side by side with new ideas. We have to own up to weak spots as much as we cheer the wins. Ethical standards need to hold firm even as business pushes get stronger.

These points lay out the tough spot and the chance in front of us. How we respond will decide if digital PPIs live up to their big changes or just turn into another tech trend that overpromises. I hold out hope that sticking to key ideas will help. Those ideas include strong research, right conduct, respect for cultures, and true care for how complicated people are. With that, the field can handle this tricky ground.

We sit at a turning point right now. Tools stand ready to bring proven well-being help to billions. Science offers paths to good results. Plans exist to keep things right and fair. What we need most is the shared drive to handle this carefully. We should value lasting good over quick wins. Voices from overlooked groups must shape the designs. We have to admit what stays unclear. Loyalty to the core idea that started positive psychology must endure. That idea centres on helping people thrive.

The path forward looks involved and unclear. It matters a great deal though. Teams from many areas need to join in. Think psychology, design, tech, ethics, public health, and the communities hit most. We must accept our limits with some modesty. At the same time, boldness to try new things despite doubts fits in. Both old ways and fresh starts deserve respect. Long-gathered knowledge pairs with chances from recent tech.

At the heart, we must recall the reason for this push. Human thriving holds real value. Pain needs our focus. Every person should get a shot at a good life. If we lock in on the goal of true, lasting, fair well-being for all kinds of people in all kinds of places.

REFERENCES

Bakker, D., Kazantzis, N., Rickwood, D., & Rickard, N. (2016). Mental health smartphone apps: Review and evidence-based recommendations for future developments. *JMIR Mental Health*, *3*(1), e7. DOI: 10.2196/mental.4984 PMID: 26932350

Bauer, M., Glenn, T., Monteith, S., Bauer, R., Whybrow, P. C., & Geddes, J. (2017). Ethical perspectives on recommending digital technology for patients with mental illness. *International Journal of Bipolar Disorders*, *5*(1), 6. DOI: 10.1186/s40345-017-0073-9 PMID: 28155206

Beauchamp, T. L., & Childress, J. F. (2019). *Principles of biomedical ethics* (8th ed.). Oxford University Press.

Bhardwaj, A., Sharma, S., & Singh, R. (2021). Ethical implications of digital mental health interventions: A review. *Indian Journal of Psychological Medicine*, *43*(4), 333–340. DOI: 10.1177/02537176211008583

Bolier, L., Haverman, M., Westerhof, G. J., Riper, H., Smit, F., & Bohlmeijer, E. (2013). Positive psychology interventions: A meta-analysis of randomized controlled studies. *BMC Public Health*, *13*(1), 119. DOI: 10.1186/1471-2458-13-119 PMID: 23390882

Brown, T. (2008). Design thinking. *Harvard Business Review*, *86*(6), 84–92. PMID: 18605031

Choi, N. G., & Dinitto, D. M. (2013). The digital divide among low-income homebound older adults: Internet use patterns, eHealth literacy, and attitudes toward computer/Internet use. *Journal of Medical Internet Research*, *15*(5), e93. DOI: 10.2196/jmir.2645 PMID: 23639979

Creswell, J. W., & Plano Clark, V. L. (2017). *Designing and conducting mixed methods research* (3rd ed.). SAGE Publications.

Diener, E., & Chan, M. Y. (2011). Happy people live longer: Subjective well-being contributes to health and longevity. *Applied Psychology. Health and Well-Being*, *3*(1), 1–43. DOI: 10.1111/j.1758-0854.2010.01045.x PMID: 26286968

Engel, G. L. (1977). The need for a new medical model: A challenge for biomedicine. *Science*, *196*(4286), 129–136. DOI: 10.1126/science.847460 PMID: 847460

Firth, J., Torous, J., Nicholas, J., Carney, R., Pratap, A., Rosenbaum, S., & Sarris, J. (2019). The efficacy of smartphone-based mental health interventions for depressive symptoms: A meta-analysis. *World Psychiatry; Official Journal of the World Psychiatric Association (WPA), 18*(3), 325–336. DOI: 10.1002/wps.20673 PMID: 31496095

Firth, J., Torous, J., Nicholas, J., Carney, R., Rosenbaum, S., & Sarris, J. (2017). Can smartphone mental health interventions reduce symptoms of anxiety? A meta-analysis of randomized controlled trials. *Journal of Affective Disorders, 218*, 15–22. DOI: 10.1016/j.jad.2017.04.046 PMID: 28456072

Grady, C. (2015). Enduring and emerging challenges of informed consent. *The New England Journal of Medicine, 372*(9), 855–862. DOI: 10.1056/NEJMra1411250 PMID: 25714163

Graham, A. L., Cobb, N. K., Raymond, L., Sill, S., & Young, J. (2011). Effectiveness of an internet-based worksite smoking cessation intervention at 12 months. *Journal of Occupational and Environmental Medicine, 53*(7), 821–828. DOI: 10.1097/JOM.0b013e318220c5b3 PMID: 17693778

Hollis, C., Falconer, C. J., Martin, J. L., Whittington, C., Stockton, S., Glazebrook, C., & Davies, E. B. (2017). Annual research review: Digital health interventions for children and young people with mental health problems–a systematic and meta-review. *Journal of Child Psychology and Psychiatry, and Allied Disciplines, 58*(4), 474–503. DOI: 10.1111/jcpp.12663 PMID: 27943285

Horne, R., Bell, K., Marin, D., & Weinman, J. (2015). Understanding patients' adherence-related beliefs about medicines prescribed for long-term conditions: A meta-analytic review. *Annals of Behavioral Medicine, 49*(1), 1–15. DOI: 10.1007/s12160-014-9649-2 PMID: 24841509

Horvath, A. O., Del Re, A. C., Flückiger, C., & Symonds, D. (2011). Alliance in individual psychotherapy. *Psychotherapy (Chicago, Ill.), 48*(1), 9–16. DOI: 10.1037/a0022186 PMID: 21401269

Huppert, F. A., & So, T. T. (2013). Flourishing across Europe: Application of a new conceptual framework for defining well-being. *Social Indicators Research, 110*(3), 837–861. DOI: 10.1007/s11205-011-9966-7 PMID: 23329863

Keyes, C. L. (2002). The mental health continuum: From languishing to flourishing in life. *Journal of Health and Social Behavior, 43*(2), 207–222. DOI: 10.2307/3090197 PMID: 12096700

Krebs, P., Prochaska, J. O., & Rossi, J. S. (2010). A meta-analysis of computer-tailored interventions for health behavior change. *Preventive Medicine*, *51*(3–4), 214–221. DOI: 10.1016/j.ypmed.2010.06.004 PMID: 20558196

Lattie, E. G., Stiles-Shields, C., & Graham, A. K. (2019). An overview of and recommendations for more accessible digital mental health services. *Nature Reviews Psychology*, *1*(2), 87–100. DOI: 10.1038/s44159-021-00003-1 PMID: 38515434

Luxton, D. D., Kayl, R. A., & Mishkind, M. C. (2011). mHealth data security: The need for HIPAA-compliant standardization. *Telemedicine Journal and e-Health*, *18*(4), 284–288. DOI: 10.1089/tmj.2011.0180 PMID: 22400974

Miner, A. S., Milstein, A., Schueller, S., Hegde, R., Mangurian, C., & Linos, E. (2016). Smartphone-based conversational agents and responses to questions about mental health, interpersonal violence, and physical health. *JAMA Internal Medicine*, *176*(5), 619–625. DOI: 10.1001/jamainternmed.2016.0400 PMID: 26974260

Mittelstadt, B. D., Allo, P., Taddeo, M., Wachter, S., & Floridi, L. (2016). The ethics of algorithms: Mapping the debate. *Big Data & Society*, *3*(2), 1–21. DOI: 10.1177/2053951716679679

Mohr, D. C., Weingardt, K. R., Reddy, M., & Schueller, S. M. (2017). Three problems with current digital mental health research... and three things we can do about them. *Psychiatric Services (Washington, D.C.)*, *68*(5), 427–429. DOI: 10.1176/appi.ps.201600541 PMID: 28412890

Nebeker, C., Torous, J., & Bartlett Ellis, R. J. (2019). Building the case for actionable ethics in digital health research supported by artificial intelligence. *BMC Medicine*, *17*(1), 137. DOI: 10.1186/s12916-019-1377-7 PMID: 31311535

Norman, D. A. (2013). *The design of everyday things: Revised and expanded edition*. Basic Books.

Obar, J. A., & Oeldorf-Hirsch, A. (2020). The biggest lie on the internet: Ignoring the privacy policies and terms of service policies of social networking services. *Information Communication and Society*, *23*(1), 128–147. DOI: 10.1080/1369118X.2018.1486870

Parks, A. C., & Biswas-Diener, R. (2013). Positive interventions: Past, present, and future. In Kashdan, T. B., & Ciarrochi, J. (Eds.), *Mindfulness, acceptance, and positive psychology* (pp. 140–165). Context Press.

Parks, A. C., Schueller, S. M., & Tasimi, A. (2012). Positive psychology in digital contexts. *The American Psychologist*, *67*(6), 577–589. DOI: 10.1037/a0029121

Patel, V., Weiss, H. A., Chowdhary, N., Naik, S., Pednekar, S., Chatterjee, S., De Silva, M. J., Bhat, B., Araya, R., King, M., Simon, G., Verdeli, H., & Kirkwood, B. R. (2010). Effectiveness of an intervention led by lay health counsellors for depressive and anxiety disorders in primary care in Goa, India (MANAS): A cluster randomised controlled trial. *Lancet*, *376*(9758), 2086–2095. DOI: 10.1016/S0140-6736(10)61508-5 PMID: 21159375

Pressman, S. D., & Cohen, S. (2005). Does positive affect influence health? *Psychological Bulletin*, *131*(6), 925–971. DOI: 10.1037/0033-2909.131.6.925 PMID: 16351329

Ramsetty, A., & Adams, C. (2020). Impact of the digital divide in the age of COVID-19. *Journal of the American Medical Informatics Association : JAMIA*, *27*(7), 1147–1148. DOI: 10.1093/jamia/ocaa078 PMID: 32343813

Riva, G., Banos, R. M., Botella, C., Wiederhold, B. K., & Gaggioli, A. (2012). Positive technology: Using interactive technologies to promote positive functioning. *Cyberpsychology, Behavior, and Social Networking*, *15*(2), 69–77. DOI: 10.1089/cyber.2011.0139 PMID: 22149077

Ryff, C. D. (2014). Psychological well-being revisited: Advances in the science and practice of eudaimonia. *Psychotherapy and Psychosomatics*, *83*(1), 10–28. DOI: 10.1159/000353263 PMID: 24281296

Ryff, C. D., Singer, B. H., & Dienberg Love, G. (2004). Positive health: Connecting well-being with biology. *Philosophical Transactions of the Royal Society of London. Series B, Biological Sciences*, *359*(1449), 1383–1394. DOI: 10.1098/rstb.2004.1521 PMID: 15347530

Sanders, E. B. N., & Stappers, P. J. (2008). Co-creation and the new landscapes of design. *CoDesign*, *4*(1), 5–18. DOI: 10.1080/15710880701875068

Schueller, S. M., Tomasino, K. N., & Mohr, D. C. (2017). Integrating human support into behavioral intervention technologies: The efficiency model of support. *Clinical Psychology : a Publication of the Division of Clinical Psychology of the American Psychological Association*, *24*(1), 27–45. DOI: 10.1111/cpsp.12173

Seligman, M. E. P. (2011). *Flourish: A visionary new understanding of happiness and well-being*. Free Press.

Seligman, M. E. P., & Csikszentmihalyi, M. (2000). Positive psychology: An introduction. *The American Psychologist*, *55*(1), 5–14. DOI: 10.1037/0003-066X.55.1.5 PMID: 11392865

Seligman, M. E. P., Steen, T. A., Park, N., & Peterson, C. (2005). Positive psychology progress: Empirical validation of interventions. *The American Psychologist*, *60*(5), 410–421. DOI: 10.1037/0003-066X.60.5.410 PMID: 16045394

Sheldon, K. M., & Lyubomirsky, S. (2006). How to increase and sustain positive emotion: The effects of expressing gratitude and visualizing best possible selves. *The Journal of Positive Psychology*, *1*(2), 73–82. DOI: 10.1080/17439760500510676

Sin, N. L., & Lyubomirsky, S. (2009). Enhancing well-being and alleviating depressive symptoms with Positive Psychology Interventions: A practice-friendly meta-analysis. *Journal of Clinical Psychology*, *65*(5), 467–487. DOI: 10.1002/jclp.20593 PMID: 19301241

Steptoe, A., Deaton, A., & Stone, A. A. (2015). Subjective well-being, health, and aging. *Lancet*, *385*(9968), 640–648. DOI: 10.1016/S0140-6736(13)61489-0 PMID: 25468152

Torous, J., Myrick, K. J., Rauseo-Ricupero, N., & Firth, J. (2021). Digital mental health and COVID-19: Using technology today to accelerate the curve on access and quality tomorrow. *JMIR Mental Health*, *8*(3), e18848. DOI: 10.2196/18848 PMID: 32213476

Veinot, T. C., Mitchell, H., & Ancker, J. S. (2018). Good intentions are not enough: How informatics interventions can worsen inequality. *Journal of the American Medical Informatics Association : JAMIA*, *25*(8), 1080–1088. DOI: 10.1093/jamia/ocy052 PMID: 29788380

Watts, S., Marchand, A., Bouchard, S., Gosselin, P., Langlois, F., Belleville, G., & Dugas, M. J. (2020). Telepsychotherapy for generalized anxiety disorder: A randomized controlled trial. *Cognitive Behaviour Therapy*, *49*(3), 192–205. DOI: 10.1080/16506073.2019.1699741

Yardley, L., Morrison, L., Bradbury, K., & Muller, I. (2015). The person-based approach to intervention development: Application to digital health-related behavior change interventions. *Journal of Medical Internet Research*, *17*(1), e30. DOI: 10.2196/jmir.4055 PMID: 25639757

Chapter 3
Delivering Health in the Gig Economy:
Telemedicine as a Tool for Access, Inclusion, and Well-Being

Pooja Kalbalia
http://orcid.org/0000-0002-3739-3165
St. Joseph's University, India

Kailash Koushik
Christ University, India

ABSTRACT

Quick commerce delivery workers in Southeast Asia face significant health risks from long working hours, environmental exposure, and limited access to healthcare. This narrative review explores how telemedicine can address these challenges by analysing literature from South and Southeast Asia. Thematic analysis highlights three key areas: barriers to adoption (low digital literacy, poor internet connectivity, financial limitations, and mistrust), policy and platform gaps (fragmented regulations, weak accountability, and data security concerns), and climate-linked vulnerabilities (heat stress, pollution, and mental health strain). Findings suggest that telemedicine offers affordable consultations, mental health support, and flexible digital platforms that are well-suited to the unpredictable schedules of gig workers. However, broader adoption requires policy integration, literacy training, and inclusive initiatives. While evidence remains emergent, telemedicine shows strong potential as a scalable, preventive health solution for quick commerce workers in Southeast Asia.

DOI: 10.4018/979-8-2600-3085-1.ch003

INTRODUCTION

The platform-based gig economy has swiftly reshaped global labour markets and is widely portrayed as the future of work, providing flexible employment opportunities to millions worldwide (Kalbalia & Koushik, 2025b) .The quick commerce sector, characterised by on-demand delivery services for groceries, food, and everyday essentials, has rapidly transformed consumer behaviour and economic landscapes in Southeast Asia (Bajwa et al., 2018; Kalbalia & Koushik, 2025c).Driven by advancements in mobile technology and digital platforms, this industry caters to the increasing demand for speed and convenience in urban areas (Liyanage et al., 2019). However, the foundations of this evolving sector rest on the labour of gig workers, a workforce that engages in short-term, flexible jobs often facilitated by digital platforms (Stanford, 2017). While the sector's growth has reshaped retail and logistics, the working conditions of delivery personnel remain a critical and often overlooked issue, particularly in health and safety (Mayhew & Quinlan, 2006; Nikulin et al., 2022).

Gig workers in quick commerce endure demanding conditions intensified by environmental, structural, and systemic challenges (Kalbalia & Koushik, 2025a). Climate change plays a significant role in worsening their hardships, as extreme weather events such as heatwaves, heavy rainfall, and monsoons become more frequent and severe (Schulte & Chun, 2009). These environmental factors directly impact delivery workers, who often work outdoors or travel long distances under harsh conditions (Jiang et al., 2024). Heat stress, dehydration, and exposure to polluted air are common occupational hazards, while sudden weather changes pose safety risks. Such factors not only compromise the immediate health of these workers but also have long-term implications for their physical and mental well-being (Abokhashabah et al., 2021; Applebaum et al., 2016).

Beyond environmental challenges, structural issues within the gig economy further worsen the vulnerabilities of delivery workers (Anwar & Graham, 2021; Kalbalia et al., 2024). Their work typically involves long hours and irregular schedules, often dictated by fluctuating consumer demand (Lambert et al., 2012). This unpredictability leaves workers unable to establish stable routines, including accessing timely healthcare. Furthermore, the absence of employer-provided benefits such as health insurance, sick leave, or other social protections means that many workers must bear the full burden of healthcare costs out of pocket (Flouris et al., 2018; Koutsimpogiorgos et al., 2020). These challenges create an unwarranted environment where even minor health issues can spiral into significant economic and physical hardships. The gap between the needs of these workers and the healthcare resources available to them highlights an urgent need for innovative solutions.

Telemedicine emerges as a promising avenue to address the healthcare challenges faced by quick commerce delivery workers. Telemedicine leverages digital technology to provide remote healthcare services, including consultations, diagnosis, monitoring, and treatment (Shen et al., 2021). Telemedicine offers a practical alternative for delivery workers, whose work schedules and income levels often prevent them from accessing traditional healthcare facilities. It enables workers to seek medical advice and support without travelling, reducing time and financial barriers. Moreover, telemedicine can address specific health challenges associated with their work, such as climate-related illnesses or stress-induced mental health conditions (Alanzi, 2021).

Telemedicine's potential to transform healthcare access lies in its ability to deliver timely, personalised, and scalable interventions. For example, climate-specific health alerts integrated into telemedicine platforms can provide workers with real-time information on heat stress or air quality, enabling them to take preventive measures (Katzman et al., 2022). Similarly, remote mental health counselling can help workers manage job-related stress and anxiety, which are prevalent in the gig economy (Yassa et al., 2022). Preventive services such as regular health check-ups and acute illness management can further enhance the overall well-being of this workforce. By bridging the gap between healthcare services and needs of delivery workers, telemedicine can play a critical role in building resilience among this vulnerable group.

While telemedicine has great potential, its implementation in quick commerce platforms faces various challenges. In Southeast Asia, workers' uneven access to digital infrastructure and low levels of digital literacy remain significant barriers (Nutbeam & Lloyd, 2020). While smartphone penetration is high in urban areas, reliable internet connectivity is not guaranteed across all regions. Additionally, many workers may lack the skills or confidence to use telemedicine apps effectively, necessitating targeted efforts to improve digital literacy (Fitzpatrick, 2023; Stanberry, 2000). On the part of platform providers, financial constraints and regulatory uncertainties often deter investment in telemedicine services. Companies operating on tight profit margins may hesitate to allocate resources to worker healthcare unless clear incentives or mandates exist. These challenges underline the need for a collaborative approach to scale telemedicine solutions.

Opportunities to overcome these barriers are equally substantial. Mobile-based telemedicine platforms tailored to the specific needs of gig workers can ensure accessibility and affordability (Hui et al., 2022). Collaboration with local healthcare providers, community organisations, and non-governmental organisations can create cost-effective healthcare delivery models. For instance, partnerships can facilitate integrating telemedicine services into existing platforms while leveraging community networks to promote awareness and adoption. Digital health education programs can empower workers to use telemedicine tools effectively, enhancing engagement and outcomes (V. Sharma et al., 2024). Innovative features such as climate risk alerts and region-specific health resources can further address the unique challenges faced by delivery workers, particularly in the context of climate change (Flouris et al., 2018).

LITERATURE REVIEW

Telemedicine leverages electronic and telecommunication technologies to provide healthcare services, including remote consultations, diagnostics, and patient monitoring (Alanzi, 2021; Haleem et al., 2021). Initially developed to connect specialists to remote or underserved regions in high-income countries, telemedicine has progressively gained traction in low- and middle-income countries (LMICs) as a cost-effective and accessible alternative to traditional healthcare systems (Comlek & Ordu, 2021). Its adoption is particularly relevant in regions where limited infrastructure, insufficient medical personnel, and a scarcity of diagnostic tools hinder access to adequate healthcare (Gonzalez Garcia et al., 2019; Marsh et al., 2022).

Telemedicine in Low and Middle-Income Countries: Adoption and Potential

Conceptual frameworks supporting telemedicine adoption in LMICs highlight its capacity to bridge geographical healthcare access gaps, address human resource shortages, and improve the efficiency of medical information flow (Marshall et al., 2021). For example, telemedicine platforms facilitate remote consultations for patients who lack proximity to hospitals, saving time, reducing transportation costs, and alleviating pressure on overburdened healthcare systems (Hjelm, 2005). Furthermore, telemedicine enhances cost-efficiency by minimising unnecessary referrals and enabling effective triaging. Studies show that telemedicine systems improve primary care, preventive services, and mental health support outcomes, particularly in resource-constrained environments (Haleem et al., 2021).

The successful implementation of telemedicine depends on its alignment with cultural, linguistic, and infrastructural contexts (Jelinek et al., 2022). For instance, patient trust, digital literacy, and cultural attitudes toward remote consultations are critical in determining telemedicine adoption rates (Azahra et al., 2024). Community engagement, including the involvement of local health workers and policymakers, enhances the likelihood of alignment with regional health priorities and regulatory standards, fostering long-term sustainability (Seaton et al., 2022). However, the literature identifies challenges, including technological constraints such as unreliable internet connections, limited smartphone access, and sporadic electricity supply

(Gleiss & Lewandowski, 2022). Data privacy concerns further complicate telemedicine adoption, as sensitive patient information demands secure handling (Grande et al., 2020). Divergent regulatory frameworks, inconsistent licensing protocols, and varying standards for remote patient care add additional complexity to the equitable deployment of telemedicine systems (Alanzi, 2021).

Gig Work and Health Challenges

The gig economy, characterised by platform-based services such as quick commerce, ride-hailing, and food delivery, has transformed labour markets globally (Shah et al., 2023). While these platforms offer flexibility and income opportunities, they expose workers to precarious conditions with minimal social protections (Koutsimpogiorgos et al., 2020). Quick commerce, in particular, emphasises rapid delivery under tight deadlines, amplifying workers' occupational health risks (Mayhew & Quinlan, 2002). Research on gig workers' health highlights musculoskeletal, cardiovascular, and mental health issues resulting from prolonged physical exertion, irregular work hours, and high-stress environments (Landsbergis et al., 2001). Additionally, delivery workers navigate congested urban spaces, often exposed to traffic-related pollution and unpredictable road conditions, further compromising their well-being (Chandel, 2025; Khreis et al., 2016)

Climate Change and Occupational Health Risks

Climate change intensifies these vulnerabilities, especially in regions like South and Southeast Asia, which experience extreme weather patterns, including heatwaves, monsoons, and fluctuating precipitation (Nadeau et al., 2017). Studies reveal that rising temperatures aggravate the risks of heat-related illnesses, dehydration, and long-term chronic conditions for outdoor workers with limited control over their work environments, who are particularly susceptible to these climate-induced health hazards (Gibb et al., 2024; Schulte & Chun, 2009). Additionally, prolonged exposure to air pollution in urban settings heightens their respiratory risks.

The absence of formal labour protections further compounds these challenges. Unlike traditional employees, gig workers often lack health insurance, paid sick leave, and occupational health screenings (Lester et al., 2021; Stewart & Stanford, 2017). As independent contractors, gig workers face financial barriers to healthcare access and receive minimal support for preventive care (Pande, 2024).This precarious situation forces many workers to prioritise short-term income over long-term health, foregoing medical consultations or preventive interventions.

Regional Dynamics in Digital Health and Telemedicine

The rapid growth of mobile technologies has spurred digital health innovations in South and Southeast Asia (Khanijahani et al., 2022). India, Indonesia, the Philippines, and Vietnam are leveraging high smartphone penetration to promote mobile health (mHealth) applications and digital health platforms. Governments and non-governmental organisations are deploying telemedicine solutions to address healthcare inequities in urban and rural communities (Megasari et al., 2023). However, telemedicine adoption remains uneven due to regulatory gaps, infrastructural deficiencies, and disparities in digital literacy (Nutbeam & Lloyd, 2020).

While some nations, such as India, have implemented telemedicine guidelines, others lack comprehensive frameworks to address medical licensing, liability, and data privacy concerns. These inconsistencies impede telemedicine's integration into national healthcare systems, undermining trust among users and providers. Furthermore, infrastructural challenges, including unreliable telecommunications networks and electricity in rural areas, hinder the effectiveness of digital health tools (Du et al., 2022).

Telemedicine and Vulnerable Populations

Studies on telemedicine for vulnerable populations reveal its potential to improve healthcare access for communities facing geographic and economic barriers (Agochukwu et al., 2018; Yarney et al., 2023). For example, telemedicine has proven effective in addressing mental health needs, particularly among individuals under chronic stress, by reducing stigma and providing privacy (Ford et al., 2022). Mobile-based telemedicine models integrating community health workers have demonstrated cost-effectiveness and scalability in low-resource settings (Durojaiye et al., 2022). However, the literature highlights potential inequities in telemedicine's reach. While telemedicine services appeal due to convenience, affordability, and accessibility, individuals with limited digital access or literacy may remain excluded (Megasari et al., 2023). To mitigate this risk, targeted training, culturally sensitive communication strategies, and user-friendly interfaces are essential for broad adoption.

Despite its promise, the role of telemedicine in addressing the health challenges of gig workers in the quick commerce industry remains underexplored. Existing studies focus primarily on rural populations, chronic disease management, and maternal and child health (Khanijahani et al., 2022). The intersection of climate change, gig work, and telemedicine solutions has received limited attention, leaving a critical gap in understanding how to tailor digital health tools to the unique demands of quick commerce delivery workers. The absence of research on integrating telemedicine into platform-based work environments limits insights into effective implementation. Questions remain about how platforms can incorporate telemedicine functionalities, such as health alerts or scheduling teleconsultations, and what regulatory or financial incentives might encourage adoption. Addressing these gaps is vital to ensuring that telemedicine can be a comprehensive solution rather than a substitute measure.

METHODOLOGY

The research employs a qualitative, literature-based methodology, relying on secondary data sources to examine the integration of telemedicine into gig economy platforms. The study identifies patterns, barriers, and opportunities in telemedicine adoption by systematically reviewing academic literature, policy documents, reports, and guidelines. The research synthesises evidence from four main categories of secondary data: academic literature from databases such as PubMed and Scopus, policy documents and health strategies from governmental and intergovernmental organisations like the WHO, reports from NGOs and development agencies addressing occupational health and climate adaptation, and industry reports detailing platform-specific strategies and innovations. These sources ensure a balanced perspective, combining theoretical insights with practical relevance.

A structured data retrieval process was implemented, using keyword searches with terms like "telemedicine," "gig workers," "quick commerce," and "climate adaptation," refined by Boolean operators and filters (e.g., publication date within the last decade). Inclusion criteria encompassed English-language publications focused on Southeast Asia and relevant topics such as telemedicine, gig economy health, and climate resilience. Exclusion criteria omitted irrelevant studies, opinion pieces lacking evidence, and specialised applications unrelated to the study's context. Academic sources were assessed for peer review status and methodological rigour to ensure the quality and credibility of the selected data. Thematic analysis was employed to interpret the data, identifying recurring themes such as "barriers to telemedicine adoption," "policy fragmentation," and "climate-related health risks." A coding framework guided data organisation into broader themes and subthemes, including regulatory and policy landscapes (e.g., licensing issues, reimbursement models) and climate-related occupational health challenges (e.g., heat stress interventions, air quality monitoring). Themes were refined for coherence and relevance, connecting findings to the research questions and contextualising results within existing theoretical frameworks.

ANALYSIS AND DISCUSSION

Themes and Codes generated

1. Barriers to Telemedicine Adoption
    - o Digital infrastructure issues: unreliable internet, high data costs, limited smartphone access.
    - o Financial constraints include consultation fees, app subscriptions, and a lack of employer health benefits.
    - o Digital literacy challenges: navigation difficulties, language barriers, complex interfaces.
    - o Trust issues: scepticism about diagnosis accuracy and preference for in-person consultations.
2. Policy Fragmentation
    - o Regulatory inconsistencies: unclear licensing requirements, cross-border consultation ambiguities.
    - o Employer responsibility: gaps include a lack of gig platform health benefits and classification as independent contractors.
    - o Data security: Concerns include risks of breaches and a lack of transparency in data handling.
    - o Policy silos: limited integration of health and occupational policies.
3. Climate-Related Health Risks
    - o Heat stress risks: exposure to high temperatures, dehydration, fatigue.
    - o Air quality concerns: exposure to pollutants, respiratory health issues.
    - o Injury risks: road accidents and lack of immediate medical care.
    - o Mental health challenges: job stress, anxiety, exposure to extreme conditions.

BARRIERS TO TELEMEDICINE ADOPTION

The adoption of telemedicine has been significantly influenced by various barriers that can be categorised into digital infrastructure issues, financial constraints, digital literacy challenges, and trust issues. These barriers not only hinder the implementation of telemedicine but also affect its effectiveness and accessibility across different populations.

Digital Infrastructure Issues

A primary barrier to telemedicine adoption is inadequate digital infrastructure, including unreliable internet connectivity, high data costs, and limited smartphone access. In many regions, particularly in low-resource settings, the lack of reliable internet can severely restrict the ability of both healthcare providers and patients to engage in telemedicine services. For instance, a study highlighted that many healthcare institutions in Nigeria were only at a "beginner level of readiness" for telemedicine implementation due to insufficient digital infrastructure (Musa et al., 2023). Similarly, research in Kenya emphasised that physical ICT infrastructure and fast internet connectivity are crucial for effectively utilising telemedicine (Onsongo et al., 2023). The disparities in digital infrastructure can lead to unequal access to healthcare services, exacerbating existing health inequities (Omaghomi et al., 2023). Furthermore, the financial aspect of digital infrastructure cannot be overlooked. High data costs can deter patients from utilising telemedicine services, particularly in regions where healthcare costs are already a significant burden. The financial implications of telemedicine, including the costs associated with necessary technology and internet access, can be prohibitive for many individuals and healthcare providers, further complicating the adoption process.

Financial Constraints

Financial constraints represent another significant barrier to telemedicine adoption. Consultation fees and app subscriptions can deter patients without employer health benefits or adequate insurance coverage. A systematic review indicated that financial barriers, including the costs associated with telemedicine services, are a critical factor influencing its adoption (Kruse et al., 2018). In many cases, patients may prioritise in-person consultations over telemedicine due to perceived or actual costs, which can limit the reach of telehealth services (Pierce et al., 2021). Moreover, the lack of reimbursement policies for telemedicine services in certain regions can further complicate the financial landscape. Although there has been progress in some countries post-pandemic, reimbursement for telemedicine remains inconsistent, which can discourage healthcare providers from offering these services (Hart et al., 2022).The financial sustainability of telemedicine programs is thus contingent on establishing supportive policies that ensure equitable access to care.

Digital Literacy Challenges

Digital literacy is a crucial factor influencing the adoption of telemedicine. Many patients face challenges in navigating telemedicine platforms, which can be aggravated by language barriers and complex user interfaces. A qualitative analysis found that multilingual patients often experienced difficulties in using telemedicine services, leading to a hesitance to engage with these platforms fully (Nguyen et al., 2022). This highlights the need for user-friendly interfaces and multilingual support to enhance accessibility. Additionally, healthcare providers may lack the training to effectively utilise telemedicine technologies. A review of telemedicine guidelines in Southeast Asia identified limited digital literacy among healthcare providers as a significant challenge (P. Sharma et al., 2023). The successful implementation of telemedicine requires patient education and comprehensive training programs for healthcare professionals to ensure they are equipped to navigate and utilise telemedicine technologies effectively.

Trust Issues

Trust issues also play a critical role in the adoption of telemedicine. Many patients express scepticism regarding the accuracy of diagnoses made through telemedicine, preferring in-person consultations where they feel more assured of the quality of care (Nguyen et al., 2022). This scepticism can stem from a lack of familiarity with telemedicine technologies and concerns about a potential misdiagnosis or inadequate care. A systematic review indicated that trust in the technology and the healthcare providers delivering care through telemedicine is essential for its acceptance (Kruse et al., 2018). Moreover, the cultural context can influence trust in telemedicine. In some regions, traditional in-person consultations are deeply ingrained in healthcare practices, making it challenging for telemedicine to gain acceptance. The resistance to change among healthcare providers, driven by fears of increased medical errors and a preference for established practices, can further hinder the integration of telemedicine into existing healthcare systems (Hosseini et al., 2024).

In short, the barriers to telemedicine adoption are multifaceted. Digital infrastructure issues, financial constraints, digital literacy challenges, and trust issues create obstacles. To address these barriers, we need a comprehensive approach that improves digital infrastructure, establishes supportive financial policies, enhances digital literacy among patients and healthcare providers, and fosters trust in telemedicine technologies. By tackling these challenges, we can fully realise the potential of telemedicine to improve healthcare access and outcomes.

POLICY FRAGMENTATION IN THE GIG ECONOMY

The gig economy has emerged as a significant component of modern labour markets, characterised by short-term, flexible work arrangements facilitated by digital platforms. However, this new economic model is fraught with policy fragmentation, which manifests in various forms, including regulatory inconsistencies, employer responsibility gaps, data security concerns, and policy silos. These issues affect gig workers' rights, protections, and overall well-being.

Regulatory Inconsistencies

One of the most prominent issues in the gig economy is the lack of clear and consistent regulatory frameworks. Licensing requirements for gig platforms often vary significantly across jurisdictions, leading to confusion and ambiguity for workers and employers. For instance, the classification of gig workers as independent contractors rather than employees has significant implications for their access to benefits and protections (Koutsimpogiorgos et al., 2020). This classification is often upheld by platforms that leverage "clickwrap agreements," which allow them to impose unilateral terms that can change without notice, further complicating the regulatory landscape (Lei, 2021).

The absence of standardised regulations can create an environment where gig workers are left vulnerable to exploitation and inadequate protection (Ayentimi et al., 2023). Moreover, cross-border consultation ambiguities exacerbate these inconsistencies. As gig work often transcends national borders, the lack of harmonised regulations can lead to significant worker rights and protection disparities. This fragmentation is particularly evident in the European Union, where different member states have adopted varying approaches to gig work regulation, resulting in a patchwork of protections that can be difficult for workers to navigate (Tan et al., 2020). A cohesive regulatory framework that addresses these inconsistencies is critical to ensuring fair treatment for gig workers across different jurisdictions.

Employer Responsibility Gaps

Another significant area of concern is the responsibility gaps that exist between gig platforms and their workers. Many gig platforms do not provide health benefits or other essential protections typically associated with traditional employment, leaving workers to fend for themselves regarding health insurance and social security (Palhad et al., 2023). This lack of employer responsibility is particularly problematic during the COVID-19 pandemic, where gig workers have faced heightened health risks without adequate support (Harpur & Blanck, 2020). The classification of gig workers as independent contractors further complicates this issue, as it often absolves platforms of responsibilities related to worker welfare and benefits (Gussek et al., 2021).

The implications of this classification are profound, as gig workers frequently experience financial instability and job insecurity, which can adversely affect their mental and physical health (Gregory, 2021). The absence of employer-provided benefits undermines the well-being of gig workers and contributes to broader societal issues, such as increased reliance on public health systems and social safety nets (Chen et al., 2022). Addressing these gaps requires re-evaluating the legal definitions of employment and the responsibilities of gig platforms towards their workers.

Data Security Concerns

Data security is another critical issue within the gig economy, as gig platforms often collect vast amounts of personal information from their users. The risks of data breaches and the lack of transparency in data handling practices raise significant concerns about the privacy and security of gig workers (Cox et al., 2024). Many gig workers are unaware of how their data is being used or shared, which can lead to exploitation and misuse of their information (Jiaojiao & Lifei, 2023) Furthermore, the reliance on algorithms for management and decision-making in gig work can exacerbate these concerns, as the opaque nature of algorithmic processes can lead to discriminatory practices and a lack of accountability (Zhang et al., 2023). The ethical implications of data handling in the gig economy are profound, as they intersect with worker autonomy and control issues. Gig workers often find themselves at the mercy of algorithms that dictate their work conditions, pay rates, and job opportunities, raising questions about the fairness and transparency of these systems (Wood & Lehdonvirta, 2021) To mitigate these risks, there is a pressing need for robust data protection regulations that safeguard the rights of gig workers and ensure transparency in data handling practices.

Policy Silos

Finally, the fragmentation of health and occupational safety policies further complicates the landscape for gig workers. Many gig workers operate in environments that lack adequate health and safety regulations, leading to increased risks of injury and illness (Kaushik, 2024). The limited integration of health and occupational policies means that gig workers often fall through the cracks of existing regulatory frameworks, leaving them without traditional employee protections (Hadi & Pratono, 2024). This lack of integration can result in significant disparities in access to healthcare and occupational safety measures, further exacerbating the vulnerabilities faced by gig workers. A holistic approach to policy development that considers the unique challenges of gig work is essential. By integrating health, safety, and labour policies, governments can create a more supportive environment for gig workers, ensuring they receive the protections and benefits necessary for their well-being (Cropanzano et al., 2022). Such an approach would enhance the quality of work for gig workers and contribute to broader societal goals of equity and social justice.

In conclusion, the gig economy poses complex challenges related to policy fragmentation. Regulatory inconsistencies, gaps in employer responsibility, data security concerns, and policy silos create an environment where gig workers often find themselves vulnerable and unprotected. To address these issues, policymakers, platform operators, and stakeholders must work together to create a cohesive regulatory framework that safeguards the rights and well-being of gig workers. Only through comprehensive reforms can the gig economy realise its potential as a fair and equitable labour market.

CLIMATE-RELATED HEALTH RISKS

Climate change poses significant health risks across various domains, including heat stress, air quality, injury risks, and mental health challenges. Each area is interlinked, reflecting the complex interplay between environmental changes and human health.

Heat Stress Risks

Heat stress is critical as global temperatures rise, leading to increased dehydration, fatigue, and heat-related illnesses. Exposure to high temperatures can exacerbate existing health conditions and lead to acute health crises. Research indicates that extreme heat can significantly impact physiological functions, leading to heat exhaustion and heat stroke, particularly among vulnerable populations such as the elderly and those with pre-existing health conditions (Lõhmus, 2018). The National Institute for Occupational Safety and Health (NIOSH) has established criteria for safe exposure levels to heat, emphasising the need for protective measures in occupational settings (Jacklitsch et al., 2016). Furthermore, studies have shown that prolonged exposure to high temperatures can lead to increased morbidity and mortality rates, particularly in regions with inadequate healthcare infrastructure (Venugopal et al., 2015).

Air Quality Concerns

Air quality is another pressing issue linked to climate change, as rising temperatures can exacerbate the formation of ground-level ozone and other pollutants. Poor air quality is associated with various respiratory health issues, including asthma, chronic obstructive pulmonary disease (COPD), and other pulmonary disorders. The World Health Organisation (WHO) recognises air pollution as a major environmental risk to health, particularly in urban areas where industrial activities and vehicular emissions are prevalent (Illingworth, 2024). Research has demonstrated that climate change can act as a threat amplifier, worsening pre-existing health disparities and disproportionately affecting marginalised communities (Hwong et al., 2022). Moreover, the interplay between heat and air quality can create a vicious cycle where increased temperatures lead to higher pollution levels, compromising respiratory health (Cianconi et al., 2023).

Injury Risks

Increased temperatures and extreme weather events also heighten injury risks, particularly in the context of road accidents and the accessibility of medical care. As climate-related disasters become more frequent, accidents increase due to deteriorating infrastructure and hazardous conditions. For instance, heavy rainfall and flooding can lead to road washouts and increased vehicular accidents (Levison et al., 2018). Additionally, the lack of immediate medical care during extreme weather events can exacerbate injuries sustained, leading to higher morbidity rates (Shoib et al., 2023). Integrating climate adaptation strategies into urban planning is essential to mitigate these risks and enhance community resilience (Levison et al., 2018).

Mental Health Challenges

The mental health implications of climate change are profound and multifaceted. Individuals exposed to extreme environmental conditions often experience heightened levels of anxiety, stress, and depression. The concept of eco-anxiety has gained traction, reflecting the psychological distress associated with environmental degradation and climate change (Ojala et al., 2021). Research indicates that climate change can lead to helplessness and grief, particularly among young people and vulnerable populations (Gunasiri et al., 2022). The mental health impacts are not merely a consequence of direct exposure to climate events but also stem from the broader socio-economic disruptions caused by climate change, such as displacement and loss of livelihoods (Crane et al., 2022). Furthermore, the mental health consequences of climate change are compounded by existing social inequalities.

Vulnerable populations, including women and Indigenous communities, often bear the brunt of climate-related stressors due to pre-existing socio-economic disadvantages (Goudet et al., 2024). Studies have shown that women, particularly in developing countries, face unique challenges related to mental health in the context of climate change, exacerbated by gender roles and limited access to resources (Goudet et al., 2023). Integrating mental health considerations into climate change adaptation and mitigation strategies is crucial for effectively addressing these challenges.

Even though climate change poses numerous health risks, including heat stress, air quality issues, injury risks, and mental health challenges, to tackle these problems, we must integrate public health considerations into climate policy and planning comprehensively. By acknowledging the interconnectedness of these health risks, stakeholders can create more effective strategies to mitigate the impacts of climate change on human health.

LIMITATIONS

This study is subject to several limitations that should be considered when interpreting its findings. First, the reliance on secondary data through a narrative literature review limits the scope for empirical validation. While the synthesis of existing research provides valuable theoretical and contextual insights, the absence of primary data constrains the ability to capture lived experiences, behavioural nuances, and platform-specific practices of gig workers and service providers. As a result, the findings should be understood as analytical and interpretive rather than empirically causal.

Second, the lack of primary engagement with gig workers, healthcare providers, and platform companies may restrict the practical applicability and operational feasibility of the proposed telemedicine solutions. Without direct stakeholder input, it is not possible to assess workers' real-world preferences, levels of trust in telemedicine systems, or the readiness of platforms to integrate health services into existing digital infrastructures.

Third, the regional focus on Southeast Asia introduces contextual limitations. Labour regulations, healthcare systems, digital infrastructure, and climate exposure vary significantly across regions, which may limit the generalisability of the findings to other global contexts. While many of the identified challenges are common to gig workers worldwide, the policy implications and implementation pathways may differ in regions with stronger labour protections or more advanced health systems.

Additionally, although the study identifies key barriers such as digital literacy gaps, infrastructural constraints, and policy fragmentation, it does not provide a granular assessment of telemedicine implementation models within specific gig platforms. Factors such as platform governance structures, cost-sharing mechanisms, algorithmic management practices, and provider reimbursement models remain underexplored and warrant further investigation. The heterogeneity of the reviewed literature, including variations in study designs, definitions of gig work, and measurements of health outcomes, may introduce interpretive inconsistencies. While thematic analysis was employed to enhance coherence, differences in methodological quality and contextual focus across sources could influence the synthesis of findings.

Despite these limitations, the study offers a comprehensive conceptual foundation for understanding the potential role of telemedicine in addressing the health vulnerabilities of quick commerce workers and provides a basis for future empirical, policy-oriented, and intervention-based research.

CONCLUSION

The rapid expansion of quick commerce across Southeast Asia has reshaped consumption patterns, urban logistics, and labour markets, embedding speed and convenience at the core of everyday economic life. However, this transformation has come at a significant human cost, particularly for delivery workers who operate under conditions of occupational precarity, environmental exposure, and limited institutional protection. The findings of this review underscore that gig workers in quick commerce face intersecting health vulnerabilities, including physical strain, climate-related risks, and mental health challenges intensified by algorithmic management, irregular working hours, and restricted access to formal healthcare systems. These vulnerabilities are further exacerbated by the absence of employer-provided health benefits and fragmented regulatory oversight, placing the burden of health management largely on individual workers.

Within this context, telemedicine emerges as a viable and scalable intervention capable of addressing systemic gaps in healthcare access for gig workers. By enabling timely, remote, and flexible healthcare delivery, telemedicine aligns closely with the realities of a highly mobile and time-constrained workforce. The review demonstrates that telemedicine has the potential to strengthen both preventive and curative care by facilitating early diagnosis, continuous health monitoring, mental health support, and rapid response to climate-related health risks. Importantly, telemedicine should not be viewed merely as a technological substitute for in-person care, but as a complementary health infrastructure that can enhance resilience, reduce healthcare delays, and mitigate long-term health deterioration among delivery workers.

However, the realisation of telemedicine's potential is contingent upon the implementation of comprehensive and coordinated strategies that address existing structural barriers. Infrastructural limitations, digital literacy gaps, financial constraints, and policy fragmentation continue to impede equitable access and sustained adoption. Without deliberate intervention, telemedicine risks reproducing existing inequalities, particularly among workers with limited digital access or technological confidence. Therefore, embedding telemedicine within gig economy platforms requires not only technological innovation but also institutional commitment, regulatory clarity, and inclusive design principles that prioritise worker well-being.

FUNDING

This research received no specific grant from any funding agency in the public, commercial, or not-for-profit sectors.

Clinical trial number - Not applicable.

Declaration of Competing Interest

The authors declare that they have no competing financial interests or personal relationships that could have appeared to influence the current work.

REFERENCES

Abokhashabah, T., Jamoussi, B., Summan, A. S., Abdelfattah, E., & Ahmad, I. (2021). Effects of Heat Stress Exposure and Climate Change on Health and Safety of Outdoor Workers. *Current World Environment*, *16*(3), 836–847. DOI: 10.12944/CWE.16.3.15

Agochukwu, N. Q., Skolarus, T. A., & Wittmann, D. (2018). Telemedicine and prostate cancer survivorship: A narrative review. *mHealth*, *4*(0), 45–45. DOI: 10.21037/mhealth.2018.09.08 PMID: 30505843

Alanzi, T. M. (2021). Gig health vs ehealth: Future prospects in saudi arabian health-care system. *Journal of Multidisciplinary Healthcare*, *14*, 1945–1953. DOI: 10.2147/JMDH.S304690 PMID: 34326645

Anwar, M. A., & Graham, M. (2021). Between a rock and a hard place: Freedom, flexibility, precarity and vulnerability in the gig economy in Africa. *Competition & Change*, *25*(2), 237–258. DOI: 10.1177/1024529420914473

Applebaum, K. M., Graham, J., Gray, G. M., LaPuma, P., McCormick, S. A., Northcross, A., & Perry, M. J. (2016). An Overview of Occupational Risks From Climate Change. *Current Environmental Health Reports*, *3*(1), 13–22. DOI: 10.1007/s40572-016-0081-4 PMID: 26842343

Ayentimi, D. T., Abadi, H. A., & Burgess, J. (2023). Decent gig work in Sub Sahara Africa? *The Journal of Industrial Relations*, *65*(1), 112–125. DOI: 10.1177/00221856221111693

Azahra, A. S., Pirdaus, D. I., & Prabowo, A. (2024). Digital Health Literacy and Telemedicine in the Information Age: A Comprehensive Review and Future Prospects. *International Journal of Linguistics. Communication & Broadcasting*, *2*(1), 13–19. DOI: 10.46336/ijlcb.v2i1.89

Bajwa, U., Gastaldo, D., Di Ruggiero, E., & Knorr, L. (2018). The health of workers in the global gig economy. *Globalization and Health*, *14*(1), 1–4. DOI: 10.1186/s12992-018-0444-8 PMID: 30563539

Chandel, A. S. (2025). Traffic congestion in Shimla: A smart city in the Himalayan mountain landscape—analyzing socioeconomic impacts from the perspectives of drivers and passengers. *Urban, Planning and Transport Research*, *13*(1), 2502000. Advance online publication. DOI: 10.1080/21650020.2025.2502000

Chen, T., Song, W., Song, J., Ren, Y., Dong, Y., Yang, J., & Zhang, S. (2022). Measuring Well-Being of Migrant Gig Workers: Exampled as Hangzhou City in China. *Behavioral Sciences (Basel, Switzerland)*, *12*(10), 365. DOI: 10.3390/bs12100365 PMID: 36285934

Cianconi, P., Hanife, B., Hirsch, D., & Janiri, L. (2023). Is climate change affecting mental health of urban populations? In *Current Opinion in Psychiatry* (Vol. 36, Issue 3, pp. 213–218). Curr Opin Psychiatry. DOI: 10.1097/YCO.0000000000000859

Comlek, S., & Ordu, A. (2021). Interventional pain management during sars-cov-2 pandemic. *Signa Vitae*, *17*(4), 178–184. DOI: 10.22514/sv.2021.008

Cox, J. A., Read, G. J. M., Butler, G. L., & Salmon, P. M. (2024). Examining gender differences in gig worker safety. *Human Factors and Ergonomics in Manufacturing*, *34*(1), 3–15. DOI: 10.1002/hfm.21007

Crane, K., Li, L., Subramanian, P., Rovit, E., & Liu, J. (2022). Climate Change and Mental Health: A Review of Empirical Evidence, Mechanisms and Implications. In *Atmosphere* (Vol. 13, Issue 12). Atmosphere (Basel). DOI: 10.3390/atmos13122096

Cropanzano, R., Keplinger, K., Lambert, B. K., Caza, B., & Ashford, S. J. (2022). The Organizational Psychology of Gig Work: An Integrative Conceptual Review. *The Journal of Applied Psychology*, *108*(3), 492–519. DOI: 10.1037/apl0001029 PMID: 36222635

Du, Y., Zhou, Q., Cheng, W., Zhang, Z., Hoelzer, S., Liang, Y., Xue, H., Ma, X., Sylvia, S., Tian, J., & Tang, W. (2022). Factors Influencing Adoption and Use of Telemedicine Services in Rural Areas of China: Mixed Methods Study. *JMIR Public Health and Surveillance*, *8*(12), e40771. DOI: 10.2196/40771 PMID: 36563026

Durojaiye, O. C., Jibril, I., & Kritsotakis, E. I. (2022). Effectiveness of telemedicine in outpatient parenteral antimicrobial therapy (Tele-OPAT): A systematic review. In *Journal of Telemedicine and Telecare*. SAGE PublicationsSage UK: London, England. DOI: 10.1177/1357633X221131842

Fitzpatrick, P. J. (2023). Improving health literacy using the power of digital communications to achieve better health outcomes for patients and practitioners. In *Frontiers in Digital Health* (Vol. 5, p. 1264780). Frontiers Media SA. DOI: 10.3389/fdgth.2023.1264780

Flouris, A. D., Dinas, P. C., Ioannou, L. G., Nybo, L., Havenith, G., Kenny, G. P., & Kjellstrom, T. (2018). Workers' health and productivity under occupational heat strain: A systematic review and meta-analysis. *The Lancet. Planetary Health*, *2*(12), e521–e531. DOI: 10.1016/S2542-5196(18)30237-7 PMID: 30526938

Ford, J. H.II, Jolles, S. A., Heller, D., Langenstroer, M., & Crnich, C. (2022). There and back again: The shape of telemedicine in U.S. nursing homes following COVID-19. *BMC Geriatrics, 22*(1), 1–12. DOI: 10.1186/s12877-022-03046-y PMID: 35436869

Gibb, K., Beckman, S., Vergara, X. P., Heinzerling, A., & Harrison, R. (2024). Extreme Heat and Occupational Health Risks. *Annual Review of Public Health, 45*(1), 315–335. DOI: 10.1146/annurev-publhealth-060222-034715 PMID: 38166501

Gleiss, A., & Lewandowski, S. (2022). Removing barriers for digital health through organizing ambidexterity in hospitals. *Journal of Public Health (Berlin), 30*(1), 21–35. DOI: 10.1007/s10389-021-01532-y

Gonzalez Garcia, M., Fatehi, F., Bashi, N., Varnfield, M., Iyngkaran, P., Driscoll, A., Neil, C., Hare, D. L., & Oldenburg, B. (2019). A Review of Randomized Controlled Trials Utilizing Telemedicine for Improving Heart Failure Readmission: Can a Realist Approach Bridge the Translational Divide? *Clinical Medicine Insights. Cardiology, 13*, 1179546819861396. Advance online publication. DOI: 10.1177/1179546819861396 PMID: 31316270

Goudet, J.-M., Arif, F. B., Owais, H., Ahmed, H. U., & Ridde, V. (2023). Intersecting Vulnerabilities: Unraveling the Complex Relationship between Women, Climate Change, and Mental Health in Bangladeshi Communities. In medRxiv (p. 2023.06.06.23290721). Cold Spring Harbor Laboratory Press. DOI: 10.1101/2023.06.06.23290721

Goudet, J. M., Arif, F. B., Owais, H., Ahmed, H. U., & Ridde, V. (2024). Climate change and women's mental health in two vulnerable communities of Bangladesh: An ethnographic study. *PLOS Global Public Health, 4*(6 June), e0002080. DOI: 10.1371/journal.pgph.0002080

Grande, D., Luna Marti, X., Feuerstein-Simon, R., Merchant, R. M., Asch, D. A., Lewson, A., & Cannuscio, C. C. (2020). Health Policy and Privacy Challenges Associated with Digital Technology. *JAMA Network Open, 3*(7), e208285–e208285. DOI: 10.1001/jamanetworkopen.2020.8285 PMID: 32644138

Gregory, K. (2021). 'My Life Is More Valuable Than This': Understanding Risk among On-Demand Food Couriers in Edinburgh. *Work, Employment and Society, 35*(2), 316–331. DOI: 10.1177/0950017020969593

Gunasiri, H., Wang, Y., Watkins, E. M., Capetola, T., Henderson-Wilson, C., & Patrick, R. (2022). Hope, Coping and Eco-Anxiety: Young People's Mental Health in a Climate-Impacted Australia. *International Journal of Environmental Research and Public Health, 19*(9), 5528. Advance online publication. DOI: 10.3390/ijerph19095528 PMID: 35564923

Gussek, L., Schned, L., & Wiesche, M. (2021). Obsolescence in IT Work: Causes, Consequences and Counter-Measures. *Lecture Notes in Information Systems and Organisation, 48 LNISO*, 572–586. DOI: 10.1007/978-3-030-86800-0_40

Hadi, A. A. W. K., & Pratono, A. H. (2024). Ethical predicaments of gig economy: Bibliometric approach. *Optimum: Jurnal Ekonomi Dan Pembangunan, 14*(1), 40–48. DOI: 10.12928/optimum.v14i1.9316

Haleem, A., Javaid, M., Singh, R. P., & Suman, R. (2021). Telemedicine for health-care: Capabilities, features, barriers, and applications. In *Sensors International*. DOI: 10.1016/j.sintl.2021.100117

Harpur, P., & Blanck, P. (2020). Gig Workers with Disabilities: Opportunities, Challenges, and Regulatory Response. *Journal of Occupational Rehabilitation, 30*(4), 511–520. DOI: 10.1007/s10926-020-09937-4 PMID: 33146784

Hart, A., Romney, D., Sarin, R., Mechanic, O., Hertelendy, A. J., Larson, D., Rhone, K., Sidel, K., Voskanyan, A., & Ciottone, G. R. (2022). Developing Telemedicine Curriculum Competencies for Graduate Medical Education: Outcomes of a Modified Delphi Process. *Academic Medicine, 97*(4), 577–585. DOI: 10.1097/ACM.0000000000004463 PMID: 34670239

Hjelm, N. M. (2005). Benefits and drawbacks of telemedicine. In *Journal of Telemedicine and Telecare* (Vol. 11, Issue 2, pp. 60–70). SAGE PublicationsSage UK: London, England. DOI: 10.1258/1357633053499886

Hosseini, S. M., Boushehri, S. A., & Alimohammadzadeh, K. (2024). Challenges and solutions for implementing telemedicine in Iran from health policymakers' perspective. *BMC Health Services Research, 24*(1), 1–11. DOI: 10.1186/s12913-023-10488-6 PMID: 38200535

Hui, C. Y., Abdulla, A., Ahmed, Z., Goel, H., Habib, G. M. M., Hock, T. T., Khandakr, P., Mahmood, H., Nautiyal, A., Nurmansyah, M., Panwar, S., Patil, R., Rinawan, F. R., Salim, H., Satav, A., Shah, J. N., Shukla, A., Tanim, C. Z. H., Balharry, D., & Pinnock, H. (2022). Mapping national information and communication technology (ICT) infrastructure to the requirements of potential digital health interventions in low and middle-income countries. *Journal of Global Health, 12*, 04094. DOI: 10.7189/jogh.12.04094 PMID: 36579436

Hwong, A. R., Wang, M., Khan, H., Chagwedera, D. N., Grzenda, A., Doty, B., Benton, T., Alpert, J., Clarke, D., & Compton, W. M. (2022). Climate change and mental health research methods, gaps, and priorities: a scoping review. In *The Lancet Planetary Health* (Vol. 6, Issue 3, pp. e281–e291). Lancet Planet Health. DOI: 10.1016/S2542-5196(22)00012-2

Illingworth, P. (2024). Will Including Health at COP28 Mean Transformation of Global Mental Health Action? And will Mental Health Professionals transform to help achieve it? *Mental Health: Global Challenges*, *7*(1), 50–54. DOI: 10.56508/mhgcj.v7i1.187

Jacklitsch, B., Williams, W., Musolin, K., Coca, A., Kim, J.-H., & Turner, N. (2016). NIOSH criteria for a recommended standard: occupational exposure to heat and hot environments. *US Department of Health and Human Services*, Publication 2016-106.

Jelinek, R., Pandita, D., Linzer, M., Engoang, J. B. B. N., & Rodin, H. (2022). An Evidence-Based Roadmap for the Provision of More Equitable Telemedicine. *Applied Clinical Informatics*, *13*(3), 612–620. DOI: 10.1055/s-0042-1749597 PMID: 35675839

Jiang, L., Wang, J., Castaño-Rosa, R., Zhong, C., & Cao, S. (2024). Heat exposure and coping strategies for food delivery riders under urban heat extremes. *Energy and Building*, *322*, 114693. DOI: 10.1016/j.enbuild.2024.114693

Jiaojiao, L., & Lifei, M. (2023). The Dilemma and Thinking of Gig Workers in the Digital Organization Environment. *Information Systems and Economics*, *4*(6). Advance online publication. DOI: 10.23977/infse.2023.040606

Kalbalia, P., & Koushik, K. (2025a). Driving Better Health Outcomes for Gig Workers Through Strategic Health Initiatives. In *Immersive Technology for the Gig Economy* (pp. 323–346). IGI Global Scientific Publishing., DOI: 10.4018/979-8-3373-1290-3.ch012

Kalbalia, P., & Koushik, K. (2025b). Health Communication as Capability: Gig Workers' Freedoms Through Sen's Approach. *The Howard Journal of Communications*, ●●●, 1–13. DOI: 10.1080/10646175.2025.2570753

Kalbalia, P., & Koushik, K. (2025c). Regulating the gig economy: Addressing worker rights in India's quick commerce sector. In *Sustainability and Adaptability of Gig Economies in Global Business* (pp. 85–105). IGI Global., DOI: 10.4018/979-8-3693-9385-7.ch004

Kalbalia, P., Nath, N. J., & Haneefa, K. V. (2024). Utilisation and Accessibility of Healthcare Services Among Gig Workers: A Systematic Review. In *Population, Environment and Disease: Towards Health Geography* (pp. 77–95). Springer., DOI: 10.1007/978-3-031-67624-6_5

Katzman, J. G., Tomedi, L. E., Herring, D., Jones, H., Groves, R., Norsworthy, K., Martin, C., Liu, J., Kazhe-Dominguez, B., & Arora, S. (2022). Educating Community Health Professionals About the Health-Related Effects of Climate Change Through ECHO Telementoring. *Journal of Primary Care & Community Health*, *13*, 21501319221102033. Advance online publication. DOI: 10.1177/21501319221102033 PMID: 35603993

Kaushik, A. (2024). Comprehensive Impact of On-Demand Platforms: Examining the Gig Economy\'s Influence on Specialized Professionals, Work-Life Balance, and Gig Workers\' Perspectives. *International Journal for Research in Applied Science and Engineering Technology*, *12*(1), 552–559. DOI: 10.22214/ijraset.2024.58005

Khanijahani, A., Akinci, N., & Quitiquit, E. (2022). A Systematic Review of the Role of Telemedicine in Blood Pressure Control: Focus on Patient Engagement. In *Current Hypertension Reports* (Vol. 24, Issue 7, pp. 247–258). Springer. DOI: 10.1007/s11906-022-01186-5

Khreis, H., Warsow, K. M., Verlinghieri, E., Guzman, A., Pellecuer, L., Ferreira, A., Jones, I., Heinen, E., Rojas-Rueda, D., Mueller, N., Schepers, P., Lucas, K., & Nieuwenhuijsen, M. (2016). The health impacts of traffic-related exposures in urban areas: Understanding real effects, underlying driving forces and co-producing future directions. In *Journal of Transport and Health* (Vol. 3, Issue 3, pp. 249–267). Elsevier. DOI: 10.1016/j.jth.2016.07.002

Koutsimpogiorgos, N., van Slageren, J., Herrmann, A., & Frenken, K. (2020). Conceptualizing the Gig Economy and Its Regulatory Problems. *Policy & Internet*. https://doi.org/DOI: 10.31235/OSF.IO/JMQYT

Kruse, C. S., Karem, P., Shifflett, K., Vegi, L., Ravi, K., & Brooks, M. (2018). Evaluating barriers to adopting telemedicine worldwide: A systematic review. In *Journal of Telemedicine and Telecare* (Vol. 24, Issue 1, pp. 4–12). J Telemed Telecare. DOI: 10.1177/1357633X16674087

Lambert, S. J., Haley-Lock, A., & Henly, J. R. (2012). Schedule flexibility in hourly jobs: Unanticipated consequences and promising directions. *Community Work & Family*, *15*(3), 293–315. DOI: 10.1080/13668803.2012.662803

Landsbergis, P. A., Schnall, P. L., Belkic, K. L., Baker, D., Schwartz, J., & Pickering, T. G. (2001). Work stressors and cardiovascular disease. In *Work* (Vol. 17, Issue 3, pp. 191–208). John Wiley & Sons, Ltd. DOI: 10.3233/WOR-2001-00189

Lei, Y. W. (2021). Delivering Solidarity: Platform Architecture and Collective Contention in China's Platform Economy. *American Sociological Review*, *86*(2), 279–309. DOI: 10.1177/0003122420979980

Lester, G. V., Brock Baskin, M. E., & Clinton, M. S. (2021). Employer-Sponsored Benefits in the United States: The Past, Present, and Future. *Compensation and Benefits Review*, *53*(1), 24–42. DOI: 10.1177/0886368720947609 PMID: 34955602

Levison, M. M., Butler, A. J., Rebellato, S., Armstrong, B., Whelan, M., & Gardner, C. (2018). Development of a climate change vulnerability assessment using a public health lens to determine local health vulnerabilities: An Ontario health unit experience. *International Journal of Environmental Research and Public Health*, *15*(10), 2237. Advance online publication. DOI: 10.3390/ijerph15102237 PMID: 30322040

Liyanage, S., Dia, H., Abduljabbar, R., & Bagloee, S. A. (2019). Flexible mobility on-demand: An environmental scan. In *Sustainability (Switzerland)* (Vol. 11, Issue 5, p. 1262). Multidisciplinary Digital Publishing Institute. DOI: 10.3390/su11051262

Lõhmus, M. (2018). Possible biological mechanisms linking mental health and heat—a contemplative review. In *International Journal of Environmental Research and Public Health* (Vol. 15, Issue 7). Int J Environ Res Public Health. DOI: 10.3390/ijerph15071515

Marsh, Z., Nguyen, Y., Teegala, Y., & Cotter, V. T. (2022). Diabetes management among underserved older adults through telemedicine and community health workers. In *Journal of the American Association of Nurse Practitioners* (Vol. 34, Issue 1, pp. 26–31). Lippincott Williams and Wilkins. DOI: 10.1097/JXX.0000000000000595

Marshall, A. I., Lasco, G., Phaiyarom, M., Pangkariya, N., Leuangvilay, P., Sinam, P., Suphanchaimat, R., Julchoo, S., Kunpeuk, W., & Zhang, Y. (2021). Evidence on child nutrition recommendations and challenges in crisis settings: A scoping review. *International Journal of Environmental Research and Public Health*, *18*(12), 6637. DOI: 10.3390/ijerph18126637 PMID: 34203109

Mayhew, C., & Quinlan, M. (2002). Fordism in the fast food industry: Pervasive management control and occupational health and safety risks for young temporary workers. *Sociology of Health & Illness*, *24*(3), 261–284. DOI: 10.1111/1467-9566.00294

Mayhew, C., & Quinlan, M. (2006). Economic pressure, multi-tiered subcontracting and occupational health and safety in Australian long-haul trucking. *Employee Relations*, *28*(3), 212–229. DOI: 10.1108/01425450610661216

Megasari, A. L., Masbahah, , Riatma, D. L., & Fatsena, R. A. (2023). The effect of telemedicine plus application on the covid-19 patients' quality of life. *Journal of Public Health Dentistry*, *21*(2), 56–68. DOI: 10.55131/jphd/2023/210205

Musa, S., Ramatu, A., Haliru, L., Abigail, D., & Gumbi, S. (2023). Establishing a paediatric telemedicine centre in a low-resource setting: Experience and challenges from a teaching hospital in Kaduna, Nigeria. *Sri Lanka Journal of Child Health, 52*(2), 155–160. DOI: 10.4038/sljch.v52i2.10548

Nadeau, C. P., Urban, M. C., & Bridle, J. R. (2017). Climates Past, Present, and Yet-to-Come Shape Climate Change Vulnerabilities. In *Trends in Ecology and Evolution* (Vol. 32, Issue 10, pp. 786–800). Elsevier Ltd. DOI: 10.1016/j.tree.2017.07.012

Nguyen, M. L. T., Garcia, F., Juarez, J., Zeng, B., Khoong, E. C., Nijagal, M. A., Sarkar, U., Su, G., & Lyles, C. R. (2022). Satisfaction can co-exist with hesitation: Qualitative analysis of acceptability of telemedicine among multi-lingual patients in a safety-net healthcare system during the COVID-19 pandemic. *BMC Health Services Research, 22*(1), 1–9. DOI: 10.1186/s12913-022-07547-9 PMID: 35164746

Nikulin, D., Wolszczak-Derlacz, J., & Parteka, A. (2022). Working Conditions in Global Value Chains: Evidence for European Employees. *Work, Employment and Society*, *36*(4), 701–721. DOI: 10.1177/0950017020986107

Nutbeam, D., & Lloyd, J. E. (2020). Understanding and Responding to Health Literacy as a Social Determinant of Health. In *Annual Review of Public Health* (Vol. 42, pp. 159–173). Annual Reviews Inc., DOI: 10.1146/annurev-publhealth-090419-102529

Ojala, M., Cunsolo, A., Ogunbode, C. A., & Middleton, J. (2021). Anxiety, Worry, and Grief in a Time of Environmental and Climate Crisis: A Narrative Review. In *Annual Review of Environment and Resources* (Vol. 46, Issue Volume 46, 2021, pp. 35–58). Annual Reviews Inc. DOI: 10.1146/annurev-environ-012220-022716

Omaghomi, T. T. (2023). Telemedicine in rural Africa: A review of accessibility and impact. *World Journal of Advanced Research and Reviews, 21*(2), 421–431. DOI: 10.30574/wjarr.2024.21.2.0475

Onsongo, S., Kamotho, C., Rinke De Wit, T. F., & Lowrie, K. (2023). Experiences on the Utility and Barriers of Telemedicine in Healthcare Delivery in Kenya. *International Journal of Telemedicine and Applications, 2023*(1), 1487245. DOI: 10.1155/2023/1487245 PMID: 37180825

Palhad, S., Onwubu, S., Singh, R., Thakur, R., Thakur, S., & Mkhize, G. (2023). The Benefits and Challenges of the Gig Economy: Perspective of Gig Workers and Small Medium and Micro Enterprises (SMMEs) in South Africa. *African Journal of Inter/Multidisciplinary Studies, 5*(1), 1–12. DOI: 10.51415/ajims.v5i1.1051

Pande, N. (2024). WHAT ARE THE ECONOMIC IMPLICATIONS OF THE RISE OF THE GIG ECONOMY ON EMPLOYMENT STABILITY AND BENEFITS? *EPH-International Journal of Business & Management Science*, *10*(1), 53–67. DOI: 10.53555/EIJBMS.V10I1.175

Pierce, B. S., Perrin, P. B., Dow, A. W., Dautovich, N. D., Rybarczyk, B. D., & Mishra, V. K. (2021). Changes in physician telemedicine use during COVID-19: Effects of practice setting, demographics, training, and organizational policies. *International Journal of Environmental Research and Public Health*, *18*(19), 9963. DOI: 10.3390/ijerph18199963 PMID: 34639269

Schulte, P. A., & Chun, H. K. (2009). Climate change and occupational safety and health: Establishing a preliminary framework. *Journal of Occupational and Environmental Hygiene*, *6*(9), 542–554. DOI: 10.1080/15459620903066008 PMID: 19551548

Seaton, C. L., Rondier, P., Rush, K. L., Li, E. P. H., Plamondon, K., Pesut, B., Oelke, N. D., Dow-Fleisner, S., Hasan, K., Currie, L. M., Kurtz, D., Jones, C., & Bottorff, J. L. (2022). Community stakeholder-driven technology solutions towards rural health equity: A concept mapping study in Western Canada. *Health Expectations*, *25*(6), 3202–3214. DOI: 10.1111/hex.13627 PMID: 36245334

Shah, A. Q., Noronha, N., Chin-See, R., Hanna, C., Kadri, Z., Marwaha, A., Rambharack, N., & Ng, J. Y. (2023). The use and effects of telemedicine on complementary, alternative, and integrative medicine practices: A scoping review. *BMC Complementary Medicine and Therapies*, *23*(1), 1–40. DOI: 10.1186/s12906-023-04100-x PMID: 37533042

Sharma, P., Sethi, M. I. S., Liem, A., Bhatti, H. B. S., Pandey, V., & Nair, A. (2023). A Review of Telemedicine Guidelines in the South-East Asia Region. In *Telemedicine Reports* (Vol. 4, Issue 1, pp. 271–278). Telemed Rep. DOI: 10.1089/tmr.2023.0040

Sharma, V., Feldman, M., & Sharma, R. (2024). Telehealth Technologies in Diabetes Self-management and Education. In *Journal of Diabetes Science and Technology* (Vol. 18, Issue 1, pp. 148–158). SAGE Publications Inc. DOI: 10.1177/19322968221093078

Shen, Y. T., Chen, L., Yue, W. W., & Xu, H. X. (2021). Digital Technology-Based Telemedicine for the COVID-19 Pandemic. In *Frontiers in Medicine* (Vol. 8, p. 646506). DOI: 10.3389/fmed.2021.646506

Shoib, S., Hussaini, S. S., Armiya'u, A. Y., Saeed, F., Őri, D., Roza, T. H., Gürcan, A., Agrawal, A., Solerdelcoll, M., Lucero-Prisno, D. E.III, Nahidi, M., Swed, S., Ahmed, S., & Chandradasa, M. (2023). Prevention of suicides associated with global warming: Perspectives from early career psychiatrists. *Frontiers in Psychiatry*, *14*, 1251630. Advance online publication. DOI: 10.3389/fpsyt.2023.1251630 PMID: 38045615

Stanberry, B. (2000). Telemedicine: Barriers and opportunities in the 21st century. In *Journal of Internal Medicine* (Vol. 247, Issue 6, pp. 615–628). DOI: 10.1046/j.1365-2796.2000.00699.x

Stanford, J. (2017). The resurgence of gig work: Historical and theoretical perspectives. *Economic and Labour Relations Review*, *28*(3), 382–401. DOI: 10.1177/1035304617724303

Stewart, A., & Stanford, J. (2017). Regulating work in the gig economy: What are the options? *Economic and Labour Relations Review*, *28*(3), 420–437. DOI: 10.1177/1035304617722461

Tan, Z. M., Aggarwal, N., Cowls, J., Morley, J., Taddeo, M., & Floridi, L. (2020). The Ethical Debate about the Gig Economy: A Review and Critical Analysis. SSRN *Electronic Journal*. DOI: 10.2139/ssrn.3669216

Venugopal, V., Chinnadurai, J. S., Lucas, R. A. I., & Kjellstrom, T. (2015). Occupational heat stress profiles in selected workplaces in India. *International Journal of Environmental Research and Public Health*, *13*(1), 89. Advance online publication. DOI: 10.3390/ijerph13010089 PMID: 26729144

Wood, A., & Lehdonvirta, V. (2021). Platform Precarity: Surviving Algorithmic Insecurity in the Gig Economy. SSRN *Electronic Journal*. https://doi.org/DOI: 10.2139/SSRN.3795375

Yarney, L., Mintah, N. A., Ayisi, E. K., & Adzei, F. A. (2023). Narratives of Clinicians on Telemedicine and Delivery of Quality Healthcare in Ghana. *Open Journal of Social Sciences*, *11*(08), 232–256. DOI: 10.4236/jss.2023.118017

Yassa, H. A., Hussein, A. A. R. M., Makhlouf, H. A., Makhlouf, N. A., Youssef, H. M. S., Sotohy, R. S. A., & Essa, A. A. (2022). *Pros and cons of telemedicine in diagnosis and management: A cross sectional survey*. Electronic Journal of General Medicine., DOI: 10.29333/ejgm/12236

Zhang, L., Yang, J., Zhang, Y., & Xu, G. (2023). Gig worker's perceived algorithmic management, stress appraisal, and destructive deviant behavior. *PLoS ONE, 18*(11 November). DOI: 10.1371/journal.pone.0294074

Chapter 4
Art Therapy in Primary Education:
Creative Practices and Activities for Children's Well-Being

Maria Athanasekou
http://orcid.org/0000-0002-2971-9452
Hellenic Open University, Greece & Frederick University, Cyprus

ABSTRACT

Art therapy stands at the intersection of health psychology, education, and child development, offering unique ways to support resilience, meaning-making, and well-being in primary schools. Rooted in health psychology, it demonstrates how embodied creative expression promotes adaptive behavior and holistic wellness. Since children often lack the vocabulary to express complex emotions, art activities—drawing, painting, collage—enable symbolic communication and self-discovery. Research confirms benefits such as reduced anxiety, improved focus, and stronger relationships. Multisensory art-making enhances neural integration, memory, and regulation. Activities like "safe place" drawings, "strength shields," and group murals foster resilience, inclusion, and collaboration. While not a substitute for clinical therapy, arts-based interventions in classrooms provide preventative, accessible tools that promote emotional health and cultivate creativity, affirming children's innate capacity to flourish.

INTRODUCTION

Art therapy has become an increasingly significant field of practice at the intersection of psychology, education, and health sciences. While its origins lie

DOI: 10.4018/979-8-2600-3085-1.ch004

primarily in clinical contexts, art therapy has, in recent years, found a meaningful place in educational environments, especially in primary schools. This integration reflects the recognition that schools are not only sites of academic instruction but also environments where children undergo profound social, emotional, and cognitive development. For many children, primary education represents a foundational stage during which they begin to establish self-concept, regulate emotions, navigate peer relationships, and build resilience in the face of challenges. These formative years provide a unique window for interventions that support holistic well-being, and art therapy offers an ideal medium through which such support can be delivered. Art therapy can be broadly defined as the intentional use of visual and creative processes to foster psychological growth, emotional regulation, and personal meaning-making (Malchiodi, 2020). It differs from traditional art instruction because its focus is not primarily on technical skill or aesthetic achievement but rather on the symbolic and expressive potential of art-making. In the context of primary education, this distinction is critical: while arts education helps children learn techniques of drawing, painting, or crafting, art therapy-based approaches emphasize the personal stories, emotions, and internal worlds that children externalize through their creative activity (Case & Dalley, 2014). For children who may lack the verbal sophistication to articulate complex inner experiences, art offers a direct, embodied, and accessible pathway to self-expression.

The urgency of integrating art therapy into primary education stems from a growing awareness of the psychosocial challenges children face today. Issues such as anxiety, stress, social exclusion, and the pressures of academic achievement are increasingly evident in school-aged populations worldwide (Marks et al., 2018). The COVID-19 pandemic further exacerbated these challenges, disrupting children's routines, limiting social interactions, and heightening stress in family and educational environments (UNICEF, 2021). In this climate, the role of schools as spaces for promoting resilience and emotional well-being has never been more critical. Art therapy provides a preventative and responsive framework for addressing these needs, equipping children with lifelong tools for coping, meaning-making, and creative problem-solving. From a health psychology perspective, well-being in childhood must be understood not only as the absence of psychological distress but as the active cultivation of resilience, emotional self-regulation, and adaptive coping strategies (Marks et al., 2018). Art therapy aligns closely with this perspective by enabling children to explore and transform emotions symbolically, often bypassing the limitations of verbal expression. A child who struggles to articulate sadness, for instance, may depict it through color, line, or form; this externalization creates opportunities for reflection, dialogue, and healing. In this way, art therapy embodies the principles of experiential health psychology, in which behavior, meaning, and well-being are deeply interconnected. Furthermore, art therapy fits naturally within the pedagogical mission of primary education, which increasingly emphasizes the importance of social and emotional learning (SEL). SEL frameworks aim to cultivate self-awareness, emotional literacy, relationship skills, and responsible decision-making (CASEL, 2020). Art therapy-based activities—such as drawing a "safe place," creating "resilience trees," or collaborating on group murals—map directly onto these competencies, supporting the broader goal of nurturing well-rounded, emotionally intelligent learners. By embedding such practices into everyday classroom routines, educators can transform classrooms into safe spaces where academic learning and psychosocial development coexist harmoniously. The interdisciplinary relevance of art therapy is also noteworthy. It draws upon insights from developmental psychology, neuroscience, health promotion, and pedagogy. Neuroscientific research, for example, highlights how multisensory engagement in creative activity enhances neural integration, memory consolidation, and emotional regulation (Bolwerk, Mack-Andrick, Lang, Dörfler, & Maihöfner, 2014). Developmental theories, from Vygotsky's (1978) emphasis on symbolic play to Erikson's (1963) stages of psychosocial growth, affirm that creativity is a fundamental mechanism through which children make sense of their worlds. Within health psychology, art therapy represents a concrete application of the biopsychosocial model, offering embodied strategies for cultivating resilience in the face of adversity.

This chapter situates art therapy within these overlapping frameworks, presenting a comprehensive exploration of its role in primary education. Specifically, it has three central aims. First, it examines the theoretical foundations of art therapy as a practice grounded in health psychology and developmental theory. Second, it surveys neuroscientific and empirical evidence demonstrating the psychological, social, and cognitive benefits of art therapy in schools. Third, it provides practical guidance for educators and practitioners by presenting structured classroom activities that can be implemented to support children's well-being. Alongside these aims, the chapter also considers ethical and pedagogical challenges, including boundaries between therapy and education, issues of equity and inclusion, and the sustainability of integrating art therapy into school systems. Ultimately, the central argument of this chapter is that art therapy is both a therapeutic and pedagogical tool. By fostering embodied creativity and psychosocial resilience, art therapy equips children not only to cope with stressors but to thrive as emotionally intelligent, socially connected, and resilient individuals. It expands the scope of health psychology into educational practice and demonstrates that children's well-being is best nurtured when creativity, meaning-making, and emotional support are recognized as integral to the learning process. The following sections explore these dimensions in depth, beginning with a review of the theoretical foundations of art therapy within health psychology.

THEORETICAL FOUNDATIONS: ART THERAPY AND HEALTH PSYCHOLOGY, HISTORICAL OVERVIEW OF ART THERAPY IN SCHOOLS

Art therapy as a structured field emerged in the mid-20th century, but the use of artistic activities for emotional and cognitive development in children has deeper historical roots. In educational contexts, early instances of art integration were not explicitly therapeutic but rather pedagogical, aiming to enhance creativity and personal expression (Junge & Linesch, 1993). The post–World War II era marked a significant expansion in the therapeutic use of art within schools, influenced by the broader recognition of child psychology and the need for psychosocial support in post-traumatic environments (Malchiodi, 2012).

By the 1960s and 1970s, art therapy gained institutional legitimacy, coinciding with the rise of humanistic psychology and progressive education movements that emphasized the whole child—emotional, social, and cognitive development (Rubin, 2016). Schools began employing art therapy not only for children with identified emotional or behavioral difficulties but also as a preventive practice for general well-being. This development reflected a shift from perceiving education as solely academic instruction toward a more holistic perspective incorporating emotional health (Case & Dalley, 2014).

The integration of art therapy into primary education contexts also paralleled broader societal changes. Increasing awareness of mental health in children, coupled with legislation on inclusive education, supported the introduction of art-based interventions into schools. The UNESCO framework on arts in education highlighted the role of creativity and artistic engagement in fostering cultural and emotional resilience (UNESCO, 2006). Thus, the historical trajectory of art therapy in schools demonstrates a gradual evolution from informal, expressive practices to professionalized therapeutic interventions embedded within educational structures.

Distinction Between Therapeutic and Educational Uses of Art

Although art-making is widely acknowledged as beneficial for children's development, the distinction between therapeutic and educational uses of art is crucial for both ethical and professional clarity. In educational contexts, art education traditionally focuses on skill development, aesthetic appreciation, and fostering creativity (Eisner, 2002). Its primary goals are pedagogical: nurturing imagination, teaching artistic techniques, and supporting cognitive growth through engagement with artistic media. By contrast, art therapy operates within a psychotherapeutic framework, wherein the creative process is used as a means of expression, self-discovery, and emotional healing (Malchiodi, 2012). The emphasis lies not on the aesthetic quality of the artwork but on the process and meaning-making that emerges. For example, in therapeutic settings, a child's drawing of a family might serve as a diagnostic tool to reveal underlying anxieties, relational conflicts, or unmet emotional needs (Case & Dalley, 2014). In contrast, in an art classroom, a similar drawing would likely be evaluated based on compositional balance or storytelling ability.

Nevertheless, the boundaries are not rigid. Contemporary educational practice increasingly integrates socio-emotional learning, where creative activities serve both educational and therapeutic purposes. This overlap has generated what some scholars term "therapeutic education" (Ecclestone & Hayes, 2009), where art activities are employed to cultivate resilience, empathy, and emotional intelligence within standard curricula. The key distinction lies in intent and context: therapeutic art aims for psychological healing within a clinical or quasi-clinical framework, whereas educational art primarily supports cognitive and aesthetic development, with well-being as a secondary outcome. Ethical considerations underscore this distinction. While trained art therapists adhere to clinical guidelines and confidentiality protocols, teachers employing creative methods in the classroom are not expected to perform therapeutic functions. Nonetheless, educational systems increasingly recognize the value of collaboration between teachers and therapists to ensure that children's emotional needs are adequately addressed (Rubin, 2016).

Health Psychology and the Biopsychosocial Model

The theoretical foundation of art therapy in education can be further understood through the lens of health psychology, particularly the biopsychosocial model (Marks et al., 2018). This model posits that health and well-being are determined by the dynamic interaction of biological, psychological, and social factors. In contrast to reductionist biomedical approaches, the biopsychosocial perspective emphasizes holistic health, making it especially relevant for educational and therapeutic contexts involving children. Biologically, art therapy supports sensory-motor development and enhances neuroplasticity through multimodal stimulation. Engaging in drawing, painting, or sculpting activates brain regions associated with fine motor skills, visual-spatial processing, and emotional regulation (Kaimal et al., 2017). Psychologically, the process of artistic expression provides an avenue for self-reflection, symbolic communication, and the externalization of inner experiences, all of which contribute to emotional regulation and resilience (Malchiodi, 2012). Socially, art therapy fosters group interaction, peer empathy, and cooperative learning, thereby enhancing children's sense of belonging and reducing social isolation (Case & Dalley, 2014).

In school contexts, the biopsychosocial model justifies the integration of art therapy not only for children with identified mental health needs but also as a preventive measure for general well-being. For example, group art projects encourage collaboration and social identity formation, while individual projects support self-expression and psychological resilience. Teachers who adopt this perspective recognize that academic success is not independent of emotional and social well-being, and that creativity can serve as a mediating factor between stressors and adaptive coping. Marks et al. (2018) argue that interventions addressing only one domain—biological, psychological, or social—are insufficient in promoting holistic health. In primary education, this insight underscores the necessity of combining academic instruction with emotional support systems. Art therapy exemplifies this integration, offering a multisensory, symbolic, and relational practice that speaks to all three domains of the biopsychosocial model simultaneously.

Creativity and Resilience in Developmental Psychology

Developmental psychology provides a further theoretical foundation for understanding the role of art therapy in primary education, especially through the contributions of Vygotsky, Erikson, and Piaget. Each theorist highlights different aspects of how creativity and resilience function within child development. Vygotsky (1978) emphasized the sociocultural foundations of creativity, positing that imaginative activity is central to cognitive development. For him, art-making is not merely a leisure activity but a developmental tool that mediates between individual expression and cultural frameworks. Through the "zone of proximal development," children engage in artistic activities that scaffold new skills with the guidance of adults or peers. Art therapy in schools aligns with this theory by providing structured yet flexible environments where children can experiment creatively while receiving supportive feedback. Erikson's (1963) psychosocial stages of development further illuminate the connection between art, resilience, and identity. In the primary school years, children navigate the stage of "industry versus inferiority," where competence and self-esteem are critical. Artistic activities provide opportunities to demonstrate competence, overcome challenges, and experience mastery, thereby reinforcing resilience. Moreover, art therapy allows children to process psychosocial conflicts symbolically, which can strengthen their capacity to navigate future developmental tasks. Piaget (1951) focused on cognitive development, highlighting the role of symbolic play and representation in children's learning. For Piaget, creativity and resilience are embedded in the child's ability to accommodate and assimilate new experiences into existing cognitive schemas. Art-making offers a unique medium for this process: drawings, for example, provide external representations of internal concepts, bridging the gap between concrete and abstract thought. In therapeutic settings, such symbolic representation can also help children process traumatic or confusing experiences, facilitating adaptive coping.

Across these theoretical perspectives, creativity is consistently framed as a mechanism for resilience. Art therapy thus operates not only as a clinical intervention but also as a developmental support, enabling children to cultivate adaptive strategies in the face of stressors. Research supports this view, showing that participation in creative activities is positively correlated with psychological resilience, emotional regulation, and social competence (Eisner, 2002).

Synthesis and Implications

Taken together, the historical trajectory of art therapy in schools, the distinction between therapeutic and educational uses of art, the biopsychosocial framework of health psychology, and developmental psychology theories of creativity and resilience provide a robust theoretical foundation for art therapy in primary education. The convergence of these perspectives underscores the multidimensional role of art-making in children's lives: as a tool for cognitive growth, emotional regulation, identity formation, and social integration.

The implications for practice are significant. Schools that embrace art therapy within a biopsychosocial framework recognize that children's well-being is not ancillary to education but integral to it. By distinguishing between therapeutic and educational uses of art, educators and therapists can collaborate more effectively, ensuring that interventions are both ethically sound and developmentally appropriate. Drawing on developmental psychology, practitioners can tailor interventions to align with children's cognitive and psychosocial stages, thereby maximizing their impact.

Ultimately, art therapy in primary education is not simply an ancillary activity but a theoretically grounded practice that bridges education and health. Rooted in historical precedent, informed by psychology, and guided by contemporary health models, it holds the potential to support children's holistic development and long-term resilience.

Neuroscientific and Embodied Perspectives in Art Therapy

Multisensory Learning and Memory Consolidation

Multisensory learning, which engages multiple sensory modalities—such as visual, auditory, and tactile inputs—has been shown to enhance memory consolidation and cognitive processing. This approach is particularly beneficial in educational settings, where it supports deeper learning and long-term retention. For instance, research indicates that incorporating tactile and kinesthetic experiences into learning activities can significantly improve memory performance, especially in young children (Firstanti Wardany et al., 2021). By stimulating various sensory pathways, multisensory learning creates richer neural representations, facilitating stronger and more durable memory traces.

In the context of art therapy, engaging multiple senses through activities like drawing, sculpting, or painting not only fosters creativity but also reinforces memory consolidation. The act of creating art involves complex sensorimotor interactions that enhance neural connectivity and support the integration of new information. This multisensory engagement is particularly beneficial for children, as it aligns with their developmental needs and learning styles.

Art and Neural Integration

The relationship between art-making and neural integration has been explored in several studies. Bolwerk et al. (2014) conducted a study examining the effects of visual art production on brain connectivity. They found that participants who engaged in art-making activities exhibited increased functional connectivity in brain regions associated with self-reflection and emotional regulation. This enhanced connectivity was linked to improvements in psychological resilience, suggesting that art-making can facilitate neural integration and support mental health.

Further research supports these findings, indicating that art production activates brain networks involved in emotional processing and cognitive flexibility. For example, engaging in art activities has been shown to reduce activity in the amygdala, a region associated with stress and anxiety, while enhancing connectivity in areas related to executive function and self-regulation (Bolwerk et al., 2014). These neural changes underscore the therapeutic potential of art in promoting mental well-being.

Embodied Cognition: Tactile, Kinesthetic, and Visual Engagement

Embodied cognition posits that cognitive processes are deeply rooted in the body's interactions with the world. This perspective emphasizes the role of sensory and motor experiences in shaping thought and learning. In educational contexts, embodied learning strategies that incorporate movement, touch, and visual engagement have been shown to enhance understanding and retention of information. In art therapy, embodied cognition is particularly relevant. Activities that involve tactile exploration, such as clay modeling or textile work, engage the sense of touch and promote sensory integration. Kinesthetic activities, like dance or gesture-based art, involve bodily movement, supporting motor coordination and spatial awareness. Visual engagement through drawing or painting stimulates the visual cortex and encourages creative expression. These embodied experiences are not merely peripheral to cognitive processes but are integral to how individuals perceive, understand, and interact with the world. By incorporating embodied practices into art therapy, therapists can facilitate deeper emotional processing and cognitive integration, supporting overall well-being.

Stress Reduction and Neuroplasticity Through Creative Activity

Engaging in creative activities, including art-making, has been associated with reductions in stress and enhancements in neuroplasticity. Studies have shown that creative expression can lower levels of cortisol, a hormone associated with stress, and increase the production of brain-derived neurotrophic factor (BDNF), a protein that supports neuroplasticity and cognitive function (Kaimal et al., 2017).

Art therapy leverages these effects by providing individuals with opportunities to express emotions, process trauma, and develop coping strategies through creative means. The act of creating art can serve as a form of emotional release, reducing stress and promoting relaxation. Additionally, the neural changes associated with creative activity support cognitive flexibility and resilience, enabling individuals to adapt to challenges and recover from adversity.

These findings highlight the importance of incorporating creative practices into therapeutic settings, particularly for children and adolescents, who may benefit from non-verbal forms of expression to navigate complex emotions and experiences. The brain, often described as the *hard drive* of human existence, regulates emotional responses and determines whether memories of events are encoded or forgotten. At the same time, lived experiences leave imprints on the body and mind. As Ζωγάκη (2020) notes, *"experience leaves a mark. This observation has been confirmed experimentally thanks to the recent discoveries of neurobiology, which demonstrate that the plasticity of neural networks allows the recording of experience."* Neural plasticity is thus regarded as a central component of memory formation and learning mechanisms and remains a significant focus of neurobiological research.

Positive emotions are primarily associated with the activity of four neurotransmitters: dopamine, oxytocin, serotonin, and endorphins. Artistic engagement and aesthetic experiences activate these neurochemical systems, generating feelings of joy and pleasure. The beneficial effects of art on human well-being have been widely documented. During the COVID-19 pandemic, for instance, many individuals turned to creative practices such as photography, music, painting, and drawing as coping mechanisms to counteract stress and anxiety, demonstrating the therapeutic role of art during times of crisis (Athanasekou, 2020, Zarghami, 2021).

Art's benefits extend beyond psychological relief to measurable physiological outcomes. Research has shown that as little as 45 minutes of art-making can reduce stress, improve critical thinking, and support memory. A Drexel University study published in *Art Therapy* under the title *Reduction in Cortisol Levels and Participants' Responses After Art Production* demonstrated that artistic activity significantly lowers cortisol levels, a biological marker of stress (Kaimal, Ray, & Muniz, 2016). Similarly, a University of Westminster study found that individuals who spent their lunch break in an art gallery reported lower stress levels, with significant reductions in cortisol concentrations just 35 minutes after their visit (Athanasekou, 2021).

Viewing art also triggers strong emotional responses. Neurobiologist Semir Zeki's research using brain scans revealed that observing art activates the brain's reward system, releasing dopamine—the neurotransmitter linked to love and pleasure (Athanasekou, 2021). Furthermore, visits to galleries have been shown to relieve mental fatigue in ways comparable to spending time in nature, highlighting art's restorative potential.

Engaging in creative and complex artistic tasks stimulates the brain by fostering new neural connections and enhancing communication between the two hemispheres. Studies on visual art production indicate that these processes contribute to mental resilience—the ability to adapt to challenges and adversity. Moreover, creating art reduces stress and negative emotions, producing effects similar to those experienced through meditation. Much like prayer or mindfulness practice, artistic engagement redirects attention toward details and sensory perception, temporarily suspending everyday concerns (Athanasekou, 2020).

Art therapy has also been applied effectively in clinical contexts, particularly for individuals with dementia or chronic health conditions. In dementia care, creative expression enhances cognitive function, strengthens memory, and reduces symptoms of depression and anxiety. Dr. Arnold Bresky has reported up to 70% improvement in memory among dementia and Alzheimer's patients using art therapy interventions (Athanasekou, 2021).

EMPIRICAL EVIDENCE FOR ART THERAPY IN SCHOOLS - PSYCHOLOGICAL AND EMOTIONAL OUTCOMES

Art therapy has demonstrated significant positive effects on children's psychological and emotional well-being within educational settings. A systematic review by Moula et al. (2020) highlighted that children participating in art therapy reported improvements in self-esteem, self-confidence, self-expression, mood, communication, understanding, resilience, and reductions in aggressive behavior. These outcomes suggest that art therapy provides a valuable avenue for emotional expression and regulation, particularly for children facing emotional challenges.

Further supporting these findings, a study by Shukla (2022) found that art therapy interventions, including activities such as painting and collage-making, led to enhanced self-esteem in participants. The process of creating art allowed children to experience a sense of accomplishment and competence, reinforcing positive self-perceptions.

Social and Interpersonal Outcomes

Beyond individual emotional benefits, art therapy has also been associated with improved social and interpersonal outcomes. Research by Lauss and Helm (2024) indicated that integrating arts into classrooms fosters positive social relationships among pupils by promoting creative expression and social skills such as empathy, mutual support, and teamwork. These social competencies are crucial for creating a conducive learning environment and enhancing peer interactions.

Additionally, a study by Malchiodi, 2020 (2020) demonstrated that art therapy enhanced the ability of children with Autism Spectrum Disorder (ASD) to engage and assert themselves in social interactions, leading to improved social inclusion and reduced social withdrawal. This underscores the potential of art therapy to facilitate social integration for children with diverse needs.

Cognitive and Academic Outcomes

The impact of art therapy on cognitive and academic outcomes has been a subject of interest in recent studies. Narimani et al. (2018) investigated the effects of painting-based art therapy on executive functions and visual-motor coordination in dyslexic students. The results indicated improvements in executive functions, such as planning and problem-solving, and enhanced visual-motor coordination, suggesting that art therapy can support cognitive development in children with learning disabilities.

However, a mixed-methods study by Moula et al. (2022) found no significant differences in reading, writing, and math scores between children attending art therapy and those receiving standard educational support. Despite this, both groups met national minimum expectations for learning, indicating that while art therapy may not directly influence academic performance, it contributes to overall cognitive engagement and development.

Practical Applications: Classroom Activities

Art therapy in primary education can be translated into structured, developmentally appropriate classroom activities that simultaneously address emotional, social, and cognitive outcomes. These activities enable children to express themselves creatively, develop resilience, and integrate emotional literacy into academic learning. Among the diverse approaches utilized in classroom settings, seven activities have been identified as particularly effective: Safe Place Drawing, Resilience Trees, Strength Shields, Group Murals, Storytelling with Art, Clay Modeling for Release, and Emotion Masks (Moula et al., 2020; Malchiodi, 2020, 2020). Each of these exercises not only provides a medium for creative expression but also aligns with principles of child-centered pedagogy and socio-emotional learning (Kaimal et al., 2017).

Safe Place Drawing involves the creation of a visual representation of a personal safe space to promote emotional regulation and self-soothing (Shukla, 2022). Children are encouraged to reflect on locations or experiences where they feel secure and calm, and then translate these perceptions into a drawing, using materials such as paper, colored pencils, crayons, or markers. The activity begins with a discussion about the concept of a "safe place," prompting children to consider sensory elements such as color, sound, and texture. Through the drawing process, children externalize feelings of safety and comfort, which can then be further explored through guided reflection or small-group sharing. Facilitation of Safe Place Drawing typically spans thirty to forty-five minutes, with adaptations made for developmental level, such as providing templates or prompts for younger children and encouraging freeform, detailed expression for older participants (Moula et al., 2020). Case observations reveal that children frequently express underlying anxieties and stressors through this activity, as in the example of an eight-year-old who depicted a bedroom with exaggerated bright colors and floating clouds, verbalizing feelings of both security and underlying concern about school transitions. Integration with literacy and health education can be achieved by having children compose descriptive paragraphs about their safe space or by discussing coping strategies associated with feelings of safety, while social studies lessons can explore the role of safe physical and emotional environments (Kaimal et al., 2017).

Resilience Trees provide a visual metaphor for personal strengths and coping mechanisms, enabling children to conceptualize resilience in tangible terms (Malchiodi, 2020, 2020). In this activity, children draw a tree, labeling the roots with supportive people or past experiences, the trunk with personal qualities, and branches with coping strategies or goals. The use of visual symbols and decorations such as stickers or magazine cutouts reinforces meaning and allows children to personalize their representation. Facilitators guide children through a discussion of the various components of the tree, encouraging them to articulate the sources of their resilience. Younger children may benefit from pre-printed symbols and structured guidance, whereas older children can integrate complex metaphors or abstract representations (Moula et al., 2020). In one observed case, a ten-year-old drew roots labeled "Mom, soccer, reading," a trunk of "determination," and branches representing strategies like "asking for help" and "deep breathing." Reflecting on the tree facilitated articulation of coping mechanisms, supporting both emotional development and self-awareness. The activity can be linked with social studies through examination of familial and community support systems, health education through discussions of emotional resilience, and literacy through narrative writing about the tree's components (Kaimal et al., 2017).

Strength Shields emphasize identification and reinforcement of personal qualities, serving to enhance self-esteem (Shukla, 2022). Children design a shield divided into segments that represent individual strengths, skills, or positive traits, and decorate these sections using visual symbolism. Facilitators may encourage discussion about the choices made, fostering peer recognition and mutual affirmation. Adaptations allow for simplification through prompts or templates for younger children, while older children can explore symbolic metaphors or complex visual design (Malchiodi, 2020, 2020). In one illustrative case, a nine-year-old student labeled her shield with "kindness, curiosity, soccer skills" and added a sun symbol to represent optimism, sharing the creation with peers and reinforcing positive self-perceptions and self-confidence. Curriculum integration can occur through literacy by composing acrostic poems based on personal strengths, social studies through reflection on individual identity and social roles, and health education by linking self-esteem with healthy decision-making and adaptive behaviors (Moula et al., 2020).

Group Murals provide a collaborative approach, emphasizing teamwork, negotiation, and collective creativity (Kaimal et al., 2017). Children work together to produce a large visual artwork on a shared theme, such as "Our Ideal School" or "Dream Community." This activity begins with planning, brainstorming, and the allocation of responsibilities, fostering negotiation and decision-making skills. Throughout the creative process, facilitators encourage reflection and discussion on artistic choices and collaboration. Younger children may focus on cooperative painting or drawing within allocated spaces, while older children can coordinate complex thematic elements (Malchiodi, 2020, 2020). One observed example involved a group of fifth graders negotiating space and responsibilities while depicting a shared vision of a community park, library, and school. The activity not only promoted artistic collaboration but also enhanced empathy, problem-solving, and communication skills. Group murals can be integrated into social studies through exploration of civic engagement, into health education by discussing cooperative behavior, and into literacy through written narratives accompanying mural elements (Moula et al., 2020).

Storytelling with Art merges narrative development with artistic expression, supporting emotional processing, literacy skills, and perspective-taking (Shukla, 2022). Children create sequential visual narratives, such as comic strips or storyboards, in response to prompts like "A Day I Overcame a Challenge." They are encouraged to combine drawings with captions, dialogue, or speech bubbles, thereby integrating visual and verbal modes of expression. Facilitation involves guidance on narrative coherence, pacing, and emotional content. Younger children may dictate captions to facilitate engagement, whereas older children can construct more elaborate storylines incorporating symbolism and metaphor. In one case, a seven-year-old illustrated a personal story of losing a soccer game but learning perseverance, using the narrative as a springboard for verbal reflection on coping strategies and emotional understanding. Curriculum integration occurs naturally with literacy through sequencing and narrative skills, with social studies through exploration of personal experiences within social contexts, and with health education by reinforcing resilience and emotional regulation strategies (Kaimal et al., 2017; Moula et al., 2020).

Clay Modeling for Release utilizes tactile and kinesthetic engagement to allow children to externalize emotions and reduce stress (Malchiodi, 2020, 2020). Children are invited to create abstract forms or figures in clay that represent their feelings, with reflective discussion guided by prompts such as "What does your sculpture represent?" or "How did it feel to create it?" Facilitators provide alternative materials and ensure a safe, comfortable environment, particularly for children with sensory sensitivities. Time allocation ranges from forty to sixty minutes, with younger children receiving more structured guidance and older children encouraged to explore symbolic or abstract representations (Shukla, 2022). In practice, a child sculpted a twisted spiral representing anxiety about transitioning schools, using the reflection process to articulate feelings and develop coping strategies. Integration with literacy can be achieved through reflective journaling, with health education addressing stress management and self-expression, and science lessons exploring material properties and sensory experiences (Moula et al., 2020).

Emotion Masks encourage children to identify and represent complex emotions using visual symbolism (Kaimal et al., 2017). Participants select an emotion and design a mask using materials such as paper plates, cardboard, paints, markers, and decorative materials. The activity fosters exploration of emotional expression and empathy, and can be extended into role-play exercises to practice perspective-taking in social situations. Facilitation involves discussion of color, shape, and texture choices, with adaptations for age and developmental level; younger children focus on simple representations, whereas older children can employ abstract symbolism. In one observed example, a ten-year-old created a mask depicting frustration through jagged edges and dark colors, which facilitated discussion with peers about strategies for managing anger and recognizing emotional cues in others. Curriculum integration includes literacy through story creation from the mask's perspective, health education through emotional regulation strategies, and social studies through examination of cultural expressions of emotion (Moula et al., 2020; Malchiodi, 2020, 2020).

Across all activities, facilitators play a critical role in providing age-appropriate guidance, maintaining a safe and supportive environment, and observing both individual and group responses. Materials should be non-toxic, sensory-appropriate, and flexible to accommodate children with diverse needs. Typical session durations range from forty to ninety minutes, allowing flexibility for attention span, developmental stage, and engagement level (Kaimal et al., 2017; Shukla, 2022). Observation and reflective discussion are integral to all activities, providing insights into children's emotional, social, and cognitive development. Integration with the curriculum ensures that these activities are not isolated experiences but part of a holistic educational approach, supporting literacy, social studies, and health education objectives while promoting socio-emotional learning, creativity, and resilience (Moula et al., 2020).

Collectively, these seven activities illustrate the practical application of art therapy in primary classrooms. They provide structured opportunities for emotional expression, resilience-building, social skill development, and cognitive engagement. Through case observations, it is evident that children respond positively to these interventions, demonstrating enhanced self-esteem, improved emotion regulation, stronger peer relationships, and increased engagement in learning processes. By embedding creative activities within the educational curriculum, teachers and therapists can support holistic child development, bridging therapeutic and educational objectives in a manner that is both engaging and developmentally appropriate (Malchiodi, 2020, 2020; Kaimal et al., 2017; Moula et al., 2020; Shukla, 2022).

Inclusion and Diversity in Art Therapy Practices

Art therapy in educational contexts must be approached with careful attention to inclusion and diversity to ensure that all children, regardless of ability, background, or previous experiences of trauma, can benefit from creative expression. Children with special educational needs (SEN) often face barriers in conventional classroom environments, including challenges in communication, social interaction, and self-regulation. Art therapy provides a non-verbal, experiential modality that can circumvent these barriers, offering alternative pathways for self-expression and engagement (Malchiodi, 2020, 2020; Moula et al., 2020). Through the use of visual, tactile, and kinesthetic media, children with developmental delays, learning differences, or sensory processing difficulties can convey thoughts and emotions that may be difficult to articulate verbally. For example, children with Autism Spectrum Disorder (ASD) have shown improvements in social interaction and emotional expression when engaged in structured art therapy activities, such as collaborative murals or emotion-focused mask-making exercises, which support both self-awareness and social inclusion (Malchiodi, 2020, 2020).

Trauma-informed approaches are critical for ensuring that art therapy practices do not inadvertently retraumatize children who have experienced adverse events, including abuse, neglect, or chronic stress. Trauma-sensitive facilitation emphasizes predictability, safety, and choice, allowing children to engage in artistic processes at their own pace. Techniques such as Safe Place Drawing or Resilience Trees can be particularly effective in providing children with a sense of control and emotional containment, while reflective discussions support the externalization and processing of complex feelings. Educators and therapists must recognize potential triggers in materials, themes, or group interactions, adapting sessions to reduce anxiety and promote a supportive environment (Malchiodi, 2012). The inclusion of grounding exercises, sensory regulation strategies, and the option to opt out of certain activities enhances safety and fosters trust, which is essential for meaningful therapeutic engagement.

Cultural sensitivity is another foundational consideration in inclusive art therapy. Schools often reflect diverse student populations, encompassing multiple ethnicities, languages, and cultural traditions. Art therapy interventions must be adapted to respect cultural norms and values, ensuring that materials, prompts, and interpretive frameworks are meaningful and relevant to all participants (Cohen-Yatziv & Regev, 2019). For instance, when facilitating activities such as Group Murals or Storytelling with Art, incorporating culturally significant symbols, narratives, and aesthetic forms allows children to explore identity, heritage, and shared community experiences while fostering cross-cultural empathy among peers. Furthermore, understanding cultural variations in emotional expression is essential for accurately interpreting children's artwork and supporting their socio-emotional development (Kapitan, 2016). Sensitivity to cultural and linguistic diversity promotes equitable participation, helping to prevent marginalization of students whose cultural or communicative styles differ from the mainstream classroom norms.

Ensuring equity and accessibility is particularly important in resource-limited schools, where constraints in materials, space, and trained personnel may limit opportunities for art therapy implementation. Creative adaptation strategies, such as using recycled or low-cost materials, can provide children with meaningful artistic experiences without compromising therapeutic intent (Malchiodi, 2012). Teachers and facilitators can also adopt group-based or peer-supported approaches to maximize engagement when individual resources are limited. In addition, integrating art therapy into the broader curriculum, such as embedding creative activities in literacy, social studies, or health education, enhances accessibility while reinforcing academic objectives (Moula et al., 2020). Professional development for educators in inclusive, trauma-informed, and culturally sensitive practices further strengthens the capacity to deliver equitable art therapy interventions, ensuring that all children benefit from the socio-emotional and cognitive gains associated with creative expression.

Moreover, the principles of Universal Design for Learning (UDL) can guide inclusive art therapy practice by providing multiple means of representation, engagement, and expression (CAST, 2018). For example, offering children a choice of media, allowing alternative ways to communicate ideas (drawing, clay modeling, storytelling), and scaffolding activities according to developmental level enhances participation for children with diverse abilities. Inclusion also extends to classroom culture, encouraging peer support, collaborative work, and recognition of individual contributions to collective projects. When these practices are combined with trauma-informed and culturally sensitive approaches, art therapy becomes a vehicle for equity, promoting both individual well-being and social cohesion.

In summary, the successful integration of art therapy into primary education requires deliberate attention to inclusion and diversity. Children with special educational needs benefit from non-verbal, experiential modes of expression that support emotional regulation, social engagement, and resilience (Malchiodi, 2020, 2020; Moula et al., 2020). Trauma-informed facilitation ensures safety, choice, and predictability, reducing the risk of retraumatization and fostering trust (Malchiodi, 2012). Cultural sensitivity and adaptation make interventions meaningful and equitable across diverse populations, while resource-conscious strategies and UDL-informed practices enhance accessibility and participation in schools with limited materials or personnel (CAST, 2018; Cohen-Yatziv & Regev, 2019). By embedding these principles into everyday art therapy activities, educators can create inclusive, supportive, and culturally responsive environments that foster emotional well-being, resilience, and social-emotional development for all children.

Ethical and Pedagogical Considerations

The integration of art therapy within primary education requires careful attention to both ethical and pedagogical frameworks to ensure that children benefit from creative interventions while minimizing potential risks. A critical consideration is the boundary between therapeutic and pedagogical roles. While art therapy promotes emotional expression, socio-emotional growth, and resilience, classroom teachers may not possess the specialized training required for clinical therapeutic intervention (Malchiodi, 2012). Establishing clear distinctions between teaching and therapy prevents role confusion and ensures that art-based activities support learning objectives without inadvertently crossing into clinical treatment. Teachers should facilitate creative exercises as part of socio-emotional learning (SEL) or curriculum-aligned activities while recognizing when referral to a qualified art therapist is necessary for more complex psychological or behavioral concerns (Cohen-Yatziv & Regev, 2019).

Confidentiality and voluntary participation are foundational ethical principles in educational art therapy. Children must feel safe in expressing personal thoughts and emotions without fear of disclosure or judgment. Clear communication regarding the purpose of activities, the voluntary nature of participation, and the limits of confidentiality is essential . For example, while reflective discussions or group sharing may enhance social learning, children should have the option to opt out or contribute at their own comfort level. Maintaining confidentiality is particularly crucial when addressing sensitive topics, such as trauma, grief, or family dynamics, and facilitators must carefully manage documentation, storage of artwork, and communication with parents or school staff in accordance with ethical guidelines (Malchiodi, 2012).

Teacher training and referral systems are integral to ethical practice. Educators implementing art therapy–inspired interventions must receive professional development in trauma-informed pedagogy, child development, and inclusive practices (Malchiodi, 2020, 2020; Moula et al., 2020). Training should emphasize recognizing signs of distress, supporting diverse learning needs, and employing safe facilitation techniques. Teachers should also be familiar with referral pathways to school counselors, psychologists, or licensed art therapists when a child requires individualized or clinical support beyond the classroom setting. Such systems ensure that children receive appropriate care while maintaining the integrity of the educational environment and preventing the overextension of teaching staff into therapeutic roles (Cohen-Yatziv & Regev, 2019).

Avoiding harm and ensuring safe facilitation extend to both physical and psychological safety. Physical safety involves the provision of non-toxic, age-appropriate materials and the organization of the classroom to prevent accidents during art activities (Shukla, 2022). Psychological safety requires that facilitators foster an environment of trust, respect, and predictability, particularly for children with trauma histories or special educational needs. Activities should be carefully structured to avoid triggering distressing memories or intense emotional responses, with alternatives or modifications provided for children who may find certain materials, prompts, or group dynamics challenging . Reflection and debriefing are essential components, allowing children to process their experiences and enabling facilitators to monitor emotional responses, adjust activities, and provide additional support when needed (Malchiodi, 2012).

The ethical application of art therapy in classrooms also involves attention to developmental appropriateness and cultural sensitivity. Activities must be tailored to children's cognitive, emotional, and motor abilities to prevent frustration or exclusion. Facilitators should also consider cultural norms around emotional expression, symbolism, and artistic styles, ensuring that interventions are inclusive and respectful of diverse identities and backgrounds (Cohen-Yatziv & Regev, 2019). Awareness of cultural, linguistic, and socio-economic factors contributes to equity and supports engagement across the student population. For instance, offering multiple means of expression—such as drawing, clay modeling, or storytelling—can accommodate varied abilities and preferences, aligning with principles of Universal Design for Learning (CAST, 2018).

In addition, ethical facilitation entails the ongoing monitoring of the teacher-student dynamic to avoid inadvertent power imbalances or undue pressure. Children should perceive art activities as exploratory, playful, and supportive rather than evaluative or performance-based. Feedback should be constructive, non-judgmental, and centered on effort, creativity, and reflection rather than artistic skill or accuracy. Such approaches reinforce positive self-concept, promote intrinsic motivation, and reduce anxiety associated with creative tasks (Kaimal et al., 2017).

Finally, an ethical pedagogical framework requires continuous reflection on practice. Facilitators must evaluate both intended and unintended outcomes of art therapy–based activities, including emotional, social, and cognitive effects. Documentation, supervision, and professional collaboration enhance accountability and help to refine interventions for safety, effectiveness, and inclusivity (Moula et al., 2020). By prioritizing ethical considerations alongside pedagogical goals, educators can provide art-based interventions that support holistic child development while safeguarding well-being, promoting autonomy, and fostering a safe and inclusive learning environment.

In summary, the ethical and pedagogical implementation of art therapy in primary education hinges on clearly delineating roles between teaching and therapy, ensuring voluntary participation and confidentiality, providing adequate teacher training and referral mechanisms, and maintaining both physical and psychological safety. Attention to developmental, cultural, and individual diversity further reinforces inclusivity, equity, and effectiveness. By integrating these considerations into classroom practice, educators can offer creative activities that enhance socio-emotional development, support resilience, and complement academic learning, all within an ethically responsible framework (Malchiodi, 2020, 2020; Malchiodi, 2012; Moula et al., 2020).

Policy and Sustainability

The integration of art therapy into primary education requires strategic alignment with educational policy frameworks, cross-sector collaboration, and sustainable implementation strategies. Embedding art therapy within school curricula necessitates recognition at the policy level of the value of creative interventions for children's socio-emotional, cognitive, and social development. Policy initiatives should define clear objectives for art-based programs, including measurable outcomes related to emotional well-being, resilience, social inclusion, and academic engagement (Cohen-Yatziv & Regev, 2019). Such frameworks ensure that art therapy is not treated as an ancillary activity but as an integral component of holistic education. This may involve inclusion in national or regional educational standards, mental health promotion policies, or social-emotional learning (SEL) guidelines, thereby providing legitimacy and structured support for program implementation (Malchiodi, 2020, 2020).

Cross-sector collaboration between education, health, and social services is essential for the effective delivery and sustainability of school-based art therapy initiatives. Partnerships between schools, licensed art therapists, mental health professionals, and community organizations create networks that provide both expertise and resources (Moula et al., 2020). For example, collaboration with child psychologists or social workers ensures that students with complex needs are identified, referred, and supported appropriately, while health professionals can provide guidance on trauma-informed practices and inclusion of children with special educational needs . Such integrated approaches facilitate comprehensive care and ensure that art therapy interventions address the multidimensional needs of students. Collaborative networks also allow for shared evaluation and research, promoting evidence-based practice and continuous improvement of programs.

Teacher training and professional development constitute a critical element in the sustainability of art therapy in schools. Educators require foundational knowledge in developmental psychology, socio-emotional learning, trauma-informed practice, and inclusive pedagogy, as well as practical skills in facilitating art-based activities (Kaimal et al., 2017; Malchiodi, 2012). Training programs may include workshops, supervised practice, and mentorship with licensed art therapists, enabling teachers to integrate therapeutic principles within educational contexts safely and effectively. Additionally, dual-training models that prepare professionals to serve both pedagogical and therapeutic roles can increase program capacity and resilience. Long-term sustainability also depends on the availability of supervision and ongoing professional support, ensuring that staff maintain fidelity to ethical standards and evidence-based practices while adapting to evolving student needs (Shukla, 2022).

Funding and resource allocation are central to the long-term viability of school-based art therapy programs. Sustainable funding models may involve governmental education budgets, grants from mental health agencies, partnerships with non-profit organizations, or community-based sponsorships (Malchiodi, 2020, 2020). Cost-effective strategies, such as the use of low-cost or recycled materials and group-based interventions, can maximize impact while minimizing financial burden (Moula et al., 2020). Additionally, evidence of program efficacy—through assessment of emotional, social, and academic outcomes—supports advocacy for continued funding, demonstrating that art therapy contributes to both individual well-being and broader educational objectives. Integrating program evaluation into routine practice, including systematic collection of qualitative and quantitative data, ensures accountability and informs policy decisions regarding resource allocation and program expansion.

Sustainability is further enhanced by institutionalizing art therapy within school culture and infrastructure. Embedding creative practices into regular curricula,

SEL programs, and wellness initiatives ensures that they are not dependent solely on individual champions or temporary projects (Cohen-Yatziv & Regev, 2019). Schools may establish dedicated spaces for art therapy, integrate creative activities into lesson plans, and schedule regular sessions as part of weekly routines. Such structural integration supports continuity, normalizes creative self-expression, and reinforces the pedagogical and therapeutic value of art-based interventions. In addition, fostering community engagement—through exhibitions, parent workshops, and collaborative projects—strengthens the visibility and perceived legitimacy of art therapy, contributing to its sustainability and long-term adoption.

In conclusion, the sustainability of art therapy in primary education depends on deliberate integration into educational policy, robust cross-sector collaboration, comprehensive training models, and stable funding mechanisms. Policy recognition provides legitimacy and structure for implementation, while partnerships with health and social services ensure holistic support for students. Training and supervision of educators and therapists maintain quality and ethical practice, and resource planning coupled with institutional integration supports long-term continuity. By aligning art therapy initiatives with systemic educational priorities, schools can create enduring programs that enhance children's emotional, social, and cognitive development while fostering inclusive, supportive, and resilient learning environments (Malchiodi, 2020, 2020; Kaimal et al., 2017; Moula et al., 2020; Shukla, 2022).

CONCLUSION

The integration of art therapy into primary education represents a transformative approach to fostering children's emotional, social, and cognitive development. Across the preceding sections, it has become evident that art therapy offers a unique intersection between pedagogy and mental health, providing children with non-verbal, experiential modalities to express emotions, develop resilience, and enhance social engagement. The historical development of art therapy within educational settings demonstrates both its therapeutic potential and its capacity to complement traditional academic objectives (Malchiodi, 2020, 2020; Moula et al., 2020). Distinguishing between therapeutic and educational applications underscores the importance of clarity in implementation, ensuring that classroom teachers facilitate creative processes while recognizing the boundaries of clinical intervention (Malchiodi, 2012).

The theoretical foundations of art therapy, informed by developmental psychology and health psychology, highlight the centrality of creativity, resilience, and the biopsychosocial model in understanding child development (Marks et al., 2018; Vygotsky, 1978; Erikson, 1968; Piaget, 1972). Engaging in artistic activities allows children to process complex emotions, navigate social dynamics, and consolidate learning experiences, promoting both self-regulation and executive functioning. Neuroscientific perspectives reinforce these insights, demonstrating that multisensory engagement, embodied cognition, and creative expression contribute to neural integration, memory consolidation, and stress reduction (Bolwerk et al., 2014; Kaimal et al., 2017). Such findings provide a compelling evidence base for incorporating art therapy into everyday educational practice, emphasizing the importance of both individual and collective creative experiences.

Empirical research further supports the value of art therapy in schools, revealing measurable gains in psychological, social, and cognitive domains. Children participating in structured art therapy activities exhibit improvements in self-esteem, emotion regulation, empathy, peer relationships, and attention, demonstrating that creative engagement fosters holistic development (Malchiodi, 2020, 2020; Moula et al., 2020). Comparative studies indicate that art therapy can complement or even exceed the outcomes of other social-emotional learning interventions, particularly for children facing trauma, anxiety, or special educational needs (Cohen-Yatziv & Regev, 2019; Shukla, 2022). These findings collectively affirm that art therapy serves not only as a therapeutic tool but also as a pedagogical strategy capable of enhancing engagement, inclusion, and academic readiness.

Practical applications of art therapy within classrooms illustrate the feasibility and adaptability of these approaches. Activities such as Safe Place Drawing, Resilience Trees, Strength Shields, Group Murals, Storytelling with Art, Clay Modeling for Release, and Emotion Masks provide structured yet flexible opportunities for self-expression, reflection, and social learning (Moula et al., 2020; Malchiodi, 2020, 2020). Facilitators play a pivotal role in guiding these experiences, ensuring developmental appropriateness, ethical practice, and integration with curricular objectives. Case observations demonstrate that children respond positively to these interventions, exhibiting enhanced resilience, improved social skills, and deeper engagement in academic and creative tasks. When integrated into literacy, social studies, and health education curricula, art therapy becomes a multifaceted tool that bridges cognitive, emotional, and social domains, promoting comprehensive learning outcomes (Kaimal et al., 2017).

Inclusion and diversity remain central to ethical and effective implementation. Art therapy offers pathways for children with special educational needs, trauma histories, and diverse cultural backgrounds to participate meaningfully in creative activities (Malchiodi, 2020, 2020; Cohen-Yatziv & Regev, 2019). Trauma-informed facilitation, culturally sensitive adaptations, and resource-conscious strategies ensure equitable access and psychological safety, fostering participation, empowerment, and self-efficacy. Universal Design for Learning principles further enhance inclusivity, offering multiple means of representation, engagement, and expression to accommodate diverse abilities and learning styles (CAST, 2018). These strategies collectively underscore the potential of art therapy to reduce disparities, promote social cohesion, and strengthen the well-being of all students.

Ethical and pedagogical considerations are fundamental to sustainable and responsible practice. Maintaining clear boundaries between pedagogy and therapy, ensuring voluntary participation, protecting confidentiality, and providing professional training and referral pathways safeguard children's welfare while enabling teachers to facilitate art-based activities effectively (Malchiodi, 2012; Shukla, 2022). Attending to physical and psychological safety, cultural sensitivity, and developmental appropriateness reinforces the ethical integrity of interventions and enhances the potential for positive outcomes. Moreover, systemic reflection and evaluation allow educators and administrators to refine practices, document impact, and support evidence-based advocacy for continued program development (Moula et al., 2020).

Policy and sustainability are crucial to the long-term integration of art therapy in education. Recognition at the policy level, cross-sector collaboration, structured teacher training, and secure funding mechanisms ensure continuity, quality, and scalability (Malchiodi, 2020, 2020; Kaimal et al., 2017). Embedding art therapy within curricular standards and school culture normalizes creative expression as part of everyday learning, fostering a holistic approach to child development that values emotional and social well-being alongside academic achievement. Collaborative networks between educators, mental health professionals, and community organizations provide additional support, allowing programs to adapt to emerging needs while maintaining fidelity to ethical and evidence-based practices (Moula et al., 2020).

Looking forward, the vision for art therapy in primary education encompasses systemic change toward holistic well-being. Schools should be recognized not only as sites of academic instruction but also as environments that nurture emotional resilience, creativity, and social competence. Art therapy offers a practical, evidence-informed pathway for realizing this vision, reinforcing the notion that creative expression is integral to children's mental health and educational success. By fostering inclusive, trauma-sensitive, culturally responsive, and ethically sound practices, art therapy can transform classrooms into spaces of emotional safety, empowerment, and collaborative learning (Cohen-Yatziv & Regev, 2019).

In conclusion, art therapy in primary education represents a convergence of pedagogy, psychology, and creative practice that offers measurable benefits for children's holistic development. Evidence from developmental theory, neuroscience, empirical research, and classroom practice converges to support the integration of art therapy as both a health-promoting and educational tool (Bolwerk et al., 2014; Moula et al., 2020). Ensuring inclusion, ethical practice, and sustainability requires policy support, teacher training, cross-sector collaboration, and resource allocation, yet the potential rewards—a generation of children with enhanced emotional literacy, resilience, social competence, and creative capacity—justify the investment. By advocating for systemic adoption, continuous professional development, and cultural responsiveness, educators, therapists, and policymakers can establish art therapy as a central component of holistic primary education, promoting the well-being, equity, and flourishing of all children (Malchiodi, 2020; Shukla, 2022). The integration of art therapy into educational ecosystems is not merely an enrichment of the curriculum; it is a necessary evolution toward schools that prioritize the comprehensive development of the whole child, combining creativity, empathy, and resilience as foundational competencies for lifelong well-being.

REFERENCES

Αθανασέκου, Μ. (2020). επιμ. και συγγραφή, Γιατί με αφορά η τέχνη. Οι πολλές της διαστάσεις και πως αξιοποιούνται στη ζωή μας», Ηδυέπεια.

Αθανασέκου, Μ. (2021). *Η σχέση της τέχνης με την ψυχολογία - Η πρόσληψη της νοητικής υστέρησης και η απεικόνισή της στη ζωγραφική από τον 15ο έως τον 19ο αιώνα, στο βιβλίο Αργυριάδης, Α., Λόγος, αναπηρία, θεραπευτικές και εκπαιδευτικές παρεμβάσεις –Νέα δεδομένα και τάσεις στην Ειδική Αγωγή, σελ.* Εκδόσεις Ηδυέπεια.

Bolwerk, A., Mack-Andrick, J., Lang, F. R., Dörfler, A., & Maihöfner, C. (2014). How art changes your brain: Differential effects of visual art production and cognitive art evaluation on functional brain connectivity. *PLoS One*, *9*(7), e101035. DOI: 10.1371/journal.pone.0101035 PMID: 24983951

Case, C., & Dalley, T. (2014). *The handbook of art therapy* (3rd ed.). Routledge. DOI: 10.4324/9781315779799

CASEL. (2020). *SEL framework*. Collaborative for Academic, Social, and Emotional Learning. https://casel.org/sel-framework/

CAST. (2018). *Universal design for learning guidelines version 2.2.* http://udlguidelines.cast.org

Cohen-Yatziv, L., & Regev, D. (2019). The effectiveness of art therapy with children: A review of the empirical literature. *Frontiers in Psychology*, *10*, 2375. DOI: 10.3389/fpsyg.2019.02375

Ecclestone, K., & Hayes, D. (2009). *The dangerous rise of therapeutic education.* Routledge. DOI: 10.4324/9780203870563

Eisner, E. W. (2002). *The arts and the creation of mind.* Yale University Press.

Erikson, E. H. (1963). *Childhood and society* (2nd ed.). Norton.

Junge, M. B., & Linesch, D. (1993). Our own voices: New paradigms for art therapy research. *Art Therapy: Journal of the American Art Therapy Association*, *10*(1), 3–11. DOI: 10.1080/07421656.1993.10758986

Kaimal, G., Ray, K., & Muniz, J. (2017). Reduction of cortisol levels and participants' responses following art making. *Art Therapy: Journal of the American Art Therapy Association*, *33*(2), 74–80. DOI: 10.1080/07421656.2016.1166832 PMID: 27695158

Kapitan, L. (2016). *Introduction to art therapy research* (2nd ed.). Routledge.

Lauss, J., & Helm, C. (2024). The role of the arts in the classroom: Does integration of the arts promote social relationships in the classroom? *ResearchGate*. https://www.researchgate.net/publication/387452576

Malchiodi, C. A. (2012). *Handbook of art therapy* (2nd ed.). Guilford Press.

Malchiodi, C. A. (2020). *Trauma and expressive arts therapy: Brain, body, and imagination in the healing process*. Guilford Press.

Marks, D. F., Murray, M., Evans, B., & Estacio, E. V. (2018). *Health psychology: Theory, research and practice* (5th ed.). Sage.

Moula, Z., Powell, J., & Karkou, V. (2020). *A systematic review of child-focused outcomes and experiences in arts therapies*. Edge Hill University. https://research.edgehill.ac.uk/files/23144225/Systematic_review_Final_version.pdf

Narimani, M., Abolghasemi, A., & Ilbeigy Ghalenei, R. (2018). Effect of art therapy (painting) on executive functions and visual motor coordination in dyslexic children. *Middle Eastern Journal of Disability Studies, 8,* 50. https://jdisabilstud.org/article-1-645-en.html

Piaget, J. (1951). *Play, dreams and imitation in childhood*. Routledge & Kegan Paul.

Piaget, J. (1972). *Psychology and pedagogy*. Viking Press.

Rubin, J. A. (2016). *Approaches to art therapy: Theory and technique* (3rd ed.). Routledge. DOI: 10.4324/9781315716015

Sani, Y., Wardany, O. F., Herlina, H., & Vernanda, G. (2021). The implementation of embodied learning: A literature review. *Edukasi, 15*(1), 1–10. DOI: 10.15294/edukasi.v15i1.30008

Shukla, A. (2022). Role of art therapy in the promotion of mental health. *PubMed Central*. https://pubmed.ncbi.nlm.nih.gov/

UNESCO. (2006). *Road map for arts education*. UNESCO.

UNICEF. (2021). *The state of the world's children 2021: On my mind – Promoting, protecting and caring for children's mental health*. United Nations Children's Fund. https://www.unicef.org/reports/state-worlds-children-2021

Vygotsky, L. S. (1978). *Mind in society: The development of higher psychological processes*. Harvard University Press.

Ζωγάκη, Ε. (2020). Όψεις του πραγματικού: οι εικαστικές τέχνες και η ματιά του θεατή. Οπτική αντίληψη, αισθητικές θεωρίες και καλλιτεχνικές συμβάσεις. Στο Αθανασέκου (Επιμ.) *Γιατί με αφορά η τέχνη (σελ.331-347)*. Αθήνα: Ηδυέπεια.

Zarghami, M. (2021). Psychiatric aspects of coronavirus (2019-nCoV) infection. *Iranian Journal of Psychiatry and Behavioral Sciences*, *14*(1), 2019–2021.

Chapter 5
Embodied Creativity:
Art, Meaning, and Behaviour in the Practice of Health Psychology

Maria Athanasekou
http://orcid.org/0000-0002-2971-9452
Hellenic Open University, Greece & Frederick University, Cyprus

ABSTRACT

Health psychology examines links between psychological processes, health, and social context. Within this field, art functions as a mediator of resilience, identity, and behavioural change. Creative expression is an embodied practice through which people process experience and develop coping strategies. Engagement in visual arts, music, dance, or writing bridges cognition, emotion, and bodily awareness, turning illness into meaning (Stuckey & Nobel, 2010; Fuchs, 2018). Dance, for example, aligns movement and rhythm to reduce stress (Koch et al., 2014), while visual art externalises trauma (Kaimal & Ray, 2017). Such practices resonate with enactive approaches to cognition (Varela et al., 1991). Meaning-making is central in illness (Park, 2010); art provides symbolic language for suffering and agency (Puig et al., 2006). It fosters resilience, self-efficacy, and social connectedness (Forgeard & Elstein, 2014). Thus, art enriches health psychology as embodied creativity, offering holistic tools for wellbeing and behavioural change.

1. INTRODUCTION

Health psychology is a multidisciplinary field that examines how psychological, behavioural, and social factors influence physical health and wellbeing (Taylor, 2018). It is concerned not only with understanding illness and disease processes but also with promoting preventive behaviours, coping strategies, and overall quality

DOI: 10.4018/979-8-2600-3085-1.ch005

of life. Traditionally, health psychology has focused on cognitive and behavioural mechanisms, exploring how beliefs, attitudes, and health-related behaviours contribute to physical and mental outcomes (Schunk & DiBenedetto, 2020). However, human experiences of health and illness are fundamentally embodied, affective, and socially situated, suggesting the need for broader conceptual and methodological tools within the discipline.

Within this context, art has emerged as a powerful medium for understanding and facilitating health-related processes. Artistic engagement encompasses a range of creative activities—including visual arts, music, dance, theatre, and writing—that enable individuals to process emotions, negotiate identity, and find meaning in challenging experiences (Stuckey & Nobel, 2010). The integration of art into health psychology reflects an increasing recognition that health outcomes are shaped not only by cognitive and behavioural processes but also by affective, somatic, and symbolic experiences (Fuchs, 2018). In this sense, art serves as both a reflective and an active mechanism for enhancing wellbeing, bridging subjective experience with behavioural change.

Central to this chapter is the concept of *embodied creativity*, which positions artistic engagement as an integrated experience of mind, body, and environment. Embodied creativity emphasizes that creative expression is not solely a cognitive process but involves dynamic interactions between neurological, physiological, and social systems (Koch & Fuchs, 2011). Through embodied practices, such as dance, painting, or music-making, individuals externalize internal states, regulate emotions, and construct personal narratives that foster resilience and adaptive coping (Koch, Kunz, Lykou, & Cruz, 2014). In doing so, artistic practices provide a unique lens through which health psychology can examine the lived experience of illness and wellness.

Historically, the therapeutic potential of art has been recognized in various forms, including art therapy, music therapy, and expressive writing interventions (Malchiodi, 2020). These practices have been shown to reduce stress, enhance emotional regulation, and improve social connectedness, highlighting the dual capacity of art to support both individual and collective wellbeing (Camic, 2010; Haeyen, van Hooren, van der Veld, & Hutschemaekers, 2015). Recent theoretical developments in cognitive science, particularly enactive and embodied approaches, further illuminate how creativity arises through bodily interaction with the environment, underscoring the inseparability of cognitive, emotional, and somatic dimensions of experience (Varela, Thompson, & Rosch, 1991).

The objective of this chapter is to explore the role of art as an integrative and embodied modality within health psychology. Specifically, it aims to demonstrate how creative engagement facilitates meaning-making, promotes adaptive behaviours, and enhances resilience. By conceptualizing art as embodied creativity, the chapter underscores the significance of integrating artistic practices into both clinical interventions and community health initiatives. It proposes that art is not merely an adjunct to traditional therapeutic models but a fundamental medium through which individuals and communities can cultivate psychological resilience, navigate illness, and construct meaningful life narratives.

The chapter is structured into several sections. Following this introduction, the theoretical foundations of embodied creativity in health psychology are examined, including historical perspectives and contemporary cognitive-scientific insights. Subsequent sections explore the mechanisms through which art fosters meaning-making, behavioural change, and resilience. Practical applications in clinical and community settings are then discussed, highlighting the translational potential of artistic engagement. Finally, the chapter concludes by identifying future research directions and implications for policy and practice, emphasizing the transformative potential of integrating art into health psychology.

2. THEORETICAL FOUNDATIONS

Health psychology has traditionally been concerned with understanding how psychological processes influence physical health and illness, emphasizing cognition, behaviour, and social context (Taylor, 2018). The field seeks to identify mechanisms that promote adaptive coping, adherence to medical regimens, and overall wellbeing. However, an emerging body of literature highlights that human experiences of health and illness are inherently embodied, dynamic, and socially mediated (Fuchs, 2018). This recognition has created fertile ground for integrating artistic practices into health psychology, providing both theoretical and practical tools for understanding and supporting human health.

2.1 Historical Perspectives on Art in Health

The therapeutic use of art has a long and diverse history, spanning from ancient ritual practices to contemporary clinical applications. In early cultures, creative expression—through painting, music, or dance—was often intertwined with healing rituals, functioning as a medium for communal meaning-making, emotional expression, and spiritual wellbeing (Malchiodi, 2020). The formal development of art therapy in the 20th century marked a systematic approach to using artistic engagement as a psychological intervention. Pioneers such as Adrian Hill and Margaret Naumburg emphasized art as a means for self-expression and as a diagnostic tool to access unconscious processes (Malchiodi, 2020). Over the decades, expressive therapies expanded to include music, drama, and movement modalities, establishing a foundation for integrating art within psychological and medical care.

Despite the historical roots of artistic therapy, early approaches often prioritized the interpretive or diagnostic dimensions of art over its embodied, relational, and experiential qualities. In contemporary health psychology, theoretical frameworks increasingly acknowledge the importance of the body, social context, and affective processes in shaping health outcomes (Fuchs, 2018; Koch & Fuchs, 2011). This shift underscores the relevance of *embodied creativity* as both a theoretical and practical construct.

2.2 Embodied Cognition and Enactive Approaches

The concept of embodied cognition has become central to understanding human experience in health psychology. Embodied cognition posits that cognitive processes are deeply rooted in sensorimotor, affective, and bodily states, rather than existing solely as abstract, disembodied functions of the brain (Barsalou, 2008). According to this view, perception, thought, and action are inseparably intertwined, such that bodily engagement in the world shapes and informs cognitive and emotional experience.

Building on this framework, enactive approaches in cognitive science emphasize that cognition emerges through active engagement with the environment, rather than being a mere internal computation (Varela, Thompson, & Rosch, 1991). From an enactive perspective, knowledge and meaning are co-constructed through bodily interactions, social engagement, and sensory experience. This perspective aligns closely with health psychology's focus on adaptive behaviour and experiential learning, suggesting that creative practices—which involve bodily, emotional, and cognitive processes—can serve as vehicles for health-related insight, meaning-making, and behavioural change.

2.3 Creativity as an Embodied Phenomenon

Recent theoretical work positions creativity itself as an embodied process, arising from dynamic interactions among the brain, body, and environment (Koch & Fuchs, 2011; Halprin, 2003). Unlike traditional views that conceptualize creativity as a purely cognitive or intellectual endeavor, the embodied perspective highlights the role of sensorimotor activity, emotional attunement, and environmental engagement in generating novel ideas, forms, or experiences. Artistic practices such as dance, music, and painting exemplify this notion: in each modality, bodily action, sensory perception, and emotional resonance coalesce to produce meaningful creative expression (Koch et al., 2014). Embodied creativity provides a theoretical bridge between psychological processes and health outcomes. By engaging in creative practice, individuals enact and externalize internal states, which facilitates emotional regulation, narrative reconstruction, and the development of adaptive coping strategies. For example, movement-based practices such as dance therapy integrate proprioception, rhythm, and social attunement to foster stress reduction and enhance psychological resilience (Koch et al., 2014). Similarly, visual arts involve fine motor engagement, sensory perception, and symbolic representation, allowing individuals to translate complex affective experiences—such as anxiety or grief—into tangible forms (Kaimal et al., 2016). In each case, creativity is both a cognitive and embodied act, demonstrating how health psychology can benefit from integrating artistic modalities into research and practice.

2.4 Integrating Embodied Creativity into Health Psychology

Incorporating embodied creativity into health psychology entails a reconceptualization of both theory and intervention. Traditional models often emphasize cognition and behaviour as primary targets of change, whereas embodied creativity underscores the significance of somatic, affective, and relational dimensions. This integration aligns with the biopsychosocial model, expanding it to encompass artistic and symbolic processes as integral to wellbeing (Engel, 1977). It also provides a framework for understanding how art supports meaning-making, resilience, and adaptive behaviour.

By framing creativity as an embodied, enactive, and socially situated phenomenon, health psychology can better account for the complex, multi-dimensional nature of human health. Art becomes more than a therapeutic adjunct: it functions as a medium through which individuals enact coping strategies, reconstruct personal narratives, and cultivate resilience in the face of physical and psychological challenges. Moreover, this approach allows researchers and clinicians to explore mechanisms of change that extend beyond verbal or cognitive interventions, including sensorimotor engagement, affective processing, and social participation.

3. ART AS EMBODIED PRACTICE IN HEALTH PSYCHOLOGY

Art, in its many forms, offers a unique and holistic approach to understanding and promoting health. Unlike conventional cognitive or behavioural interventions, artistic engagement integrates affective, somatic, and symbolic dimensions, enabling individuals to process complex experiences, regulate emotions, and cultivate resilience (Stuckey & Nobel, 2010). By situating art within the framework of embodied creativity, health psychology recognizes that creative practice is not merely an intellectual exercise but a dynamic interplay between body, mind, and environment (Koch & Fuchs, 2011).

3.1 Mechanisms of Embodied Creativity

Embodied creativity operates through multiple, interrelated mechanisms that contribute to psychological and physiological well-being:

Artistic engagement contributes to psychological health through a multidimensional set of processes that integrate bodily, emotional, cognitive, social, and symbolic dimensions. Within health psychology, art is increasingly recognized as a mode of embodied creativity that fosters resilience, wellbeing, and adaptive coping. The following section examines five core mechanisms through which art contributes to psychological functioning.

Sensorimotor Engagement

Artistic practices involve the body in ways that foster awareness, regulation, and integration of internal states. When individuals engage in painting or sculpting, they activate fine motor skills, spatial perception, and tactile feedback, which together promote attentional focus and mindful presence (Kaimal et al., 2016). These activities require a synchronization of hand, eye, and sensory perception, supporting a state of flow that reduces stress and cultivates embodied awareness. Dance and movement therapies provide another form of sensorimotor engagement, integrating rhythm, gross motor activity, and proprioception. Research shows that dance movement therapy contributes to stress reduction, improved body image, and heightened bodily attunement, particularly among populations dealing with trauma or chronic illness (Koch et al., 2014). Sensorimotor involvement thus situates art as more than symbolic expression; it becomes a practice that grounds psychological healing in embodied processes.

Emotional Expression and Regulation

Creative practices also facilitate the externalization and modulation of emotion. Many individuals encounter difficulties verbalizing complex affective states such as grief, fear, or trauma. Art provides a safe, symbolic medium for these experiences to be expressed in constructive ways. For instance, the use of color, line, or shape can represent feelings otherwise inaccessible through language, offering both catharsis and insight (Malchiodi, 2020). Regulation occurs as participants explore different intensities of expression, experimenting with materials or movements that gradually transform emotional states. In music and dance, synchronization with rhythm creates opportunities for attunement and self-regulation. By modulating expressive intensity, individuals develop strategies for managing affect, thereby reinforcing psychological resilience.

Cognitive and Reflective Processing

Art also contributes to reflective and metacognitive processes. Creative expression invites participants to consider not only the product but also the process of art-making. Through journaling, storytelling, or narrative art, individuals reconstruct experiences, reframing them within broader life narratives. This process supports cognitive flexibility and adaptive coping strategies. Puig, Lee, Goodwin, and Sherrard (2006) found that narrative and visual art interventions enable individuals to reframe traumatic experiences, increasing their sense of agency and coherence. Reflection on the meaning of creative choices—such as color selection or symbolic imagery—enhances self-awareness and supports identity development. In this sense, artistic engagement becomes both a reflective practice and a form of narrative restructuring, aligning closely with therapeutic models in health psychology.

Social and Relational Dynamics

Art is rarely an isolated activity; many modalities unfold in participatory or group-based contexts. Shared artistic practices foster collaboration, empathy, and social connectedness. In group art therapy, for example, participants co-create works that symbolize collective identity, reducing feelings of isolation and cultivating a sense of belonging (Camic, 2010). Collaborative creativity fosters trust, encourages dialogue, and enables individuals to recognize themselves within a larger social fabric. These relational dynamics have direct implications for health, as social support and connectedness are consistently linked to improved wellbeing and recovery. By embedding individuals within creative communities, art strengthens both interpersonal bonds and collective resilience.

Symbolic Meaning-Making

Finally, art provides a symbolic framework through which individuals interpret and communicate lived experience. Symbols, metaphors, and narratives within artistic expression allow existential concerns to be externalized and reinterpreted. For instance, Frankl (1963) emphasized the human capacity to find meaning even under extreme adversity; in creative work, metaphors and images serve as vehicles for constructing coherence and continuity. Art enables identity reconstruction when illness or trauma disrupts prior self-concepts, offering new ways of articulating personal narratives. Meaning-making is particularly critical in health contexts, where uncertainty, vulnerability, and mortality often challenge established frameworks of understanding. Artistic expression, by engaging symbolic dimensions, provides a language through which individuals can navigate these existential terrains.

Across sensorimotor, emotional, cognitive, social, and symbolic dimensions, artistic engagement functions as an integrative practice that addresses multiple levels of human experience. In health psychology, these mechanisms illuminate how art contributes to wellbeing by fostering embodied regulation, emotional resilience, reflective processing, social connection, and existential meaning-making. Recognizing art as a multidimensional resource expands therapeutic possibilities, situating creativity at the heart of holistic health interventions.

3.2 Dance and Movement Therapy

Dance and movement therapy (DMT) represents a compelling example of embodied creativity, integrating physical activity, emotional expression, and social attunement within therapeutic contexts. By engaging the body as a medium of expression, DMT allows participants to explore affective states, process experiences, and cultivate agency through movement. In clinical settings, DMT has demonstrated measurable benefits, including reductions in stress, improvements in mood, and enhanced social engagement across diverse populations, such as trauma survivors, older adults, and individuals managing chronic illnesses (Koch et al., 2014). These outcomes reflect the holistic nature of dance as both a somatic and symbolic practice. At the core of DMT is the engagement with rhythm, posture, and gesture, which transforms the body into an instrument of expression. Participants learn to articulate internal experiences through movement, externalizing emotions that may be difficult to verbalize. The process of moving in synchrony with music or guided exercises facilitates self-regulation, allowing individuals to modulate intensity, pace, and spatial dynamics to reflect their internal states. By embodying emotions physically, participants gain insight into their affective experiences and develop strategies for coping with stress or trauma. This interplay between movement and emotion exemplifies the concept of embodied creativity, in which cognition, affect, and somatic awareness converge. Group-based movement therapy adds an essential social dimension. Mirroring exercises, synchronous patterns, and collaborative choreography foster empathy and attunement, creating a safe communal space for emotional processing and relational exploration. These shared experiences encourage participants to perceive and respond to others' emotional cues, strengthening interpersonal bonds and reducing feelings of isolation. In turn, the social connectivity established within DMT sessions contributes to overall psychological resilience, promoting a sense of belonging and collective support. Furthermore, the reflective aspect of DMT enhances metacognitive awareness. Participants often engage in post-session reflection, discussing their experiences and insights gained through movement. This process reinforces self-awareness, identity exploration, and problem-solving, providing opportunities to integrate embodied experiences into broader life contexts. By bridging body, emotion, and cognition, dance and movement therapy exemplifies a multidimensional intervention that supports psychological well-being. In conclusion, DMT embodies creativity in its fullest sense: it engages the body as a medium for emotional expression, nurtures social connectedness through shared movement, and facilitates cognitive and reflective processing. Through these intertwined mechanisms, participants develop enhanced coping skills, heightened body awareness, and greater resilience, illustrating the profound potential of embodied artistic practices in promoting mental health and holistic well-being.

3.3 Visual Arts

Visual arts, encompassing painting, drawing, sculpture, and mixed media, provide tangible forms through which individuals can externalize internal states. The act of creating art engages fine motor skills, visual-spatial processing, and sensory perception, producing an immersive, embodied experience (Kaimal et al., 2016). Clinical studies demonstrate that visual art interventions can alleviate anxiety, reduce depressive symptoms, and enhance quality of life in patients with chronic illnesses, including cancer and cardiovascular conditions (Czamanski-Cohen & Weihs, 2023). By externalizing complex emotions, participants gain perspective on their experiences, facilitating narrative reconstruction and adaptive coping. Visual art also allows for experimentation and transformation, enabling individuals to actively shape and modify symbolic representations of their experiences, fostering a sense of agency and empowerment.

3.4 Music and Sound-Based Interventions

Music, rhythm, and sound constitute a powerful form of embodied creativity, engaging multiple systems simultaneously to promote psychological and physiological wellbeing. Music therapy integrates auditory perception, motor coordination, and emotional processing, creating a holistic experience that fosters emotional regulation, relaxation, and social connectedness (Bradt & Dileo, 2014). By participating in music-making—whether through singing, playing instruments, or rhythmic movement—individuals activate neural networks associated with reward, attention, and memory, supporting both cognitive and affective functioning (Koelsch, 2014). This multisensory engagement exemplifies how art can function as a vehicle for embodied therapeutic intervention. The benefits of music therapy extend across diverse clinical populations. For patients experiencing pain, anxiety, or depression, music offers an accessible and flexible form of expression and engagement. Rhythmic elements provide predictable structures that can reduce arousal and induce relaxation, while melodic and harmonic patterns evoke emotional responses that facilitate catharsis and affect regulation. Active participation—such as improvisation or collaborative music-making—empowers individuals to express complex emotions safely and nonverbally. These processes enhance self-awareness and foster a sense of agency, allowing participants to experience mastery and control within therapeutic contexts. Group-based music interventions add an important social dimension, promoting cohesion, empathy, and shared meaning. Ensemble playing, choral singing, or percussive exercises create opportunities for synchronous interaction, which strengthens interpersonal attunement and mutual support. Such shared musical experiences contribute to collective resilience, particularly in populations facing social isolation, chronic illness, or psychological trauma. Participants often report increased feelings of belonging, motivation, and emotional connectedness, highlighting music's role as both an individual and communal resource.

In addition, music therapy supports cognitive and reflective processes. Engaging with musical structure—such as rhythm, dynamics, and improvisation—encourages attention, pattern recognition, and problem-solving. Reflection on musical experiences further reinforces insight into personal emotions, coping strategies, and relational dynamics. In this sense, music functions as a multidimensional medium, bridging body, mind, and social context.

In conclusion, music therapy exemplifies embodied creativity by simultaneously activating sensory, motor, emotional, and cognitive processes. Through active participation and shared engagement, music facilitates emotional regulation, social connection, and cognitive processing, while promoting resilience and wellbeing. By integrating auditory and movement-based experiences, music therapy demonstrates the capacity of art to support holistic mental health interventions, emphasizing the interconnectedness of body, mind, and community in the pursuit of psychological flourishing.

3.5 Writing and Narrative Practices

Expressive writing and narrative-based interventions constitute a symbolic, cognitive, and embodied approach to health promotion. By translating internal experiences into written form, individuals engage both cognitive and emotional processes while grounding reflection in the embodied act of writing. This modality allows participants to organize thoughts, clarify emotions, and reconstruct personal narratives in ways that enhance coherence and meaning, particularly when addressing traumatic, stressful, or emotionally charged experiences (Pennebaker & Seagal,

1999). The physical act of writing—whether by hand or digitally—also engages fine motor coordination, rhythm, and attentional focus, linking cognitive reflection with sensorimotor processes, a feature that aligns with embodied theories of creativity.

Research demonstrates that structured expressive writing can produce measurable health benefits. Frattaroli (2006) reviewed studies indicating that individuals who engage in regular writing about their experiences show reductions in physiological stress markers, improved immune system functioning, and enhanced psychological well-being. These outcomes suggest that writing is not merely a reflective or symbolic act, but also a behavior with tangible effects on body systems. The process of externalizing thoughts and emotions enables cognitive reappraisal and emotional regulation, providing participants with tools to manage distress and navigate complex emotional states. In addition to physiological benefits, expressive writing fosters metacognitive and narrative processing. Participants develop insight into their own experiences by reflecting on thematic patterns, emotional responses, and personal values. Such reflection supports adaptive coping strategies and facilitates identity negotiation, allowing individuals to reconcile past adversity with present strengths and future goals. Narrative interventions help construct coherent life stories, giving shape to otherwise fragmented or overwhelming experiences. In therapeutic settings, these practices have been applied to diverse populations, including individuals coping with trauma, chronic illness, or significant life transitions, demonstrating broad applicability and effectiveness.

In conclusion, expressive writing and narrative interventions exemplify a multidimensional approach to health that integrates cognitive, emotional, and embodied processes. By facilitating organization, reflection, and meaning-making, these practices support adaptive coping, promote psychological resilience, and yield measurable benefits for both mental and physical health. Writing, therefore, functions as a potent, accessible tool for holistic health promotion, bridging personal experience, reflective insight, and embodied engagement.

3.6 Integration of Modalities and Multisensory Approaches

Contemporary health interventions increasingly adopt multimodal approaches that integrate visual art, movement, music, and expressive writing to optimize embodied engagement and therapeutic outcomes. By combining multiple modalities, these programs engage participants across cognitive, emotional, and somatic domains, providing a richer, more holistic experience than single-modality interventions alone. For instance, art therapy programs may incorporate movement-based warm-ups, guided visual art tasks, and reflective writing exercises within a single session, allowing participants to explore feelings, narratives, and bodily states simultaneously (Malchiodi, 2020). The integration of multiple sensory and expressive channels fosters a dynamic interaction among mind, body, and environment, enhancing the depth and sustainability of therapeutic benefits.

Multimodal interventions align with the principle of embodied creativity, which posits that health-promoting processes are most effective when cognitive, emotional, somatic, and social dimensions are engaged in concert. Through visual art, participants can externalize internal experiences and explore symbolic meaning; through movement, they cultivate bodily awareness and emotion regulation; through music, they engage auditory, rhythmic, and social systems; and through writing, they integrate reflective and narrative processing. This synergistic engagement supports adaptive coping, emotional resilience, and cognitive flexibility, while also promoting a sense of agency and personal mastery. Group-based multimodal programs additionally foster social connection and relational learning. Collaborative creative activities encourage participants to synchronize movements, share artistic insights, and provide supportive feedback, which strengthens empathy, trust, and collective resilience. These social processes are critical for health outcomes, as social connectedness and perceived support are strongly associated with psychological and physical wellbeing. By embedding interventions within communal and participatory contexts, multimodal programs create opportunities for both individual and collective growth.

Research suggests that multimodal approaches can be particularly beneficial for populations experiencing trauma, chronic illness, or psychological distress. The combination of sensory, emotional, cognitive, and social engagement allows for multiple entry points into healing, accommodating diverse needs, preferences, and abilities. Participants can choose the modality that resonates most strongly with them while benefiting from the integrated, supportive structure of the program. Multimodal interventions exemplify embodied creativity in practice. By engaging multiple expressive and reflective channels simultaneously, these programs foster resilience, adaptive coping, and meaningful engagement with health-related challenges. The dynamic integration of mind, body, and environment underscores the potential of multimodal approaches as comprehensive tools for promoting holistic wellbeing.

4. MEANING-MAKING THROUGH ARTISTIC ENGAGEMENT

Meaning-making is a central concept in health psychology, particularly in contexts of illness, trauma, and life transitions. Individuals facing health challenges often experience disruption in their sense of self, purpose, and coherence, leading to emotional distress and maladaptive coping (Park, 2010). Artistic engagement provides a symbolic and embodied medium through which people can navigate these challenges, articulate otherwise inexpressible experiences, and reconstruct personal narratives. By integrating cognitive, affective, and somatic dimensions, art allows individuals to create coherence, continuity, and agency in their lives.

4.1 The Role of Symbolism in Artistic Expression

Art functions as a symbolic language that conveys complex psychological and existential experiences. Unlike verbal communication, which is constrained by linguistic structures, artistic expression can capture nuances of emotion, bodily sensation, and subjective meaning (Stuckey & Nobel, 2010). Symbols in art—whether colors, shapes, movements, or musical motifs—serve as proxies for inner states, enabling participants to externalize feelings such as fear, grief, or hope. This symbolic process fosters self-reflection, emotional insight, and cognitive integration, supporting adaptive coping and resilience.

For example, a patient undergoing cancer treatment might use abstract painting to represent feelings of vulnerability or uncertainty. The choice of color, texture, and form reflects both conscious and unconscious experiences, allowing for a visual dialogue between inner states and external expression. By engaging with these symbolic forms, the individual gains perspective on their emotions, facilitating emotional regulation and the reconstruction of a coherent narrative (Kaimal et al., 2016).

4.2 Narrative Reconstruction and Identity Negotiation

Narrative approaches in health psychology emphasize the role of personal storytelling in maintaining psychological well-being. Illness and trauma often disrupt an individual's life narrative, creating discontinuity between past, present, and anticipated future (Frank & Frank, 1991). Artistic practices, particularly expressive writing, visual art, and performance, provide tools for narrative reconstruction, allowing individuals to integrate challenging experiences into their broader life story (Puig et al., 2006).

Through art, individuals can explore multiple perspectives, reframe experiences, and assert agency over their narratives. For instance, trauma survivors may use movement therapy to enact symbolic representations of power and autonomy, gradually restoring a sense of self-efficacy and control. Similarly, expressive writing allows individuals to organize fragmented experiences, articulate emotions, and identify patterns of resilience, facilitating identity reconstruction and meaning-making (Pennebaker & Seagal, 1999).

4.3 Existential and Philosophical Dimensions

Art also engages existential processes central to human experience, such as the search for meaning, purpose, and coherence. Viktor Frankl's logotherapy emphasizes that humans can find meaning even under extreme adversity, suggesting that purpose and value are critical determinants of psychological resilience (Frankl, 1963). In health psychology, art functions as a practical extension of this insight, offering embodied and symbolic avenues for exploring existential concerns.

Through artistic engagement, individuals confront the realities of illness, mortality, and vulnerability, while simultaneously expressing hope, agency, and creative potential. For example, patients with chronic or life-threatening conditions may use collaborative art projects to express collective narratives of survival, thereby cultivating both personal and communal meaning. Artistic practices thus bridge suffering and resilience, providing frameworks for individuals to negotiate existential uncertainty, integrate emotional experiences, and reaffirm a sense of purpose.

4.4 Therapeutic and Behavioural Implications

Meaning-making through art has tangible implications for psychological and behavioural outcomes. Engaging in creative expression fosters emotional regulation, self-efficacy, and adaptive coping strategies, all of which are associated with improved health outcomes (Forgeard & Elstein, 2014). For instance, individuals who participate in structured art therapy or community-based creative programs report reduced stress, enhanced mood, and increased adherence to medical regimens (Camic, 2010).

Moreover, the skills and insights gained through artistic meaning-making can generalize to other domains of life. By witnessing their capacity to create, transform, and interpret complex experiences, participants develop confidence and agency that extend beyond artistic contexts. This generalization may manifest in proactive health behaviours, such as maintaining treatment adherence, engaging in physical activity, or seeking social support. In this sense, art functions as both a reflective and active medium for behaviour change, complementing traditional cognitive-behavioural and health psychology interventions.

4.5 Collective Meaning and Socially Situated Art

Beyond individual processes, artistic engagement supports collective meaning-making, particularly in community and group settings. Participatory arts programs—such as community murals, collaborative music projects, and group dance—create shared experiences of expression, dialogue, and social cohesion (Clift & Camic, 2016).

Collective art-making enables communities to process shared challenges, negotiate collective identities, and cultivate resilience in the face of social or health crises.

For example, community-based art initiatives for populations affected by trauma or chronic illness provide opportunities for storytelling, cultural expression, and mutual support. These programs not only facilitate individual meaning-making but also reinforce social networks, reduce isolation, and foster a sense of collective efficacy. By bridging individual and communal experiences, art acts as a conduit for integrated psychological and social wellbeing. Artistic engagement in health psychology serves as a multifaceted medium for meaning-making. Through symbolic expression, narrative reconstruction, and existential exploration, individuals can process complex experiences, reconstruct identity, and develop adaptive coping strategies. Moreover, the social dimensions of art amplify these benefits by fostering collective meaning, social cohesion, and communal resilience. Integrating art as a tool for meaning-making underscores the holistic, embodied, and socially situated nature of human health, expanding the theoretical and practical scope of health psychology.

5. BEHAVIOURAL AND HEALTH OUTCOMES

Artistic engagement functions not only as a reflective practice but also as an active behavioural intervention that can influence health outcomes directly. Within health psychology, behavioural outcomes encompass both observable actions—such as adherence to treatment regimens or engagement in healthy behaviours—and internalized capacities, such as self-efficacy, problem-solving, and adaptive coping (Bandura, 1997). By integrating art-based interventions into clinical and community settings, individuals are provided with tools to enact behavioural change while simultaneously fostering psychological resilience and wellbeing.

5.1 Art as an Active Coping Strategy

Engaging in artistic practices constitutes an active coping mechanism that allows individuals to manage stress, regulate emotions, and process challenging experiences. Active coping strategies are associated with better psychological outcomes compared to avoidant or passive approaches (Folkman & Moskowitz, 2004). Creative engagement, whether through visual arts, music, dance, or writing, enables individuals to confront emotional distress, experiment with problem-solving strategies, and gain a sense of agency over their experiences.

For instance, studies on art therapy with patients undergoing chronic illness treatment indicate that regular participation in creative activities reduces anxiety, enhances mood, and promotes adherence to medical protocols (Geue et al., 2010). Similarly, dance therapy has been linked to improved emotional regulation and stress reduction, supporting the adoption of healthier behavioural patterns, such as increased physical activity and social engagement (Koch et al., 2014).

5.2 Self-Efficacy and Mastery Through Creative Practice

Self-efficacy—the belief in one's ability to achieve desired outcomes—is a central construct in health psychology, influencing both motivation and behaviour (Bandura, 1997). Artistic engagement inherently fosters self-efficacy by providing opportunities for mastery, experimentation, and creative problem-solving. Individuals who observe their capacity to generate meaningful creations develop confidence in their ability to manage challenges beyond the artistic context.

For example, a patient participating in a structured painting program may experience increased confidence in expressing emotions, translating this skill to improved communication with healthcare providers or adherence to treatment routines. Research indicates that improvements in self-efficacy through creative engagement are associated with better health behaviours, including exercise adherence, dietary management, and proactive healthcare utilization (Creswell et al., 2015).

5.3 Enhancing Health Behaviours and Lifestyle Choices

Creative engagement supports the adoption of adaptive health behaviours by integrating affective, cognitive, and motivational processes. Participatory art programs have been shown to enhance physical activity, social participation, and lifestyle management among diverse populations, including older adults, individuals with chronic conditions, and mental health patients (Camic et al., 2014). These outcomes suggest that art-based interventions can function as a behavioural activation strategy, promoting engagement with health-promoting routines while simultaneously addressing psychological needs.

In particular, community-based interventions demonstrate that artistic involvement fosters social accountability and peer support, reinforcing sustained behavioural change. For example, group music or dance programs encourage regular attendance, coordination, and adherence to structured activities, which can generalize to other domains such as rehabilitation exercises or medical appointments (Clift & Morrison, 2011).

5.4 Physiological and Health-Related Outcomes

Beyond psychological and behavioural effects, artistic engagement has measurable impacts on physiological health outcomes. Evidence suggests that creative practices can modulate stress-related biomarkers, immune function, and cardiovascular health. Studies on art-making and music therapy show reductions in cortisol levels, blood pressure, and heart rate, indicating tangible stress reduction (Kaimal et al., 2016; Chanda & Levitin, 2013). Similarly, engagement in expressive writing has been linked to improved immune response and faster recovery from medical procedures (Smyth, 1998).

These findings support the notion that artistic engagement produces biopsychosocial benefits, aligning with health psychology's emphasis on the interplay between psychological processes, behaviour, and physiological outcomes. By influencing both subjective experiences and measurable health markers, art-based interventions demonstrate comprehensive potential for enhancing wellbeing.

5.5 Integrating Art Into Behavioural Health Interventions

Incorporating artistic engagement into health psychology interventions provides a versatile tool for promoting behavioural change and improving health outcomes. Art-based interventions can complement cognitive-behavioural therapy, motivational interviewing, and other evidence-based approaches, enriching treatment protocols by addressing affective, symbolic, and embodied dimensions (Slayton et al., 2010). For example, combining art therapy with health education programs for chronic illness management enhances participant engagement, adherence to lifestyle modifications, and emotional coping.

Furthermore, technological advances—including digital art platforms, virtual reality, and online music programs—expand the accessibility and scalability of art-based interventions. These innovations allow for individualized and group-based engagement, fostering behaviour change in both clinical and community contexts. Artistic engagement serves as an active mechanism for behavioural and health outcomes by promoting adaptive coping, self-efficacy, health behaviours, and physiological wellbeing. Through mastery, symbolic expression, and social participation, creative practices enable individuals to enact meaningful change in their lives, translating psychological growth into tangible health benefits. Integrating art into health psychology interventions bridges the gap between emotional experience and behaviour, providing a holistic approach to health promotion that aligns cognitive, affective, and somatic processes.

6. RESILIENCE AND SOCIAL DIMENSIONS

Resilience—the capacity to adapt, recover, and thrive despite adversity—is a central construct in health psychology. It encompasses emotional, cognitive, behavioural, and social processes that enable individuals to navigate stressors and maintain wellbeing (Masten, 2014). Artistic engagement offers a unique avenue for cultivating resilience, both at the individual and collective levels, by integrating embodied, affective, cognitive, and social experiences. This section explores how art functions as a tool for building resilience, highlighting its role in personal empowerment, emotional regulation, social cohesion, and community wellbeing.

6.1 Individual Resilience Through Embodied Creativity

Engaging in art fosters individual resilience by providing structured opportunities for self-expression, mastery, and adaptive coping. Embodied creativity allows participants to externalize complex emotions, confront difficult experiences, and reframe challenges in ways that enhance psychological flexibility and problem-solving abilities (Forgeard & Elstein, 2014).

For example, dance and movement therapy enable individuals to enact narratives of empowerment, control, or transformation, helping them regain a sense of agency after trauma or illness (Koch et al., 2014). Similarly, visual art interventions allow participants to manipulate materials and forms in ways that symbolize personal growth, change, or resilience, promoting a sense of accomplishment and self-efficacy (Kaimal et al., 2016). Through these embodied processes, art reinforces the capacity to tolerate uncertainty, manage stress, and engage adaptively with health-related challenges.

6.2 Emotional Regulation and Coping

Artistic practices enhance resilience by supporting emotional regulation, a key mechanism for adaptive coping. Creative engagement allows individuals to process intense affective experiences, modulate arousal, and gain insight into emotional states (Stuckey & Nobel, 2010). Music, for example, engages auditory, motor, and affective systems simultaneously, reducing stress and promoting mood stabilization (Bradt & Dileo, 2014). Expressive writing similarly provides a structured outlet for emotional exploration, enabling individuals to organize and reinterpret traumatic or stressful experiences (Pennebaker & Seagal, 1999).

By facilitating emotional processing in a safe and controlled context, artistic engagement reduces vulnerability to maladaptive coping strategies such as avoidance, rumination, or substance use. This capacity for emotional regulation strengthens resilience and equips individuals with tools to navigate ongoing or future stressors.

6.3 Social Dimensions of Resilience

Resilience is not solely an individual trait; it is also socially constructed and relationally mediated. Participatory art programs provide shared spaces for collaborative creation, dialogue, and mutual support, fostering social connectedness and collective coping. Group-based artistic activities, such as choir singing, collaborative murals, or community theater, promote interpersonal attunement, empathy, and trust, strengthening networks that buffer against psychological distress.

Socially mediated resilience extends to health outcomes by enhancing adherence to behavioural interventions, encouraging communal problem-solving, and providing social reinforcement for adaptive behaviours. For example, older adults participating in group art programs demonstrate improved social engagement, reduced loneliness, and greater motivation to maintain healthy routines (Camic et al., 2014). By linking individual creative expression with collective support, art facilitates resilience across multiple levels of experience.

6.4 Community and Cultural Resilience

Artistic engagement contributes to community resilience by enabling shared meaning-making, cultural expression, and collective coping in response to social or health crises. Community arts initiatives allow groups to articulate collective experiences, process grief or trauma, and celebrate shared identities, fostering a sense of cohesion and collective efficacy (Clift & Morrison, 2011).

For example, participatory arts programs following natural disasters or public health crises have demonstrated the capacity to support communal recovery, reduce stigma, and strengthen social networks. By embedding resilience in cultural and social frameworks, these initiatives illustrate the systemic benefits of artistic engagement beyond individual outcomes.

6.5 Integrating Resilience Into Health Psychology Practice

Health psychology interventions can harness artistic engagement to promote resilience at individual, group, and community levels. Integrative programs that combine embodied creativity with cognitive-behavioural techniques, mindfulness, or social skills training offer a multidimensional approach to fostering adaptive capacities. Clinicians and researchers are encouraged to design interventions that balance personal expression with collaborative participation, optimizing both psychological and social resilience.

Furthermore, resilience-oriented art programs align with preventive and public health goals. By promoting proactive coping, emotional flexibility, and social cohesion, art-based interventions can reduce vulnerability to stress-related disorders, improve quality of life, and strengthen community health outcomes. Artistic engagement serves as a powerful vehicle for cultivating resilience in health psychology. Through embodied creativity, emotional regulation, social participation, and community-based initiatives, art supports the development of adaptive capacities across individual and collective domains. By integrating resilience-focused artistic practices into clinical, educational, and community settings, health psychologists can enhance coping, wellbeing, and social cohesion, demonstrating the holistic potential of art in fostering psychological and behavioural health.

7. CLINICAL AND COMMUNITY APPLICATIONS

Integrating art into health psychology requires practical frameworks that translate theoretical insights into clinical and community-based interventions. Artistic engagement offers versatile applications across diverse populations and health contexts, from individual therapy to community resilience programs. This section examines how embodied creativity can be systematically incorporated into health psychology practice, highlighting program design, intervention strategies, and evidence-based outcomes.

7.1 Clinical Applications

Art-based interventions in clinical settings provide complementary tools for enhancing traditional therapeutic approaches, including cognitive-behavioural therapy (CBT), psychodynamic therapy, and psychoeducation. By engaging patients at sensory, affective, cognitive, and symbolic levels, art facilitates holistic healing processes that address both psychological and somatic dimensions of health.

7.1.1 Art Therapy in Mental Health

Art therapy is widely employed in mental health care to support emotional expression, trauma processing, and coping skill development. Visual arts, music, and movement therapies allow patients to externalize internal states, providing a non-verbal medium for processing experiences that may be difficult to articulate (Malchiodi, 2020). For example, trauma survivors participating in art therapy programs have demonstrated reductions in anxiety, depression, and post-traumatic stress symptoms, along with enhanced self-efficacy and resilience (Haeyen, van Hooren, van der Veld, & Hutschemaekers, 2015).

7.1.2 Enhancing Health Behaviour Change

Art can also be integrated with behavioural health interventions to promote treatment adherence, lifestyle modification, and self-management of chronic illness. For instance, combining expressive writing with educational programs for patients with diabetes or cardiovascular disease enhances engagement with dietary and exercise regimens, reinforcing the motivational and cognitive aspects of behaviour change (Creswell et al., 2015). Similarly, dance therapy interventions for older adults or patients with mobility limitations encourage physical activity while simultaneously addressing social and emotional wellbeing (Koch et al., 2014).

7.1.3 Multimodal Integrative Interventions

Clinical programs increasingly employ multimodal approaches that combine visual arts, music, dance, and narrative practices. These integrative interventions engage multiple sensory, cognitive, and emotional pathways, maximizing therapeutic impact. For example, a cancer support program may incorporate group painting, guided movement, and reflective journaling, fostering emotional regulation, identity reconstruction, and resilience simultaneously (Puig et al., 2006).

7.2 Community-Based Applications

Beyond individual therapy, artistic engagement functions as a vehicle for public health promotion, social cohesion, and community resilience. Community-based art programs can address health disparities, promote mental wellbeing, and cultivate collective empowerment.

7.2.1 Participatory Arts Programs

Participatory arts programs invite individuals to contribute creatively to shared projects, such as community murals, theater productions, music ensembles, or collaborative dance. These initiatives facilitate social connection, shared meaning-making, and collective coping, particularly in populations affected by trauma, chronic illness, or social marginalization.

For example, community choirs for older adults have been associated with improved mental health, reduced isolation, and strengthened social networks, illustrating how collective artistic engagement can reinforce individual and communal resilience (Clift & Morrison, 2011). Similarly, community mural projects in underserved neighborhoods provide platforms for self-expression, cultural representation, and advocacy, fostering empowerment and social cohesion.

7.2.2 Public Health and Preventive Strategies

Art-based programs can serve preventive and health-promoting functions by encouraging lifestyle changes, stress management, and social support. Integrating creative engagement into schools, workplaces, and community centers promotes wellbeing before clinical intervention becomes necessary. For instance, music and movement programs in schools have been shown to reduce stress, enhance social-emotional skills, and improve academic engagement (Hallam, 2010). These preventive strategies highlight the scalability of art-based interventions in public health frameworks.

7.3 Program Design and Implementation

Effective integration of art into health psychology requires careful program design that attends to the specific needs of participants, the chosen modalities, session frequency, setting, and evaluation strategies. Thoughtful planning ensures that artistic interventions are not only engaging but also therapeutically meaningful, supporting cognitive, emotional, social, and physiological outcomes. Several key principles guide the design and implementation of effective art-based programs.

Programs should be carefully adapted to the psychological, physical, and social characteristics of the target population. Selecting artistic modalities that align with therapeutic goals is critical. For example, movement-based interventions may be particularly effective for individuals seeking to enhance body awareness and reduce stress, whereas narrative or expressive writing may better support trauma processing and identity reconstruction. Tailoring interventions to participant needs maximizes engagement, relevance, and therapeutic impact, allowing art to serve as a flexible and responsive tool within health psychology.

Ensuring accessibility for diverse populations is a fundamental principle. Programs should accommodate individuals with varying abilities, cultural backgrounds, and resource availability. This may involve providing adaptive materials, offering multiple modalities, or designing sessions that can be delivered in community or clinical settings with limited infrastructure. Inclusive design not only promotes equity and participation but also reinforces the social and relational benefits of creative engagement, supporting broader public health goals.

Art interventions are most effective when integrated with established therapeutic models. Creative activities can complement cognitive-behavioral, psychodynamic, or mindfulness-based approaches, reinforcing desired behavioural, emotional, and cognitive outcomes. By aligning artistic engagement with evidence-based frameworks, practitioners ensure that interventions are grounded in validated principles while also harnessing the unique strengths of embodied creativity.

Systematic evaluation is essential for assessing program effectiveness and guiding continuous improvement. Both qualitative and quantitative methods can be employed to measure psychological, behavioural, and physiological outcomes. For instance, self-report measures, observational checklists, and biometric indicators can provide comprehensive insights into participants' experiences and progress. Regular assessment enables practitioners to refine program design, optimize modality selection, and document the therapeutic value of art-based interventions.

The successful integration of art into health psychology relies on programs that are tailored, inclusive, evidence-informed, and systematically evaluated. Adhering to these principles ensures that artistic interventions promote holistic wellbeing, foster adaptive coping, and provide meaningful engagement across cognitive, emotional, and somatic dimensions. Thoughtful design and rigorous assessment allow art to function as a powerful complement to traditional therapeutic approaches, enriching both individual and collective health outcomes.

7.4 Technology-Enhanced Artistic Interventions

Digital platforms, virtual reality, and online collaborative tools extend the reach and adaptability of art-based interventions. Virtual art therapy, online music ensembles, and digital storytelling platforms enable participation across geographical and physical barriers, promoting accessibility and continuity of care (Fancourt et al., 2019). Technology-enhanced interventions also allow for personalized feedback, interactive engagement, and real-time monitoring of outcomes, expanding the scope and impact of art in health psychology. Clinical and community applications of artistic engagement demonstrate the versatility and efficacy of embodied creativity as a health psychology tool. At the individual level, art facilitates emotional expression, coping, self-efficacy, and behavioural change. At the community level, participatory art promotes social cohesion, collective resilience, and public health. Thoughtful program design, integration with evidence-based practice, and the use of technology enhance accessibility, scalability, and measurable outcomes. By bridging individual and collective health processes, artistic engagement embodies a holistic and multidimensional approach to psychological and behavioural wellbeing.

8. FUTURE DIRECTIONS AND RESEARCH IMPLICATIONS

As health psychology continues to evolve, the integration of art-based interventions offers promising avenues for both theoretical advancement and practical application. While existing research supports the benefits of artistic engagement for emotional, behavioural, and social outcomes, several areas warrant further exploration to optimize efficacy, accessibility, and understanding of underlying mechanisms. This section outlines key directions for future research, methodological considerations, and emerging trends in the field.

8.1 Mechanisms of Action

A primary research priority in the integration of art within health psychology is to elucidate the mechanisms through which creative engagement influences psychological and health outcomes. While empirical evidence consistently demonstrates that art-based interventions can reduce stress, enhance resilience, and improve behavioral adherence, the pathways linking artistic practice to these outcomes remain incompletely understood. Addressing these gaps is essential for advancing theory, refining interventions, and maximizing the therapeutic potential of art across diverse populations. Future research should focus on three interrelated domains: neurobiological mechanisms, psychological and cognitive processes, and embodied somatic pathways. Art engagement activates multisensory, motor, and affective neural networks, suggesting that neuroplasticity may underlie observed improvements in emotion regulation, stress management, and adaptive coping (Chanda & Levitin, 2013). Neuroimaging studies have begun to reveal that participation in music, visual arts, and dance stimulates brain regions associated with reward, attention, executive function, and interoceptive awareness. However, further research is needed to delineate the modality-specific effects of artistic engagement on neural circuitry and to determine how these changes correlate with behavioral and emotional outcomes. Longitudinal studies, combining neuroimaging with physiological measures such as heart rate variability and cortisol levels, could clarify the temporal dynamics of neural adaptation and provide insight into the mechanisms through which art fosters psychological resilience and health-promoting behaviors. Art-based interventions may influence multiple psychological constructs that mediate health outcomes. Creative engagement has been shown to enhance self-efficacy, promote problem-solving, increase cognitive flexibility, and facilitate narrative integration (Bandura, 1997; Pennebaker & Seagal, 1999). These cognitive and metacognitive processes enable individuals to restructure experiences, manage stress, and engage adaptively with health-related challenges. Yet, causal pathways remain underexplored. Longitudinal and experimental designs are necessary to determine which psychological constructs are most salient in mediating the benefits of artistic practice. Investigating the interplay between emotion, cognition, and self-perception may reveal how art strengthens coping strategies, supports identity development, and fosters sustained behavioral change. Embodied creativity emphasizes the dynamic interaction between body, cognition, and affect, highlighting the importance of somatic engagement in therapeutic processes (Fuchs, 2018). Movement-based art forms such as dance, rhythmic improvisation, and tactile visual art involve sensorimotor integration, proprioception, and kinesthetic awareness, which can contribute to emotional processing, regulation, and resilience. Future studies should examine how somatic experiences influence psychological outcomes, including stress reduction, adaptive coping, and behavioral adherence. Research integrating motion capture, physiological monitoring, and qualitative analysis could elucidate how bodily engagement amplifies the cognitive and emotional benefits of creative practice, offering a more comprehensive understanding of the embodied mechanisms underlying art-based interventions. Advancing knowledge in these three domains—neurobiological, psychological, and embodied—will enhance the theoretical foundation of health psychology and guide the development of more precise, effective, and personalized interventions. By clarifying the mechanisms through which art affects the mind, body, and behavior, future research can optimize therapeutic applications, support evidence-based program design, and strengthen the integration of creative modalities into clinical and community health contexts. A comprehensive, mechanistic understanding of art's impact will ultimately empower practitioners to leverage creativity as a multidimensional tool for fostering resilience, wellbeing, and adaptive health behaviors across populations.

8.2 Intervention Design and Standardization

While the diversity of artistic modalities represents a significant strength, it also introduces challenges related to intervention standardization, replication, and scalability. One key area for future research involves the development of structured and replicable intervention protocols that can be implemented across clinical and community settings. Such protocols must balance consistency with flexibility, allowing for individualized adaptations that account for participants' psychological, cultural, and physical needs. Standardized yet adaptable frameworks would facilitate rigorous evaluation, enhance reproducibility, and support broader dissemination of art-based practices. Another critical consideration is understanding dose-response relationships in artistic engagement. Research is needed to determine the optimal frequency, duration, and intensity of participation required to achieve meaningful psychological and health outcomes. Clarifying these parameters would guide clinicians and program designers in structuring interventions that maximize benefits while remaining feasible and sustainable. Studies examining variations in engagement across modalities and populations could provide evidence-based guidelines for tailoring interventions to specific clinical or community contexts. Comparative effectiveness research represents a third priority. Randomized controlled trials are necessary to evaluate how different artistic modalities perform relative to one another, to combinations of modalities, and to traditional behavioral or pharmacological treatments. Such investigations would clarify the unique and additive contributions of art-based interventions, identify the mechanisms underlying observed benefits, and provide evidence to inform clinical decision-making. Addressing these challenges—through careful protocol development, dose optimization, and comparative evaluation—will strengthen the scientific foundation of art-based interventions in health psychology. By establishing standardized, evidence-informed practices, researchers and practitioners can enhance the reliability, accessibility, and scalability of creative programs, ensuring that artistic engagement functions as a robust tool for promoting resilience, wellbeing, and adaptive health behaviors across diverse populations.

8.3 Technology and Digital Innovations

Technological advancements are rapidly expanding opportunities for delivering art-based interventions at scale. Virtual reality, mobile applications, and online collaborative platforms have the potential to increase accessibility, particularly for populations facing mobility, geographic, or socioeconomic barriers (Fancourt et al., 2019). Digital modalities allow participants to engage with artistic activities from remote locations, providing flexibility and continuity that can complement in-person interventions. Future research should investigate the efficacy of digital art interventions compared with traditional in-person programs, examining psychological, behavioral, and physiological outcomes. Additionally, the integration of artificial intelligence and adaptive feedback mechanisms may allow for personalized engagement, tailoring artistic experiences to individual preferences, abilities, and therapeutic goals. Digital platforms also facilitate real-time monitoring of participant engagement, emotional states, and health outcomes, supporting evidence-informed and adaptive intervention strategies. While much of the existing research has focused on clinical populations, future studies should explore the impact of artistic engagement across a broader range of demographics and health contexts. For individuals with chronic illness or undergoing rehabilitation, art-based interventions may serve as effective tools for coping with pain, neurological conditions, or post-injury recovery. In the context of mental health, creative practices can provide long-term benefits for individuals experiencing depression, anxiety, or post-traumatic stress disorder, with research needed to examine efficacy across age groups and cultural backgrounds. Community-based programs offer opportunities for preventive health promotion, targeting stress reduction, social cohesion, and engagement in health-promoting behaviors within non-clinical populations. Expanding research across these diverse contexts will strengthen the generalizability and applicability of art-based interventions.

Adopting multilevel and interdisciplinary approaches further enhances understanding of art's role in health psychology. Collaboration with neuroscience, sociology, education, and public health enables examination of effects at the individual, group, and societal levels. At the individual level, art supports emotional regulation, self-efficacy, and adaptive behavior change. Group-level engagement fosters social support, collective resilience, and a sense of community cohesion. At the societal level, art contributes to public health outcomes, cultural engagement, and equitable access to health-promoting interventions. Integrating these levels within the biopsychosocial framework of health psychology allows for a comprehensive understanding of how artistic engagement functions across psychological, behavioral, and social domains. Methodologically, future research must balance rigor with respect for the qualitative and experiential nature of art. Mixed-methods designs combining quantitative measures, such as biomarkers or behavioral outcomes, with qualitative analyses, including narrative, thematic, or phenomenological approaches, can capture the multidimensional effects of artistic engagement. Longitudinal designs are needed to assess the durability of emotional, cognitive, and physiological benefits over time. Research should also account for cultural, social, and contextual factors, ensuring that interventions are meaningful and relevant across diverse populations. Finally, expanding the evidence base has important policy and practice implications. Integrating art into healthcare systems, schools, and community centers can promote widespread access to creative health interventions. Training health professionals in expressive modalities ensures that programs are delivered effectively and safely. Moreover, evidence-informed allocation of funding and resources can support accessible, scalable, and sustainable art-based interventions, reinforcing the potential of creativity as a tool for holistic health promotion. Future research in art and health psychology should focus on clarifying mechanisms of action, standardizing interventions, leveraging technology, expanding populations and contexts, and adopting interdisciplinary, multilevel approaches. Methodologically robust, culturally sensitive, and technologically integrated studies will enhance understanding of how artistic engagement promotes emotional, behavioural, and social health outcomes. These advances will support the development of evidence-based, scalable, and accessible interventions, positioning art as a central component of holistic health psychology practice.

CONCLUSION

This chapter has explored the multifaceted role of art in health psychology, highlighting its capacity to foster behavioural change, meaning-making, and resilience through embodied creativity. Artistic engagement transcends conventional therapeutic modalities by integrating cognitive, affective, and somatic dimensions of human experience, offering a holistic approach to health and wellbeing. Art serves as a bridge between psychological processes and lived experience, providing symbolic, emotional, and embodied means to navigate illness, trauma, and everyday stress. Through visual arts, music, dance, and writing, individuals can externalize internal states, reconstruct personal narratives, and cultivate adaptive coping mechanisms. The concept of embodied creativity emphasizes that artistic engagement is not merely cognitive or symbolic; it is a bodily practice that aligns perception, action, and affect, enabling participants to experience health-related challenges as opportunities for growth and self-expression (Fuchs, 2018; Koch & Fuchs, 2011).

At the individual level, art enhances self-efficacy, emotional regulation, and behavioural adherence, promoting proactive engagement with health behaviours and therapeutic regimens. Simultaneously, participatory art fosters social connectedness, collective meaning-making, and community resilience, underscoring the relational and cultural dimensions of health psychology. These dual pathways—individual and collective—demonstrate the comprehensive potential of art-based interventions to address psychological, behavioural, and social determinants of health. Clinical applications of art range from individualized therapy to multimodal interventions that integrate expressive modalities with evidence-based psychological treatments. Community applications expand the reach of health-promoting interventions, encouraging participatory engagement, reducing social isolation, and supporting public health goals. Technological innovations, including digital platforms and virtual reality, further enhance accessibility, scalability, and personalization, positioning artistic engagement as a versatile tool for modern health psychology.

Despite compelling evidence for its benefits, research on art in health psychology faces methodological and conceptual challenges. Future directions include elucidating mechanisms of action, standardizing intervention protocols, evaluating long-term outcomes, and exploring applications across diverse populations and cultural contexts. Interdisciplinary collaboration with neuroscience, sociology, education, and public health will advance understanding of how artistic engagement produces biopsychosocial benefits, reinforcing its integration into both clinical practice and preventive strategies. In conclusion, art—as embodied creativity—represents a fundamental dimension of human health experience. It enables individuals to engage meaningfully with their bodies, emotions, and social environments, fostering resilience, behavioural adaptation, and psychological wellbeing. By incorporating artistic practices into health psychology, researchers and practitioners gain a richer understanding of the complex interplay between mind, body, and community. The integration of art into both individual and collective interventions promises a holistic approach to health promotion, bridging the gap between scientific evidence and human experience. Ultimately, recognizing the transformative potential of art enriches the practice of health psychology, providing innovative tools to support human flourishing in clinical, community, and public health contexts.

REFERENCES

Bandura, A. (1997). *Self-efficacy: The exercise of control*. W. H. Freeman.

Barsalou, L. W. (2008). Grounded cognition. *Annual Review of Psychology*, *59*(1), 617–645. DOI: 10.1146/annurev.psych.59.103006.093639 PMID: 17705682

Bradt, J., & Dileo, C. (2014). Music interventions for mechanically ventilated patients. *Cochrane Database of Systematic Reviews*, *12*(12), CD006902. Advance online publication. DOI: 10.1002/14651858.CD006902.pub3 PMID: 25490233

Camic, P. M. (2010). Participatory art for older adults: A review of benefits and mechanisms. *Perspectives in Public Health*, *130*(6), 277–283. DOI: 10.1177/1757913910386206 PMID: 21213564

Camic, P. M., Baker, E. L., & Tischler, V. (2014). Theorizing how art gallery interventions impact people with dementia. *The Gerontologist*, *54*(6), 912–921. DOI: 10.1093/geront/gnt103 PMID: 25063936

Chanda, M. L., & Levitin, D. J. (2013). The neurochemistry of music. *Trends in Cognitive Sciences*, *17*(4), 179–193. DOI: 10.1016/j.tics.2013.02.007 PMID: 23541122

Clift, S., & Camic, P. (2016). *Oxford textbook of creative arts, health, and wellbeing: International perspectives on practice, policy, and research*. Oxford University Press.

Clift, S., & Morrison, I. (2011). Group singing fosters mental health and wellbeing: Findings from the East Kent "singing for health" network project. *Mental Health and Social Inclusion*, *15*(2), 88–97. DOI: 10.1108/20428301111140930

Creswell, J. D., Lindsay, E. K., & Moyers, T. B. (2015). How does mindfulness training affect health? A mindfulness stress buffering account. *Current Directions in Psychological Science*, *24*(6), 401–407. DOI: 10.1177/0963721414547415

Czamanski-Cohen, J., & Weihs, K. L. (2023). The role of emotion processing in art therapy (REPAT) intervention protocol. *Frontiers in Psychology, 14*, 1208901. https://doi.org/, G. L. (1977). The need for a new medical model: A challenge for biomedicine. *Science, 196*(4286), 129–136. https://doi.org/DOI: 10.3389/fpsyg.2023.1208901Engel

Fancourt, D., Aufegger, L., & Williamon, A. (2019). Low-stress and high-stress singing have contrasting effects on glucocorticoid response. *Frontiers in Psychology*, *10*, 1–13. DOI: 10.3389/fpsyg.2019.00005 PMID: 26388794

Forgeard, M. J. C., & Elstein, J. G. (2014). Advancing the clinical science of creativity. *Frontiers in Psychology*, *5*, 613. DOI: 10.3389/fpsyg.2014.00613 PMID: 24994990

Frank, A. W., & Frank, J. (1991). *At the will of the body: Reflections on illness*. Houghton Mifflin.

Frankl, V. E. (1963). *Man's search for meaning: An introduction to logotherapy*. Beacon Press.

Fuchs, T. (2018). *Ecology of the brain: The phenomenology and biology of the embodied mind*. Oxford University Press., DOI: 10.1093/oso/9780199646883.001.0001

Geue, K., Goetze, H., Buttstaedt, M., Kleinert, E., Richter, D., & Singer, S. (2010). An overview of art therapy interventions for cancer patients and the results of research. *Complementary Therapies in Medicine*, *18*(3–4), 160–170. DOI: 10.1016/j.ctim.2010.04.001 PMID: 20688262

Haeyen, S., van Hooren, S., van der Veld, W., & Hutschemaekers, G. (2015). Perceived effects of art therapy in the treatment of personality disorders, cluster B/C: A qualitative study. *The Arts in Psychotherapy*, *45*(3), 1–9. DOI: 10.1016/j.aip.2015.04.005

Hallam, S. (2010). The power of music: Its impact on the intellectual, social and personal development of children and young people. *International Journal of Music Education, 28*(3), 269–289. https://doi.org/. https://doi.org/DOI: 10.1177/0255761413490659

Halprin, D. (2003). *The expressive body in life, art, and therapy: Working with movement, metaphor, and meaning*. Jessica Kingsley Publishers.Malchiodi, C. A. (2020). *Creative interventions with traumatized children.* Guilford Press.

Kaimal, G., Ray, K., & Muniz, J. (2016). Reduction of cortisol levels and participants' responses following art making. *Art Therapy: Journal of the American Art Therapy Association*, *33*(2), 74–80. DOI: 10.1080/07421656.2016.1166832 PMID: 27695158

Koch, S. C., & Fuchs, T. (2011). Embodied arts therapies. *Frontiers in Psychology*, *2*, 1–12. DOI: 10.3389/fpsyg.2011.00124

Koch, S. C., Kunz, T., Lykou, S., & Cruz, R. (2014). Effects of dance movement therapy and dance on health-related psychological outcomes: A meta-analysis. *The Arts in Psychotherapy*, *41*(1), 46–64. DOI: 10.1016/j.aip.2013.10.004

Koelsch, S. (2014). Brain correlates of music-evoked emotions. *Nature Reviews. Neuroscience*, *15*(3), 170–180. DOI: 10.1038/nrn3666 PMID: 24552785

Masten, A. S. (2014). Global perspectives on resilience in children and youth. *Child Development*, *85*(1), 6–20. DOI: 10.1111/cdev.12205 PMID: 24341286

Park, C. L. (2010). Making sense of the meaning literature: An integrative review of meaning-making and its effects on adjustment to stressful life events. *Psychological Bulletin*, *136*(2), 257–301. DOI: 10.1037/a0018301 PMID: 20192563

Pennebaker, J. W., & Seagal, J. D. (1999). Forming a story: The health benefits of narrative. *Journal of Clinical Psychology*, *55*(10), 1243–1254. DOI: 10.1002/(SICI)1097-4679(199910)55:10<1243::AID-JCLP6>3.0.CO;2-N PMID: 11045774

Puig, A., Lee, S. M., Goodwin, L., & Sherrard, P. (2006). The efficacy of creative arts therapies to enhance emotional expression, spirituality, and psychological well-being of newly diagnosed stage I and II breast cancer patients: A preliminary study. *The Arts in Psychotherapy*, *33*(3), 218–228. DOI: 10.1016/j.aip.2006.02.004

Schunk, D. H., & DiBenedetto, M. K. (2020). Motivation and social-emotional learning in health psychology. *Journal of Health Psychology*, *25*(9), 1235–1247. DOI: 10.1177/1359105320913439

Slayton, S. C., D'Archer, J., & Kaplan, F. (2010). Outcome studies on the efficacy of art therapy: A review of findings. *Art Therapy: Journal of the American Art Therapy Association*, *27*(3), 108–118. DOI: 10.1080/07421656.2010.10129660

Smyth, J. M. (1998). Written emotional expression: Effect sizes, outcome types, and moderating variables. *Journal of Consulting and Clinical Psychology*, *66*(1), 174–184. DOI: 10.1037/0022-006X.66.1.174 PMID: 9489272

Stuckey, H. L., & Nobel, J. (2010). The connection between art, healing, and public health: A review of current literature. *American Journal of Public Health*, *100*(2), 254–263. DOI: 10.2105/AJPH.2008.156497 PMID: 20019311

Taylor, S. E. (2018). *Health psychology* (10th ed.). McGraw-Hill Education.

Varela, F. J., Thompson, E., & Rosch, E. (1991). *The embodied mind: Cognitive science and human experience*. MIT Press. DOI: 10.7551/mitpress/6730.001.0001

Chapter 6
From Brushstrokes to Brainwaves:
Art, Neuroscience, and Health Psychology in Primary Education

Maria Athanasekou
http://orcid.org/0000-0002-2971-9452
Hellenic Open University, Greece & Frederick University, Cyprus

ABSTRACT

The intersection of art, neuroscience, and health psychology offers a transformative lens on primary education, showing how creative engagement fosters cognitive, emotional, and behavioural growth. Neuroscience highlights children's heightened neuroplasticity, making them highly responsive to artistic experiences that stimulate neural networks. Arts practices activate motor, sensory, emotional, and cognitive regions, strengthening executive functions and socio-emotional regulation. Health psychology frames art as a behavioural intervention that supports resilience, coping, and wellbeing. Evidence shows that creative expression reduces stress, enhances motivation through dopamine release, and fosters prosocial behaviour. Activities like drawing and storytelling help children symbolise experiences, building self-efficacy and meaning. Art thus bridges brushstrokes and brainwaves, integrating scientific insight with humanistic values to position creativity as a cornerstone of holistic learning and resilience in education.

INTRODUCTION

The intersection of art, neuroscience, and health psychology provides a transformative lens for rethinking primary education. In recent years, scholars have

DOI: 10.4018/979-8-2600-3085-1.ch006

increasingly argued that education must move beyond the traditional emphasis on literacy and numeracy to embrace more holistic approaches to child development (Eisner, 2002; Winner et al., 2013). Early childhood is a critical period for cognitive, emotional, and social development, as the brain is uniquely malleable and responsive to environmental input (Kolb & Gibb, 2011). Consequently, the types of experiences children are exposed to during these formative years have enduring effects on their behavioural and psychological trajectories. Artistic engagement emerges as a compelling experience in this regard. Beyond its intrinsic aesthetic and cultural value, the arts have been shown to foster neuroplasticity, enhance emotional regulation, and strengthen social connections (Zaidel, 2013; Hardiman, 2016). At the same time, health psychology highlights the role of behaviours, emotions, and coping strategies in shaping lifelong health outcomes (Taylor, 2020). Together, these perspectives reveal that art is not a peripheral activity in education but a central mechanism for cultivating wellbeing, resilience, and meaning-making in children.

This chapter positions the arts as a nexus between neuroscience and health psychology in primary education. It argues that creative engagement supports both the developing brain and the developing self, enabling children to thrive cognitively, emotionally, and behaviourally.

THEORETICAL FOUNDATIONS

Neuroscience, Neuroplasticity, and Artistic Engagement in Early Childhood

Neuroscience research provides compelling evidence that the early years of development represent a critical period of heightened neuroplasticity, during which children's brains are exceptionally capable of forming and reorganizing synaptic connections in response to experiences (Kolb & Gibb, 2011). This plasticity underpins the remarkable adaptability of the young brain and establishes a biological foundation for the influence of enriched environments, including artistic engagement, on cognitive, emotional, and behavioural outcomes. Artistic activities, in particular, offer a unique and powerful stimulus because they simultaneously engage multiple neural networks—sensory, motor, emotional, and cognitive—creating conditions that promote integrated brain development (Zaidel, 2013). For instance, learning to play a musical instrument recruits auditory perception, motor coordination, and executive functioning. Children practising music must attend to rhythm, pitch, and tempo while coordinating hand movements and sustaining attention over time. These processes strengthen the prefrontal cortex, enhance working memory, and promote inhibitory control, all of which are critical for academic success and self-regulation.

Similarly, visual arts activities such as drawing and painting engage fine motor skills, visual-spatial reasoning, and symbolic thinking. By translating internal ideas into external representations, children enhance their problem-solving abilities, spatial cognition, and symbolic understanding, which are foundational for mathematics and literacy (Winner et al., 2013). Dance and movement activities further extend these benefits by combining motor planning, rhythm perception, and social coordination, thereby enhancing executive function and socio-emotional regulation (Diamond & Lee, 2011).

The field of neuroaesthetics—which investigates how artistic experiences influence brain function and psychological states—provides additional insights into the neural mechanisms of creativity (Chatterjee & Vartanian, 2014). Neuroaesthetic research shows that engaging with art can activate the reward system, including dopaminergic pathways, which reinforces motivation, positive affect, and learning readiness. These neurochemical responses are not merely transient; repeated engagement with art strengthens the neural circuits underlying attention, memory consolidation, and cognitive flexibility. Consequently, artistic experiences provide children with both short-term emotional regulation and long-term cognitive scaffolding that support academic achievement and resilience.

Moreover, artistic engagement supports embodied learning, a process whereby sensorimotor experiences are integrated with cognitive and emotional processing. For example, sculpting clay requires tactile exploration, spatial reasoning, and planning, while also offering an outlet for expressing emotions nonverbally. These activities not only reinforce neural connectivity but also facilitate self-regulation and socio-emotional growth, aligning with principles from health psychology that link behavioral engagement with psychological wellbeing (Taylor, 2020). Embodied artistic practices help children externalize feelings, process experiences, and build coping strategies, demonstrating a biopsychosocial pathway through which creativity fosters holistic development. Neuroscientific studies also highlight that the multimodal nature of art—combining auditory, visual, kinesthetic, and emotional elements—optimizes neural plasticity more effectively than unisensory experiences. Music, visual arts, drama, and dance collectively stimulate interconnected brain regions, including the prefrontal cortex, limbic system, and motor cortices, fostering both cognitive and affective integration (Hardiman, 2016; Zaidel, 2013). These interactions underscore the notion that art is not merely a leisure activity but a developmentally potent intervention, capable of shaping the architecture of the developing brain.

Finally, neuroaesthetic and educational neuroscience research provides practical implications for early childhood education. By incorporating arts-based activities into primary curricula, educators can harness neuroplasticity to enhance attention, memory, executive function, and emotional resilience. Artistic experiences create a feedback loop: children engage deeply, neural circuits strengthen, motivation increases, and learning becomes both effective and meaningful. This body of evidence demonstrates that the integration of neuroscience and art offers a scientifically grounded framework for promoting holistic child development, preparing children not only for academic success but also for lifelong cognitive, emotional, and social wellbeing.

Health Psychology and Creative Practices in Early Childhood Development

Health psychology examines how psychological and behavioural processes influence health, wellbeing, and illness across the lifespan (Taylor, 2020). In early childhood, these processes encompass emotional regulation, coping strategies, social adaptation, and the development of health-related beliefs, all of which are deeply shaped by environmental factors, including family, peers, and educational settings. Schools, in particular, provide structured contexts in which children encounter social, cognitive, and emotional challenges. These experiences play a pivotal role in shaping children's resilience—the ability to adapt positively in the face of adversity (Masten, 2014).

Resilience is not a fixed trait but a dynamic capacity that emerges through supportive interactions, structured challenges, and opportunities for self-expression. Children who cultivate resilience are better able to manage stress, regulate emotions, and navigate social complexities, laying the foundation for lifelong health and wellbeing (Masten, 2014). Artistic engagement provides a powerful mechanism for fostering these capacities. By participating in music, visual arts, drama, and movement activities, children are offered nonverbal avenues for expressing emotions, exploring experiences, and developing adaptive coping strategies (Camic & Chatterjee, 2013). For example, drawing or storytelling enables children to externalize feelings that may be difficult to articulate verbally, facilitating emotional processing and reflection. Similarly, group music-making or drama encourages collaboration, empathy, and perspective-taking, which enhance social competence and stress resilience.

Within a health psychology framework, art can therefore be conceptualized as a behavioural intervention that strengthens adaptive capacities in children. Evidence demonstrates that engagement with the arts improves affective regulation, reduces anxiety, and enhances self-efficacy, all of which are associated with positive health outcomes (Malchiodi, 2020; Sonke et al., 2017). By externalizing and symbolizing emotional experiences through creative practices, children develop problem-solving skills and emotional literacy, which in turn support healthier interpersonal interactions and academic engagement. Moreover, repeated engagement with art reinforces psychological flexibility, enabling children to adapt constructively to changing circumstances and recover more effectively from setbacks.

Health psychology also emphasizes the role of environmental and contextual factors in shaping children's behaviours and health trajectories (Bandura, 1997). In this regard, schools act as critical sites for intervention: arts-based programs can be designed to provide supportive, structured environments that encourage exploration, experimentation, and mastery. For instance, classroom-based visual arts, music, and drama programs have been shown to increase engagement, reduce stress, and enhance overall wellbeing, contributing to a positive school climate (Eisner, 2002; Hallam, 2010). Importantly, these benefits are not limited to cognitive or artistic skills but extend to socio-emotional development, helping children build constructive peer relationships and a sense of belonging.

Resilience and health-promoting behaviours cultivated through the arts also have longitudinal implications. Children who learn adaptive coping strategies and develop strong self-regulation in early education are more likely to maintain healthy patterns of thought, behaviour, and emotion throughout adolescence and into adulthood (Masten, 2014). Health psychology therefore positions artistic engagement as preventive and promotive, rather than reactive: rather than waiting for stress or maladaptive behaviours to arise, educators can proactively embed creative practices to strengthen children's psychological and behavioural resources.

Moreover, integrating health psychology with artistic engagement supports a holistic view of child development, in which cognitive, emotional, social, and behavioural growth are interconnected. Music, dance, and visual arts provide multisensory experiences that simultaneously stimulate neural, emotional, and social pathways, creating opportunities for embodied learning that integrates mind and body. In this way, art aligns with health psychology principles by promoting both individual wellbeing and environmental support systems, emphasizing the interdependence of personal capacities and contextual resources (Taylor, 2020).

In conclusion, viewing artistic engagement through the lens of health psychology highlights its potential as an essential developmental tool in primary education. Beyond fostering creativity and technical skills, the arts cultivate resilience, adaptive coping, and emotional regulation, while promoting long-term health trajectories. By embedding arts-based interventions within educational practice, schools can create environments that nurture the whole child—cognitively, emotionally, socially, and behaviourally—preparing students not only for academic achievement but also for healthy, meaningful, and resilient lives.

Art as Embodied Learning

Art in education provides multisensory, embodied experiences that engage children holistically. Drawing, painting, music, dance, and storytelling foster the integration of motor, sensory, emotional, and cognitive processes. Such embodied learning reinforces not only academic skills but also life skills, including persistence, cooperation, and problem-solving (Eisner, 2002).

Creative expression allows children to externalize emotions, regulate behaviour, and build self-efficacy. For example, music-based programs have been shown to enhance literacy and numeracy by strengthening attention and memory processes (Hallam, 2010). Similarly, visual arts activities help children develop fine motor control while also symbolising personal experiences, thus contributing to emotional processing (Malchiodi, 2020). These practices align with health psychology's emphasis on behavioural reinforcement, as repeated participation in arts activities fosters habits that support positive mental health outcomes (Sonke et al., 2017).

Resilience and Meaning-Making

Resilience is a central construct in both education and health psychology. Artistic practices contribute to resilience by providing children with nonverbal outlets for expressing emotions and reconstructing narratives of adversity (Masten, 2014; Malchiodi, 2020). Storytelling, drama, and visual arts offer children ways to symbolise uncertainty, loss, or change, helping them develop adaptive strategies for coping. In addition to resilience, art fosters meaning-making, a process by which children construct identities, values, and aspirations. Bandura's (1997) theory of self-efficacy is particularly relevant here, as creative activities provide mastery experiences that strengthen confidence across domains. Neuroscientific evidence shows that symbolic activity and self-expression activate prefrontal networks associated with planning, regulation, and self-reflection (Immordino-Yang, 2016). Thus, art nurtures not only creativity but also the psychological and neurological foundations of agency and purpose.

Educational Implications

The practical implications of integrating art into primary education are significant. Arts-based programs have been linked to reduced anxiety, improved social interaction, and greater school engagement (Eisner, 2002; Sonke et al., 2017). By embedding arts in curricula, schools can create supportive environments that promote resilience, wellbeing, and adaptive coping strategies before mental health problems escalate (Stuckey & Nobel, 2010). Moreover, arts integration aligns with culturally responsive pedagogy, offering children opportunities to connect their cultural identities with learning (Camic & Chatterjee, 2013). Health psychology underscores the importance of context in shaping behaviour, and arts practices provide flexible, inclusive avenues for meaning-making across diverse social and cultural environments.

Research Gaps and Significance

While growing evidence supports the role of art in fostering neuroplasticity and psychological wellbeing, several gaps remain. First, more longitudinal studies are needed to assess the long-term impact of arts participation on resilience and health outcomes. Second, research should address cultural variability, exploring how artistic practices rooted in specific traditions influence child development. Third, interdisciplinary methodologies that integrate neuroscientific data with educational and psychological outcomes are essential for advancing the field.

This chapter contributes to these discussions by synthesizing insights from neuroscience, health psychology, and arts education, highlighting their convergence in supporting holistic development. It argues that in the context of primary education, art should be recognized as a cornerstone of learning and wellbeing rather than a peripheral activity. By bridging brushstrokes and brainwaves, art offers a scientifically grounded and humanistically rich pathway to nurturing resilient, creative, and healthy children.

HISTORICAL AND THEORETICAL BACKGROUND

Art in Education: Historical Perspectives

The integration of art into educational practice is not a modern innovation but has deep historical roots. Ancient civilizations viewed the arts as central to child development and cultural transmission. In Ancient Greece, for example, *mousikē* encompassed music, poetry, and dance, all of which were considered essential to moral and intellectual formation. Similarly, in Confucian educational traditions, music and calligraphy were regarded as means of cultivating virtue and harmony (Wang, 2013). These early traditions underscore a long-standing recognition that art shapes not only cognitive skills but also emotional, ethical, and social dimensions of human life.

During the Renaissance, humanist educators emphasized the role of the arts in fostering creativity and imagination. This emphasis gained renewed traction in the 19th and 20th centuries, particularly with the progressive education movement, which stressed experiential and holistic learning. Figures such as John Dewey (1934/2005) argued that the arts were integral to democratic education, offering children opportunities for expression, reflection, and growth. Dewey's philosophy laid the foundation for modern perspectives that consider the arts as both an epistemological and an ontological mode of engaging with the world. In the late 20th century, educational theorists such as Elliot Eisner (2002) advanced the argument that the arts cultivate forms of thinking that are distinct from, yet complementary to, scientific reasoning. Eisner's work challenged reductionist approaches to education, positioning the arts as vehicles for imagination, empathy, and meaning-making. This historical trajectory demonstrates that art has long been considered a vital part of human development, even if its role has often been marginalized in policy and curriculum debates.

Health Psychology and Child Development

Health psychology, as a discipline, emerged in the latter half of the 20th century, focusing on the ways psychological and behavioural processes affect health and wellbeing (Taylor, 2020). Its emphasis on prevention, coping, and resilience makes it particularly relevant to childhood education. Early childhood is a formative period for developing behavioural patterns that persist into adulthood, such as stress responses, health habits, and coping mechanisms (Masten, 2014).

Health psychology provides frameworks for understanding how children's interactions with their environments—family, school, and peers—shape their developmental trajectories. Central to this perspective is the concept of resilience, defined as the capacity to adapt successfully despite adversity. Resilience is not a fixed trait but a dynamic process influenced by both internal capacities and external supports (Masten, 2014). In educational contexts, fostering resilience involves equipping children with emotional regulation strategies, problem-solving skills, and supportive relationships.

The arts intersect with health psychology by offering behavioural interventions that foster resilience, wellbeing, and meaning-making. Creative practices provide safe spaces for children to explore emotions, rehearse coping strategies, and articulate identity (Malchiodi, 2020). Moreover, health psychology highlights how these practices can influence long-term health outcomes, as positive coping skills established in childhood are predictive of healthier lifestyles in adulthood (Taylor, 2020).

Neuroscience and Learning Theories

Parallel to developments in health psychology, neuroscience has transformed understandings of learning. Brain research has shown that children's brains exhibit remarkable plasticity, meaning they are highly adaptable in response to experiences (Kolb & Gibb, 2011). This has profound implications for education, as enriched environments—such as those created by artistic engagement—stimulate synaptic growth and strengthen neural pathways. Neuroscience also underpins theories of embodied cognition, which emphasize that learning is not confined to abstract mental processes but is grounded in sensory and motor experiences. Artistic activities epitomize embodied cognition: playing an instrument engages auditory and motor systems, dancing integrates balance and rhythm, and drawing fuses fine motor control with visual-spatial reasoning. These embodied practices create deeper and more durable learning experiences than abstract instruction alone (Immordino-Yang, 2016).

The relatively new field of neuroaesthetics further bridges art and neuroscience, investigating how aesthetic experiences influence perception, emotion, and cognition (Chatterjee & Vartanian, 2014). Findings in neuroaesthetics indicate that exposure to art activates reward systems in the brain, such as the dopaminergic pathways, which enhance motivation and learning readiness . These insights substantiate educational claims that art not only enriches cultural knowledge but also enhances fundamental cognitive and emotional processes.

The Interdisciplinary Convergence

The convergence of these three fields—art education, health psychology, and neuroscience—creates a powerful interdisciplinary framework for understanding child development. Art provides the practices; health psychology provides the behavioural and emotional frameworks; and neuroscience provides the biological explanations. Together, they form a holistic approach that situates education as both a cognitive and a health-promoting process.

This convergence also responds to pressing challenges in contemporary education. Rising rates of childhood anxiety, attention disorders, and stress-related behaviours call for interventions that address not only academic achievement but also mental health and resilience (Stuckey & Nobel, 2010). The arts, when understood through this interdisciplinary lens, offer precisely such interventions—ones that are evidence-based, culturally adaptable, and developmentally appropriate.

NEUROSCIENCE OF ART AND LEARNING

Neuroplasticity and Child Brain Development

Neuroscience has fundamentally reshaped our understanding of childhood learning. Central to this shift is the concept of neuroplasticity, the brain's capacity to reorganize itself by forming new neural connections throughout life. In early childhood, this plasticity is particularly pronounced, enabling children to adapt rapidly to environmental inputs (Kolb & Gibb, 2011). Research demonstrates that enriched environments—those offering stimulation across sensory, motor, and social domains—promote synaptic growth, dendritic branching, and enhanced connectivity between neural regions.

Artistic engagement constitutes one of the most effective enriched environments for young learners. Music, visual arts, and dance not only engage multiple senses but also provide emotionally meaningful contexts that enhance synaptic activity. Studies in developmental neuroscience suggest that these multisensory experiences lead to long-term structural and functional changes in the brain. For example, children trained in music show increased cortical thickness in auditory and motor areas, alongside enhanced white matter connectivity, indicating that artistic practice can literally reshape the developing brain.

Embodied Cognition and Sensory Integration

Another key contribution of neuroscience to education is the theory of embodied cognition. Traditional models of learning have often privileged abstract, symbolic thought, but neuroscience emphasizes that cognition is grounded in bodily experience. Artistic practices exemplify embodied cognition because they integrate sensory perception with motor action, creating holistic learning experiences.

Take dance as an example: children learning choreographed movements engage motor planning regions (premotor cortex, cerebellum), spatial reasoning systems (parietal lobe), and emotion-regulating areas (amygdala, prefrontal cortex). This integration strengthens neural pathways across modalities, resulting in improved coordination, self-regulation, and memory retention. Similarly, drawing combines fine motor control, visual-spatial reasoning, and symbolic representation, thereby reinforcing executive functions while offering avenues for emotional expression (Winner et al., 2013).

Neuroscience shows that multisensory integration—the simultaneous activation of vision, hearing, touch, and movement—enhances learning outcomes. Art naturally creates such multisensory experiences, leading to more durable learning and deeper engagement compared to single-modality instruction.

Neuroaesthetics and the Arts

The emerging field of neuroaesthetics offers further insights into how artistic experiences influence the brain. Pioneered by researchers such as Zeki (2001) and Chatterjee (2014), neuroaesthetics investigates the neural mechanisms underlying aesthetic perception, creativity, and artistic production. A key finding is that engagement with art activates the brain's reward circuitry, particularly dopaminergic pathways in the ventral striatum and prefrontal cortex. This release of dopamine enhances positive affect, motivation, and readiness to learn. For children in primary education, such neurochemical reinforcement contributes to resilience and sustained attention, making them more receptive to academic instruction.

Neuroaesthetics also highlights the role of default mode network (DMN) activity during artistic engagement. The DMN, associated with self-reflection and imagination, becomes active when children engage in drawing, storytelling, or daydreaming (Immordino-Yang et al., 2012). This suggests that art supports the development of internal narrative and self-concept, processes crucial for identity formation and meaning-making.

Executive Functions and Emotional Regulation

Executive functions—such as attention, working memory, and inhibitory control—are essential for learning and behavioural regulation. Neuroscience demonstrates that these functions are enhanced by arts participation (Diamond, 2013). Musical training, for instance, has been shown to improve working memory and attentional control, while drama activities enhance perspective-taking and emotional regulation.

Importantly, artistic engagement also modulates activity in brain regions involved in emotional regulation, including the prefrontal cortex and limbic system. This is particularly valuable in primary education, where children are still developing the capacity to manage emotions such as frustration, anxiety, or excitement. Art provides structured opportunities for children to practice regulation through expression and reflection, contributing to both wellbeing and academic success.

Creativity and Neural Connectivity

Neuroscience has also illuminated how creativity—the capacity to generate novel and valuable ideas—arises from dynamic interactions between different neural networks. Beaty et al. (2016) identified that creativity depends on the interplay between the default mode network (imagination), the executive control network (planning, self-regulation), and the salience network (switching between internal and external attention). Artistic practices uniquely activate and integrate these networks, strengthening the brain's ability to flexibly switch between divergent and convergent thinking.

For children, this means that artistic engagement not only fosters creative expression but also enhances problem-solving skills, adaptability, and resilience—capacities that are increasingly recognized as essential for thriving in a rapidly changing world.

HEALTH PSYCHOLOGY AND EDUCATIONAL RESILIENCE

Health Psychology as a Framework for Education

Health psychology examines how biological, psychological, and social factors interact to influence health, wellbeing, and behaviour (Taylor, 2020). In recent decades, its principles have increasingly been applied to educational contexts, offering frameworks for understanding how children cope with stress, regulate emotions, and develop resilience in the face of challenges. For primary education, health psychology provides valuable insights into how environments can be structured to support not only cognitive achievement but also emotional wellbeing.

The biopsychosocial model is central to this perspective. Originally articulated by Engel (1977), the model argues that wellbeing emerges from the interplay of biological (e.g., neural and physiological processes), psychological (e.g., cognition, emotion, motivation), and social (e.g., peer and family relationships, classroom climate) factors. Within education, the biopsychosocial model highlights the need for integrative approaches that address children as whole beings rather than focusing narrowly on academic skills. Artistic activities align closely with this model because they simultaneously engage biological systems (through movement and sensory stimulation), psychological processes (through creativity and emotional expression), and social interaction (through collaboration and shared meaning-making).

Stress, Coping, and Emotional Regulation in Childhood

Stress is an unavoidable part of human development, but chronic or poorly managed stress can undermine learning and wellbeing. In children, stress responses are mediated by the hypothalamic-pituitary-adrenal (HPA) axis, leading to the release of cortisol. While moderate stress can enhance alertness and performance, prolonged exposure impairs memory, attention, and immune function.

Health psychology identifies coping strategies as key mediators of how stress affects development. Coping can be problem-focused (actively addressing a stressor), emotion-focused (regulating feelings), or meaning-focused (reframing experiences in light of values and purpose) (Lazarus & Folkman, 1984). In primary education, children are still learning to deploy these strategies effectively. Here, artistic practices become vital tools: drawing, storytelling, or role-play provide safe avenues for children to externalize worries, reframe challenges, and experiment with new coping mechanisms (Malchiodi, 2020).

Art's impact on emotional regulation is supported by findings in psychophysiology. Creative engagement has been shown to lower cortisol levels, reduce heart rate, and induce parasympathetic nervous system activity, all markers of stress recovery

(Kaimal et al., 2016). By cultivating habits of artistic expression, schools can equip children with lifelong strategies for regulating stress and maintaining balance.

Resilience: Building Strength Through Art

Resilience refers to the capacity to adapt positively in the face of adversity. It is not merely an innate trait but a dynamic process shaped by personal skills, supportive relationships, and environmental resources (Masten, 2014). Health psychology highlights protective factors such as optimism, self-efficacy, and social support, all of which can be cultivated through educational practices.

Artistic engagement contributes to resilience in multiple ways. First, it enhances self-efficacy, or the belief in one's ability to effect change, as articulated by Bandura (1997). Completing a drawing, mastering a dance routine, or performing a play fosters confidence and demonstrates to children that persistence yields results. Second, art builds emotional literacy, enabling children to recognize, label, and manage emotions more effectively. This emotional competence has been strongly linked to resilience and mental health. Third, collaborative arts projects foster social connectedness, which provides buffers against stress and creates a sense of belonging (Eisenberg et al., 2010).

Importantly, resilience is not only about "bouncing back" from adversity but also about "bouncing forward"—using challenges as opportunities for growth. Artistic practices align with this developmental trajectory by encouraging creativity, perspective-taking, and the reimagining of possibilities, all of which help children construct meaning from difficult experiences.

Meaning-Making and Psychological Growth

One of the most profound contributions of art in education lies in its role in meaning-making. Health psychology emphasizes that constructing meaning is central to wellbeing, particularly when individuals face uncertainty or adversity. Through symbolic expression, metaphors, and narratives, art allows children to make sense of their experiences in ways that transcend literal language.

Storytelling, for example, helps children situate themselves within broader cultural and social frameworks, strengthening identity and coherence. Visual arts enable them to represent feelings or events that may be difficult to articulate verbally, providing psychological relief and insight. Music and drama engage collective meaning-making, where shared performance fosters empathy and mutual understanding.

Meaning-making is also linked to post-traumatic growth, the positive psychological change that can follow adversity. In contexts of family disruption, illness, or migration, artistic activities provide tools for children to process trauma, imagine alternative futures, and build hopeful narratives. Integrating these practices into school curricula can transform classrooms into spaces of healing as well as learning.

Health Promotion in Educational Settings

Health psychology also emphasizes prevention and health promotion, not just treatment of problems. Schools are uniquely positioned to promote healthy behaviours and psychological resilience across entire populations of children. Embedding art into curricula supports this mission by cultivating habits that contribute to long-term wellbeing.

For instance, programs combining visual arts with mindfulness practices have been shown to reduce anxiety, improve focus, and strengthen interpersonal skills among children (Coholic & Eys, 2016). Drama-based interventions enhance empathy and conflict resolution, while music programs improve self-discipline and cooperative behaviour (Rickard & McFerran, 2012). These approaches demonstrate how art functions as a universal preventive intervention that benefits all students, not only those at risk.

By aligning artistic practices with health psychology principles, educators can create protective school environments that foster resilience, wellbeing, and academic success simultaneously. This integration is particularly critical in the 21st century, where children face complex stressors ranging from digital overload to climate anxiety (Clayton, 2020).

PRACTICAL APPLICATIONS IN PRIMARY EDUCATION

Integrating Arts into the Curriculum

While policy discussions often frame the arts as "enrichment," emerging evidence suggests that artistic engagement is foundational for children's holistic development. Integrating arts into the core curriculum of primary schools can strengthen academic learning, foster wellbeing, and cultivate resilience.

Arts integration refers to teaching and learning strategies that weave artistic practices into the instruction of academic subjects (Burnaford et al., 2007). For example, music can be used to reinforce mathematical concepts through rhythm and pattern recognition; drama can deepen comprehension of literature by allowing children to embody characters; and visual arts can enhance scientific understanding by encouraging observation, modeling, and symbolic representation. Such integration not only makes learning more engaging but also activates multiple neural systems, reinforcing memory and transfer of knowledge (Hardiman, 2016).

Educational neuroscience supports these approaches, showing that multisensory experiences consolidate learning more effectively than unisensory instruction (Immordino-Yang & Damasio, 2007). Arts-based pedagogy, therefore, aligns with how the brain naturally learns: through embodied, emotional, and socially embedded experiences.

Classroom Practices Supporting Cognitive Development

Artistic practices can be applied directly to support core cognitive skills in primary education. Visual arts promote fine motor skills, spatial reasoning, and symbolic thinking, all of which underlie early literacy and numeracy (Winner et al., 2013). Drawing activities, for example, help children strengthen their visual-spatial memory and connect symbols to concepts, preparing them for reading and writing (Cox, 2005).

Music education has been strongly associated with improvements in phonological awareness, verbal memory, and mathematical reasoning (Hallam, 2010). Rhythm exercises strengthen temporal processing, which is essential for both language acquisition and mathematical problem-solving. Dance and movement practices enhance executive functions such as inhibition, working memory, and cognitive flexibility—skills directly related to academic success (Diamond & Lee, 2011).

Drama-based education encourages narrative competence, empathy, and perspective-taking. By improvising scenarios or enacting stories, children practice flexible thinking and social cognition. These embodied practices are particularly effective for students who may struggle with traditional didactic instruction, offering alternative routes to learning.

Classroom Practices Supporting Emotional and Behavioural Development

Beyond cognitive gains, the arts are uniquely suited to support children's emotional development and behavioural regulation. Emotional literacy—understanding and managing feelings—can be taught explicitly through artistic engagement. For example, children who draw or paint emotions externalize their inner states, which teachers can then help them articulate in words (Malchiodi, 2020). Music and movement allow children to modulate arousal levels, using rhythm to either energize or calm themselves.

Art also provides structured opportunities for children to practice self-regulation. Completing an art project requires sustained attention, persistence, and planning, reinforcing behavioural patterns aligned with executive function. Moreover, the iterative nature of artistic practice—sketching, revising, rehearsing—teaches tolerance of mistakes and the value of resilience.

In terms of social behaviour, collaborative arts projects foster cooperation, empathy, and conflict resolution. A group performance or mural project requires negotiation, turn-taking, and shared responsibility. These social-emotional skills are critical not only for academic collaboration but also for long-term wellbeing (Catterall et al., 2012).

Case Studies of Arts Integration

Evidence from school-based programs illustrates the impact of arts integration on educational outcomes. A growing body of research highlights the transformative potential of arts-based programs in primary education, demonstrating that engagement with creative practices can enhance cognitive, socio-emotional, and academic outcomes. Large-scale initiatives and targeted interventions across multiple countries provide compelling evidence that integrating the arts into curricula supports not only creativity but also core learning competencies and positive attitudes toward education. One notable example is the Learning Through the Arts (LTTA) program in Canada, a comprehensive initiative that placed artists-in-residence within schools to collaborate closely with teachers in delivering arts-integrated curricula. In this model, professional artists worked alongside educators to design and implement lessons that blended visual arts, music, drama, and movement with conventional subject matter. Evaluations of the LTTA program demonstrated significant improvements in student engagement, motivation, and problem-solving abilities (Upitis & Smithrim, 2003). Importantly, these benefits were most pronounced among disadvantaged populations, suggesting that arts-based approaches can serve as a powerful equalizer in education by providing children with enriched learning experiences that might otherwise be unavailable. Through sustained participation, students developed confidence in their creative capacities, strengthened collaborative skills, and exhibited more positive attitudes toward learning overall, highlighting the capacity of arts programs to influence both academic and socio-emotional development.

In the United States, Arts for Learning Lessons provides another illustrative example of effective arts integration. This program focused on literacy development by embedding drama, dance, and music into reading instruction. For instance, children enacted stories through role-play, explored rhythm and rhyme through music, and interpreted texts visually and kinesthetically. Evaluations of the program consistently found that students in arts-integrated classrooms outperformed their peers in standardized reading assessments, demonstrating improvements in comprehension, fluency, and engagement (Deasy, 2002). By situating literacy within a multisensory, creative context, the program fostered deeper cognitive processing, facilitated memory retention, and encouraged active participation. These outcomes suggest that the arts can serve not only as vehicles for expression but also as cognitive scaffolds, enhancing the acquisition of fundamental academic skills through embodied and experiential learning. In the United Kingdom, research has also highlighted the relationship between music education and literacy development. Hallam (2010) reviewed a series of studies examining the effects of rhythm and music instruction on early reading skills and phonological awareness. Findings consistently indicated that children exposed to music programs demonstrated stronger phonemic discrimination, better auditory attention, and improved reading accuracy. The structured practice of musical rhythm, melody, and pitch engages auditory processing and working memory, which are directly linked to literacy competencies. Such evidence underscores the potential of creative practices to reinforce domain-specific academic skills, showing that music is not merely an extracurricular activity but a meaningful contributor to core curriculum outcomes.

Collectively, these programs exemplify the synergistic benefits of integrating the arts into education. First, they demonstrate that creative practices enhance engagement and motivation. Children participating in these initiatives exhibit higher levels of curiosity, sustained attention, and willingness to tackle challenging tasks. Engagement is particularly crucial for students from marginalized or disadvantaged backgrounds, for whom traditional instructional methods may fail to capture interest or accommodate diverse learning styles. Second, arts integration fosters critical thinking and problem-solving skills. By navigating creative tasks, interpreting narratives, or coordinating musical patterns, students practice flexible thinking, planning, and evaluation—abilities that generalize across academic domains. Third, these interventions support socio-emotional development. Participation in collaborative arts activities nurtures empathy, communication, and cooperation, fostering positive social relationships and adaptive coping strategies within the school context.

Beyond individual outcomes, arts-based programs contribute to broader educational environments. Schools implementing LTTA, Arts for Learning, or music and literacy initiatives report enhanced classroom climates characterized by increased teacher enthusiasm, greater student participation, and stronger connections between teachers and students (Upitis & Smithrim, 2003; Hallam, 2010). In turn, these environments reinforce the developmental benefits of arts integration, creating feedback loops in which engagement, learning, and wellbeing mutually support one another. Importantly, these examples highlight that arts-based programs are most effective when embedded within the curriculum and supported by trained educators or professional artists. Ad hoc or extracurricular exposure, while valuable, does not consistently produce the same depth of cognitive or socio-emotional gains. Sustained, intentional integration allows for meaningful connections between creative practices and subject-specific learning objectives, maximizing the impact on children's overall development.

In conclusion, evidence from Canada, the United States, and the United Kingdom demonstrates that creative practices in education are more than enrichment activities; they are strategic tools for fostering academic achievement, cognitive development, and socio-emotional wellbeing. Programs such as LTTA, Arts for Learning, and music and literacy interventions reveal that arts integration can improve engagement, strengthen problem-solving skills, and enhance literacy outcomes, particularly for students who may face educational disadvantages. These findings support the broader argument that the arts should be recognized as central components of effective, equitable, and developmentally informed primary education, providing children with opportunities to develop both the skills and dispositions necessary for lifelong learning and holistic wellbeing.

These case studies underscore the potential of arts integration to reduce educational inequalities by engaging diverse learners and offering multiple entry points into academic content.

Arts, Inclusion, and Special Educational Needs

Arts-based approaches are particularly powerful in supporting inclusive education. Children with special educational needs (SEN) often benefit from alternative modes of expression and learning that bypass linguistic or cognitive barriers.

For instance, drama therapy has been used to support children with autism spectrum disorder (ASD), improving communication, empathy, and social interaction (Corbett et al., 2014). Music therapy interventions have shown effectiveness in enhancing language development and emotional expression in children with developmental delays (Geretsegger et al., 2014). Visual arts programs provide children with attention deficit hyperactivity disorder (ADHD) opportunities for focus and self-expression in non-competitive contexts, fostering self-esteem.

Inclusive arts education also aligns with the principles of universal design for learning (UDL), which advocates for multiple means of representation, engagement, and expression. By offering varied creative pathways, educators can accommodate diverse learners and create equitable learning environments.

Teacher Training and Professional Development

The success of arts integration depends on teacher confidence and competence. Many educators report feeling unprepared to deliver arts-based instruction due to limited training in the arts during teacher education programs (Garvis & Pendergast, 2011). Professional development opportunities are therefore essential to equip teachers with both the skills and the pedagogical frameworks to embed arts effectively into the curriculum.

Collaborations between teachers and professional artists can be especially fruitful. Co-teaching models allow teachers to observe artistic processes in action while artists gain insights into educational goals. Furthermore, training that connects arts integration to neuroscience and health psychology can strengthen teachers' understanding of the developmental benefits of creative practices, increasing their motivation to sustain these approaches (Hardiman, 2016).

Policy Implications

Embedding the arts into primary education has policy implications at both national and local levels. In many systems, standardized testing regimes have marginalized the arts, framing them as expendable compared to "core" subjects (Eisner, 2002). However, the evidence presented in neuroscience and health psychology suggests that the arts are not peripheral but central to effective education.

Policies should recognize arts integration as a driver of equity, resilience, and wellbeing. Funding streams can support schools in hiring arts specialists, developing community partnerships, and sustaining arts-rich environments. In addition, curriculum frameworks should explicitly articulate the developmental benefits of the arts, rather than positioning them solely as cultural enrichment.

FUTURE DIRECTIONS

Synthesis of Key Insights

This chapter has explored the intersections of art, neuroscience, and health psychology in the context of primary education. Evidence from neuroscience demonstrates that children's brains are uniquely plastic during the early years, highly responsive to enriched and multisensory experiences (Kolb & Gibb, 2011). Artistic practices—visual art, music, dance, and drama—stimulate neural connectivity, strengthen executive functions, and enhance socio-emotional regulation (Hardiman, 2016; Winner et al., 2013).

Health psychology contributes an equally critical perspective by framing art as a behavioural and cognitive intervention that fosters resilience, coping, and wellbeing (Taylor, 2020). Artistic engagement not only reduces stress and improves mood but also supports meaning-making, identity formation, and the cultivation of adaptive health behaviours (Malchiodi, 2020; Sonke et al., 2017). Together, these perspectives position art as a cornerstone of holistic education, bridging brushstrokes with brainwaves and integrating scientific insights with humanistic values.

Implications for Educational Practice

The practical implications of this interdisciplinary synthesis are profound. First, the arts should be recognized as central rather than peripheral to primary education. Instead of framing them as enrichment or extracurricular activities, schools should embed artistic practices across the curriculum. Such integration has been shown to improve academic performance, engagement, and self-efficacy, especially for disadvantaged learners (Deasy, 2002; Upitis & Smithrim, 2003).

Second, teachers require professional development in arts-based pedagogy. Many educators lack training in how to integrate the arts effectively, resulting in underutilization of these tools (Garvis & Pendergast, 2011). Equipping teachers with neuroscientific and psychological knowledge about the benefits of art can empower them to apply creative practices more confidently and intentionally.

Third, schools should adopt a preventive health psychology framework that uses the arts to support resilience and wellbeing before problems escalate. Classroom-based art-making can lower anxiety, foster prosocial behaviours, and build emotional literacy, thereby contributing to positive school climates (Kaimal et al., 2016; Rickard & McFerran, 2012).

Implications for Policy

Educational policy must evolve to reflect the growing body of scientific evidence supporting the integration of the arts into primary education. Despite compelling findings from neuroscience, health psychology, and educational research demonstrating that creative practices enhance cognitive, emotional, and social development, many high-stakes testing regimes continue to marginalize the arts, privileging narrowly defined academic subjects such as mathematics and literacy (Eisner, 2002). This approach risks narrowing the developmental opportunities available to children, as it overlooks the evidence that arts engagement can actively support and amplify academic success, rather than detract from it. Neuroscientific studies reveal that participation in music, visual arts, and drama strengthens executive functions, attention, and memory, while health psychology demonstrates that arts-based experiences foster resilience, emotional regulation, and adaptive coping strategies (Kolb & Gibb, 2011; Taylor, 2020). Taken together, these findings indicate that the arts are integral to a holistic educational framework that promotes both academic achievement and lifelong wellbeing.

Policy frameworks should therefore mandate the integration of creative practices as a core component of national curricula, ensuring that all students have equitable access to arts education. Funding mechanisms must support the presence of arts specialists in schools and encourage partnerships between educational institutions and community organizations, thereby expanding opportunities for children to engage in diverse artistic experiences. Equity-focused initiatives are essential, as access to the arts is often stratified along socioeconomic lines, limiting opportunities for disadvantaged populations to benefit from programs that enhance cognitive, socio-emotional, and cultural development. In addition, educational policies should promote inclusive practices, ensuring that children with special educational needs can engage in arts-based learning tailored to their strengths and abilities. Evidence indicates that thoughtfully designed interventions in music, drama, and visual arts can support children with developmental differences, including autism spectrum disorder and attention-deficit/hyperactivity disorder, fostering participation, skill acquisition, and wellbeing (Geretsegger et al., 2014). By embedding creative practices into policy frameworks, governments can foster resilience, wellbeing, and lifelong learning capacities at scale, creating educational environments that support the holistic development of all children.

Despite the robust evidence supporting arts integration, important gaps remain in understanding its full potential in primary education, highlighting several key directions for future research. First, longitudinal studies are needed to examine the long-term impacts of arts engagement on resilience, health behaviours, and academic achievement. While short-term benefits are well-documented, there is limited knowledge regarding the durability of these effects across developmental stages and their influence on adult outcomes (Masten, 2014). Second, much of the existing research is concentrated in Western contexts, leaving unanswered questions about the role of culture in shaping the meaning and impact of creative practices. Comparative studies across diverse cultural settings are necessary to elucidate how sociocultural norms, values, and pedagogical traditions influence the effectiveness and interpretation of arts-based interventions (Catterall et al., 2012).

Third, the emerging field of neuroaesthetics offers promising tools for understanding the neural mechanisms underlying creative experiences (Chatterjee & Vartanian, 2014). Applying neuroaesthetic insights to educational contexts can deepen understanding of how artistic experiences interact with cognitive, emotional, and social development, potentially informing the design of curricula that optimally stimulate learning and wellbeing. Fourth, research on the role of the arts in supporting inclusion and special educational needs remains limited. Studies examining how specific modalities, such as music therapy, visual arts, or drama, can be used to enhance engagement, learning, and resilience in children with autism, ADHD, and other learning differences are critical, as is investigation into scalable strategies for implementation in classroom settings (Corbett et al., 2014). Finally, the increasing incorporation of digital and hybrid tools in education presents new avenues for investigation. Technology-mediated arts experiences—such as digital storytelling, virtual reality art creation, and online collaborative music programs—may offer novel benefits for cognitive and socio-emotional development. However, systematic research comparing digital and traditional arts interventions is necessary to understand their respective impacts on learning, resilience, and wellbeing, and to identify best practices for integrating technology while preserving the embodied and social dimensions of creative engagement.

Policy development and future research are interdependent components of a comprehensive strategy to maximize the benefits of arts integration in primary education. Policies that prioritize curriculum integration, equitable access, specialist support, and inclusivity can create conditions that allow all children to experience the cognitive, emotional, and social advantages of creative practices. Simultaneously, longitudinal, cross-cultural, neuroaesthetic, inclusion-focused, and technology-oriented research is essential to refine our understanding of how the arts contribute to holistic child development. By aligning educational policy with scientific evidence and by expanding the research base, schools can cultivate environments that not only enhance academic achievement but also foster resilience, wellbeing, and lifelong capacities for learning and flourishing in children.

CONCLUSION

At the intersection of art, neuroscience, and health psychology lies a transformative vision for primary education, one that reframes creativity not as enrichment but as a core developmental necessity. The evidence synthesized throughout this chapter demonstrates that artistic engagement nurtures the developing brain, equips children with coping strategies, and fosters resilience and wellbeing. These benefits extend well beyond immediate classroom outcomes, shaping long-term health trajectories, socio-emotional competencies, and lifelong learning capacities. Far from being an optional extra, the arts emerge as essential foundations for holistic education in the 21st century.

A growing body of neuroscientific research confirms that the early years of life are characterized by heightened neuroplasticity, during which the brain is especially responsive to environmental stimulation (Kolb & Gibb, 2011). Artistic activities—whether drawing, music, dance, or storytelling—provide precisely the kind of multisensory, emotionally rich experiences that strengthen neural connectivity. For example, music training has been linked to improvements in executive function, working memory, and attentional control. Visual arts promote fine motor coordination, visual-spatial reasoning, and symbolic thought (Winner et al., 2013). Neuroscience thus makes clear that art is not peripheral but integral to cognitive and emotional growth.

Health psychology provides a complementary perspective by framing art as a behavioural and psychological intervention. Children's coping strategies, emotional regulation, and resilience-building capacities are directly shaped by opportunities for creative expression (Taylor, 2020). When children externalize emotions through drawing, enact scenarios through drama, or express rhythm through music, they are engaging in self-regulation and meaning-making processes that support mental health and wellbeing (Malchiodi, 2020). In this sense, the arts contribute to preventive health education, reducing stress and anxiety while cultivating adaptive strategies that children can carry into adolescence and adulthood.

Equally important are the socio-emotional benefits of artistic engagement. Creative collaboration fosters empathy, perspective-taking, and cooperative behaviour—skills that are increasingly recognized as crucial for both academic achievement and social cohesion (Eisner, 2002). By integrating the arts into classroom practice, educators provide children with nonverbal modes of communication that transcend linguistic and cultural barriers. This is particularly valuable in diverse classrooms, where creative practices offer inclusive spaces for children from different backgrounds or with special educational needs to participate fully (Geretsegger et al., 2014).

The implications for educational practice are profound. Teachers must be supported to view art not as an "add-on" but as a pedagogical strategy aligned with both developmental science and health promotion. Professional development is therefore essential, equipping educators with both the confidence and the theoretical grounding to embed artistic practices across subjects (Garvis & Pendergast, 2011). Arts-based learning is not about producing artists, but about cultivating creative, resilient learners who can adapt to challenges, regulate their emotions, and engage meaningfully with the world.

At the policy level, systemic change is needed to ensure that the arts are positioned as central to national curricula. Current educational systems, often shaped by high-stakes testing, risk marginalizing the arts in favour of narrowly defined "core subjects." Yet neuroscience and health psychology demonstrate that the arts directly enhance those very capacities—attention, memory, motivation—that underpin academic performance (Hardiman, 2016). Policymakers must therefore recognize the arts as investments in both academic success and public health. This includes funding arts specialists, forging school-community partnerships, and addressing inequities in access to creative experiences (Catterall et al., 2012).

Looking ahead, the future of primary education lies in interdisciplinary integration. As neuroaesthetics expands our understanding of how artistic experiences shape the brain (Chatterjee & Vartanian, 2014), and as health psychology continues to demonstrate the importance of resilience and coping in shaping life outcomes (Masten, 2014), the case for embedding the arts in education becomes ever more compelling. Digital technologies, too, are expanding the possibilities for creative engagement, offering hybrid spaces where traditional and innovative practices can meet. The challenge will be to ensure that these opportunities remain accessible, equitable, and grounded in evidence-based practice.

Ultimately, the arts provide more than creative enrichment—they serve as lifelines of resilience and meaning-making, preparing children not only for academic success but also for healthy, fulfilling lives. When viewed through the lens of neuroscience and health psychology, artistic practices reveal themselves as tools of profound developmental importance: tools that strengthen neural pathways, foster adaptive behaviours, and cultivate the inner resources children need to thrive. In this light, art emerges not as supplemental, but as a cornerstone of 21st-century education—a bridge between science and humanity, between brain and heart, between knowledge and wellbeing.

REFERENCES

Bandura, A. (1997). *Self-efficacy: The exercise of control.* W. H. Freeman.

Beaty, R. E., Benedek, M., Kaufman, S. B., & Silvia, P. J. (2016). Default and executive network coupling supports creative idea production. *Scientific Reports, 5*(1), 10964. DOI: 10.1038/srep10964

Burnaford, G., Brown, S., Doherty, J., & McLaughlin, H. J. (2007). *Arts integration frameworks, research and practice: A literature review.* Arts Education Partnership.

Camic, P. M., & Chatterjee, H. J. (2013). Museums and art galleries as partners for public health interventions. *Perspectives in Public Health, 133*(1), 66–71. DOI: 10.1177/1757913912468523

Catterall, J. S., Dumais, S. A., & Hampden-Thompson, G. (2012). *The arts and achievement in at-risk youth: Findings from four longitudinal studies.* National Endowment for the Arts.

Chatterjee, A. (2014). Neuroaesthetics: Brain at the intersection of art and science. *Perspectives on Psychological Science, 9*(2), 113–117. DOI: 10.1177/1745691613513468

Chatterjee, A., & Vartanian, O. (2014). Neuroaesthetics. *Trends in Cognitive Sciences, 18*(7), 370–375. DOI: 10.1016/j.tics.2014.03.003

Clayton, S. (2020). Climate anxiety: Psychological responses to climate change. *Journal of Anxiety Disorders, 74*, 102263. DOI: 10.1016/j.janxdis.2020.102263

Coholic, D., & Eys, M. (2016). Benefits of an arts-based mindfulness group intervention for vulnerable children. *Child & Adolescent Social Work Journal, 33*(1), 1–13. DOI: 10.1007/s10560-015-0431-3

Corbett, B. A., Gunther, J. R., Comins, D., Price, J., Ryan, N., Simon, D., Jenson, A., & Rios, T. (2014). Brief report: Theatre as therapy for children with autism spectrum disorder. *Journal of Autism and Developmental Disorders, 44*(2), 466–472. DOI: 10.1007/s10803-013-1883-0

Cox, M. (2005). *The pictorial world of the child.* Cambridge University Press.

Deasy, R. J. (Ed.). (2002). *Critical links: Learning in the arts and student academic and social development.* Arts Education Partnership.

Diamond, A. (2013). Executive functions. *Annual Review of Psychology, 64*(1), 135–168. DOI: 10.1146/annurev-psych-113011-143750

Diamond, A., & Lee, K. (2011). Interventions shown to aid executive function development in children 4 to 12 years old. *Science*, *333*(6045), 959–964. DOI: 10.1126/science.1204529

Eisenberg, N., Spinrad, T. L., & Eggum, N. D. (2010). Emotion-related self-regulation and its relation to children's maladjustment. *Annual Review of Clinical Psychology*, *6*(1), 495–525. DOI: 10.1146/annurev.clinpsy.121208.131208

Eisner, E. W. (2002). *The arts and the creation of mind*. Yale University Press.

Engel, G. L. (1977). The need for a new medical model: A challenge for biomedicine. *Science*, *196*(4286), 129–136. DOI: 10.1126/science.847460

Garvis, S., & Pendergast, D. (2011). An investigation of early childhood teacher self-efficacy beliefs in the teaching of arts education. *International Journal of Education & the Arts*, *12*(9), 1–15. DOI: 10.59236/ijea12n9

Geretsegger, M., Elefant, C., Mössler, K. A., & Gold, C. (2014). Music therapy for people with autism spectrum disorder. *The Cochrane Library*, *6*(3), CD004381. Advance online publication. DOI: 10.1002/14651858.CD004381.pub3

Hallam, S. (2010). The power of music: Its impact on the intellectual, social and personal development of children and young people. *International Journal of Music Education*, *28*(3), 269–289. DOI: 10.1177/0255761410370658

Hardiman, M. (2016). *The brain-targeted teaching model for 21st-century schools*. Corwin Press.

Immordino-Yang, M. H. (2016). *Emotions, learning, and the brain: Exploring the educational implications of affective neuroscience*. W. W. Norton.

Immordino-Yang, M. H., Christodoulou, J. A., & Singh, V. (2012). Rest is not idleness: Implications of the brain's default mode for human development and education. *Perspectives on Psychological Science*, *7*(4), 352–364. DOI: 10.1177/1745691612447308

Immordino-Yang, M. H., & Damasio, A. (2007). We feel, therefore we learn: The relevance of affective and social neuroscience to education. *Mind, Brain and Education : the Official Journal of the International Mind, Brain, and Education Society*, *1*(1), 3–10. DOI: 10.1111/j.1751-228X.2007.00004.x

Kaimal, G., Ray, K., & Muniz, J. (2016). Reduction of cortisol levels and participants' responses following art making. *Art Therapy: Journal of the American Art Therapy Association*, *33*(2), 74–80. DOI: 10.1080/07421656.2016.1166832

Kolb, B., & Gibb, R. (2011). Brain plasticity and behaviour in the developing brain. *Journal of the Canadian Academy of Child and Adolescent Psychiatry = Journal de l'Académie Canadienne de Psychiatrie de l'Enfant et de l'Adolescent, 20*(4), 265–276.

Lazarus, R. S., & Folkman, S. (1984). *Stress, appraisal, and coping*. Springer.

Malchiodi, C. A. (2020). *Trauma and expressive arts therapy: Brain, body, and imagination in the healing process*. Guilford Press.

Masten, A. S. (2014). Global perspectives on resilience in children and youth. *Child Development, 85*(1), 6–20. DOI: 10.1111/cdev.12205

Rickard, N. S., & McFerran, K. (2012). Lifelong engagement with music: Benefits for mental health and wellbeing. *Arts & Health, 4*(2), 132–142. DOI: 10.1080/17533015.2011.584884

Sonke, J., Rollins, J., Brandman, R., & Graham-Pole, J. (2017). The state of the arts in healthcare in the United States. *Arts & Health, 9*(2), 177–190. DOI: 10.1080/17533015.2016.1211283

Stuckey, H. L., & Nobel, J. (2010). The connection between art, healing, and public health: A review of current literature. *American Journal of Public Health, 100*(2), 254–263. DOI: 10.2105/AJPH.2008.156497

Taylor, S. E. (2020). *Health psychology* (11th ed.). McGraw-Hill.

Upitis, R., & Smithrim, K. (2003). *Learning through the arts: National assessment final report*. The Royal Conservatory of Music.

Winner, E., Goldstein, T. R., & Vincent-Lancrin, S. (2013). *Art for art's sake? The impact of arts education*. OECD Publishing. DOI: 10.1787/9789264180789-en

Zaidel, D. W. (2013). Neuroesthetics is not just about art. *Frontiers in Human Neuroscience, 7*, 730. https://doi.org/10

Chapter 7
Dienes Blocks as a Pedagogical Resource for Overcoming Math's Anxiety in Early Childhood

Andonis Zagorianakos
http://orcid.org/0009-0006-3002-6609
National and Kapodistrian University, Greece

ABSTRACT

Mathematics anxiety—feelings of tension, fear, or discomfort that hinder performance—often emerges during early childhood, shaping later attitudes toward mathematics. Addressing it early is crucial to foster confidence and positive engagement. Dienes blocks, as concrete manipulatives, transform abstract concepts into tangible, visual, and tactile experiences, enabling children to explore mathematical relationships in playful, low-stress contexts. This hands-on approach supports conceptual understanding, emotional regulation, and gradual transition from concrete to abstract reasoning. Collaborative and guided activities further strengthen social interaction and autonomy, reducing affective barriers. As inclusive, multimodal resources, Dienes blocks accommodate diverse learners, including those at risk for dyscalculia or language delays. By integrating cognitive, affective, and embodied dimensions, Dienes blocks offer a powerful pedagogical means to reduce early maths anxiety and nurture enduring engagement with mathematical learning.

DOI: 10.4018/979-8-2600-3085-1.ch007

1. INTRODUCTION

Mathematics anxiety is a pervasive and well-documented phenomenon that can profoundly affect children's learning trajectories, often manifesting as early as preschool and kindergarten (Dowker, Sarkar, & Looi, 2016). Defined as a tension, apprehension, or fear that disrupts mathematical performance, mathematics anxiety has been linked to avoidance behaviors, reduced working memory capacity, and impaired problem-solving efficiency (Maloney & Beilock, 2012). The early onset of such anxiety highlights the emotional dimension of learning—an affective landscape that shapes how children perceive, engage with, and make sense of mathematical phenomena. In early childhood, mathematics is not merely a cognitive subject but a lived, embodied, and affective experience. When the emotional dimension of learning is ignored, the child's engagement with mathematics becomes alienated from its intuitive and experiential roots, leading to early disengagement and long-term underachievement.

Within this context, phenomenology offers a compelling interpretative framework. Drawing upon Edmund Husserl's foundational work, phenomenology is concerned with the structures of experience and the ways phenomena appear to consciousness (Husserl, 1931/1970). Husserl's concept of *intentionality*—that consciousness is always directed toward something—implies that mathematical objects, too, are not encountered as detached abstractions but as lived experiences constituted through the child's perceptual and motor engagement with the world. For the young learner, mathematics unfolds within the *Lebenswelt*, or the lived world, through encounters with form, quantity, rhythm, and proportion in tangible, embodied contexts. Learning, in this sense, is not the passive reception of external knowledge but an active constitution of meaning through interaction.

Merleau-Ponty (1962/2012) extends this view by emphasizing the body as the primary site of knowing. For him, perception is not a detached act of cognition but an embodied relation to the world. Through gesture, manipulation, and movement, children constitute mathematical meanings pre-reflectively—before these meanings become codified in symbols or linguistic expressions. The act of touching, stacking, or comparing Dienes blocks is not a simple mechanical behavior; it is a lived synthesis of perception and cognition. The body functions as the child's first mathematical instrument, mediating the emergence of structure and quantity through action and sensation.

This phenomenological view stands in productive tension with cognitive and constructivist theories of mathematics education, which emphasize active knowledge construction. Yet phenomenology deepens this perspective by revealing the *modes of appearance* through which mathematical phenomena are experienced. As Zagorianakos and Shvarts (2015) argue, understanding mathematical learning phenomenologically involves grasping how intuition mediates the *objectification* of abstract structures—the process through which children come to recognize stable, shareable mathematical meanings. In this view, the Dienes block is not simply a representational aid but a *phenomenal object*, through which the child intuits the essence of number and operation. When a child groups ten unit cubes into a ten-rod, this act is not merely procedural; it is an intentional engagement through which the *essence* of place value becomes pre-reflectively intuited.

Zagorianakos (2016) further elaborates this process by analyzing the *intuition of essence* in learners' engagement with mathematical phenomena. Intuition, in the Husserlian sense, is not guesswork but a mode of direct apprehension of meaning as it is constituted in experience. For the young learner, manipulating Dienes blocks enables this intuitive grasp of relationships—between one and many, part and whole, unit and group. Before the child can verbalize or symbolically represent these relationships, they are already lived through embodied interaction. The hand's movement in assembling and disassembling blocks becomes a gesture of thought. Such phenomenological insights invite educators to attend not only to the child's verbalized reasoning but to the *kinaesthetic intentionality*—the sense-making expressed through bodily action and rhythm.

Husserl (1936/1970) viewed such intentional acts as the foundation for the constitution of scientific knowledge, emphasizing that all abstraction originates in the lived experience of the world. This principle challenges traditional didactic models that introduce mathematical symbols prematurely, detaching them from perceptual and bodily grounding. Instead, phenomenology calls for a return to the *things themselves*—to the immediate, lived experience of mathematical relations as they emerge in the child's activity. In early mathematics education, this implies that manipulatives like Dienes blocks serve not as mere teaching aids but as *phenomenological mediators* between perception and abstraction.

Recent contributions by Zagorianakos (2019a, 2019b) expand phenomenology's role in mathematics education by highlighting the methodological implications for both research and teaching. Zagorianakos (2019a) outlines a phenomenological methodology that situates observation and interpretation within the lived experiences of learners, emphasizing the importance of *epoché*—the suspension of preconceived notions—to access the authentic intentional acts of the learner. In practice, this means that educators must learn to "bracket" their own assumptions about how mathematical understanding should appear, and instead attend to how it manifests through children's spontaneous engagement with materials. Similarly, Zagorianakos (2019b) proposes that phenomenology can foster a radical change in attitude toward learners' misconceptions. From this perspective, what is often labeled as an error may, in fact, reveal a valid mode of experiential sense-making. When teachers approach children's mathematical reasoning phenomenologically, they recognize it as part of an evolving lifeworld of understanding, rather than as deviation from a norm.

A further phenomenological dimension arises from the affective and intersubjective dimensions of learning. Zagorianakos (2022), drawing on Husserl's and Vygotsky's legacies, reinterprets *perezhivanie*—the lived emotional experience—as a *radical Erlebnis* that unites cognition and emotion. Within manipulative-based mathematical activity, the affective atmosphere—the joy of discovery, the frustration of difficulty, the satisfaction of success—constitutes part of the learner's intentional field. In this sense, emotional experience is not ancillary but co-constitutive of mathematical understanding. Each encounter with Dienes blocks, each act of building, trading, or balancing, is imbued with affective valence, shaping the meaning of mathematics as lived and felt.

Consequently, addressing mathematics anxiety requires more than cognitive scaffolding; it demands a phenomenologically informed pedagogy that honors the intertwining of body, affect, and thought. The manipulation of concrete materials such as Dienes blocks situates mathematics within the child's lived world, restoring the connection between sensation and abstraction. Through these embodied encounters, children not only grasp numerical relations but also transform their relationship to mathematics itself—from fear and alienation to curiosity and agency.

Phenomenology thus provides a philosophical foundation for reimagining early mathematics education: one that attends to the lived quality of learning, respects the child's intuitive intentionality, and integrates emotion as a constitutive dimension of cognition. In returning to the experiential roots of mathematical meaning, educators may find in phenomenology both a method and an ethic—a way to see mathematics not as an external system to be mastered, but as a field of lived possibilities to be discovered through the embodied joy of learning.

The present chapter unfolds along these phenomenological and pedagogical lines. Following this introduction, Section 1 revisits the theoretical foundations of mathematics anxiety, highlighting affective, cognitive, and sociocultural dimensions that influence early mathematical experiences. Section 2 presents the conceptual framework of Dienes' theory of mathematical learning and its intersection with phenomenological perspectives, emphasizing the embodied and experiential nature of concept formation. Section 3 explores the phenomenological underpinnings in depth, drawing on Husserl's notions of intentionality and the lifeworld, as well as Merleau-Ponty's insights into embodiment, perception, and the pre-reflective structure of experience. Section 4 connects these philosophical ideas with empirical research and phenomenologically oriented studies in mathematics education, including those of Zagorianakos and colleagues, to illustrate how intuition, reflection, and objectification shape learning processes. Section 5 then translates these insights into pedagogical practice by presenting detailed examples of classroom applications using Dienes blocks to address mathematics anxiety through embodied, reflective engagement. Finally, Section 6 synthesizes theoretical and practical dimensions, offering implications for teacher education, inclusive pedagogy, and future phenomenological inquiry in mathematics education.

Overall, the chapter proposes that a phenomenological perspective—anchored in the lived, embodied experience of the learner—can illuminate how mathematical understanding and emotional well-being co-emerge in early learning. It argues that overcoming mathematics anxiety requires not only better instructional design but also a renewed sensitivity to the experiential and existential dimensions of learning mathematics. Through this synthesis of phenomenology and pedagogy, the chapter seeks to reposition early mathematical education as a deeply human enterprise grounded in perception, reflection, and shared meaning.

2. THEORETICAL FRAMEWORK

2.1 Phenomenology and the Lived Experience of Learning

Phenomenology, as articulated by Edmund Husserl (1931/1970), is the philosophical study of phenomena as they are experienced from the first-person perspective. Central to Husserl's approach is the principle of intentionality, the notion that consciousness is always directed toward something, constituting the meaning of objects in relation to the perceiving subject. In the context of early mathematics education, this perspective suggests that learning is not merely a passive acquisition of numerical facts or procedural skills, but an active, lived engagement with number, quantity, and relational concepts. Children develop understanding not solely through symbolic representation, but through their embodied interactions with mathematical materials. Each encounter with a manipulable object allows the child to experience mathematical relationships directly, integrating perception, action, and reflection in ways that purely symbolic instruction cannot achieve. The child's consciousness is continuously oriented toward these objects, exploring their properties and relations, constructing meaning through the dynamic interplay of perception, manipulation, and reflection. This approach situates mathematical knowledge within the child's lived experience, bridging the gap between abstract concepts and tangible reality.

Merleau-Ponty (1962/2012) extended Husserl's insights by emphasizing the body as the primary locus of perception and cognition. Knowledge arises not from abstract computation alone, but through sensorimotor engagement with the world. When a child manipulates a Dienes block—grouping ten unit cubes into a ten-rod or decomposing a flat into smaller units—their body actively constitutes mathematical meaning. These actions are not mere motions; they are intentional acts of understanding, in which perception, touch, and spatial awareness coalesce to produce cognitive insight. Dienes blocks, therefore, are more than tactile tools; they are mediators of embodied cognition, providing a concrete anchor for abstract concepts. The blocks transform the child's interaction into a lived mathematical experience, allowing numerical structures to be perceived, felt, and acted upon. In this sense, mathematical knowledge is inseparable from bodily experience: the hand, eye, and spatial reasoning work in concert to construct meaning, forming the substrate upon which symbolic understanding can later be scaffolded.

Zagorianakos (2016, 2019b) builds upon these phenomenological foundations, emphasizing the role of intuition and pre-reflective experience in mathematics learning. From his perspective, the intuition of the "essence" of a mathematical phenomenon emerges through embodied interaction. For example, when a child exchanges ten unit cubes for a ten-rod, they gain an intuitive grasp of place value before they can articulate it symbolically. This aligns with the Husserlian notion of intentionality: the child's consciousness is directed toward the Dienes blocks as intentional objects, exploring relationships between parts and wholes, and constructing meaning through perceptual-motor engagement. The tangible manipulation of the blocks allows children to experience arithmetic operations as living phenomena; they can see addition and subtraction enacted physically, which provides the pre-reflective foundation for later symbolic reasoning.

Recent research supports the relevance of this approach. Zagorianakos (2022) emphasizes the transformative potential of Vygotskyan perezhivanie, interpreted phenomenologically as radical Erlebnis, in which affective and cognitive experiences are inseparably intertwined. When children engage with Dienes blocks in collaborative play, their emotional experiences of success, error, and discovery are as crucial as the cognitive structures they are forming. The tactile engagement, combined with social interaction and guided reflection, creates a rich context for agency, resilience, and self-efficacy. These immersive, affect-laden experiences foster deep engagement, reduce anxiety, and cultivate an enduring sense of competence, illustrating that mathematical learning is both a cognitive and emotional process.

Classroom Example 1: In a preschool classroom, a teacher presents ten individual unit cubes to children and invites them to create a tower of ten. After observing the construction, she asks, "How many cubes are in this tower? What could we do to make counting faster?" Children physically trade the ten units for a ten-rod, witnessing a tangible transformation of quantity. Through this manipulation, the concept of grouping becomes embodied: children see, feel, and act upon the mathematical structure. Later, the teacher asks, "Can anyone show another way to make ten?" prompting reflection and multiple solution pathways. This sequence exemplifies the phenomenological principle that understanding arises from intentional bodily engagement, demonstrating how guided sensorimotor exploration fosters both conceptual insight and positive affective experiences in early mathematics.

Classroom Example 2: For addition, a teacher sets out two ten-rods and five unit cubes. She asks children to predict how many cubes are represented in total before they combine them. Children physically group the units and rods, exploring how smaller units integrate into larger quantities. When a child notices that ten units can be exchanged for a ten-rod, the class pauses to reflect on this transformation, emphasizing the embodiment of number operations. Through discussion, students articulate strategies, reinforcing the reflective dimension of their engagement. Here, the Dienes blocks mediate both pre-reflective understanding—through physical manipulation—and reflective reasoning, as children verbalize and compare approaches.

Classroom Example 3: In subtraction activities, children are asked to take fifteen units and remove seven. Using Dienes blocks, they trade ten units for a ten-rod, then remove seven individual cubes. This concrete action makes the concept of subtraction visible and manipulable, transforming an abstract operation into a perceptually accessible experience. The teacher prompts, "How many are left? Can we see it in another way?" allowing students to explore multiple representations. This not only develops arithmetic understanding but also encourages students to notice patterns and relationships, deepening both cognitive and embodied comprehension.

Classroom Example 4: Pattern recognition and multiplicative reasoning can be explored with Dienes blocks. Children are asked to create repeating sequences with rods and flats, such as a pattern of one rod followed by a flat. Through physically building and rearranging these sequences, they develop a sense of iteration, grouping, and scaling. The teacher guides reflection on "Why does this pattern repeat? How many units are in each sequence?" Students experience mathematical regularity as a tangible, lived phenomenon, linking embodied perception with abstract reasoning.

These examples illustrate how Dienes blocks function as instruments of intentional, embodied cognition, supporting both the pre-reflective intuition described by Zagorianakos (2016, 2019) and later symbolic reasoning. They demonstrate that mathematical understanding arises through dynamic interactions involving the body, the materials, and the social environment. By integrating phenomenology, constructivism, and embodied cognition, teachers can create learning experiences that are cognitively rigorous, emotionally supportive, and developmentally appropriate. In this framework, mathematics becomes a living, inhabitable domain: children actively construct meaning, navigate challenges, and cultivate curiosity and confidence. Dienes blocks thus serve not only as pedagogical tools but as mediators of the child's lived mathematical experience, aligning cognition, affect, and agency in the earliest stages of learning.

2.2 Phenomenology of Anxiety and Mathematical Engagement

Phenomenology also offers a lens for understanding the emergence of mathematics anxiety in early childhood. Heidegger (1927/1962, p. 230) conceptualized anxiety as a mode of being-in-the-world where the coherence of experience is disrupted. In the mathematical context, anxiety arises when symbolic representations become alien or disconnected from lived experience. The child encounters numbers and operations as abstract, unintelligible objects, resulting in frustration, avoidance, and diminished agency. From a phenomenological perspective, the child's intentional arc—the alignment of perception, action, and understanding—is fractured.

Dienes blocks intervene effectively in this rupture. By providing tangible, manipulable representations, these blocks re-anchor mathematical relations in the child's lived body. When a child decomposes a ten-flat into ten tens or constructs hundreds from tens and units, the abstract relationships become perceivable, manipulable, and controllable. This restores intentional coherence: the body perceives, acts, and reflects, facilitating comprehension while simultaneously reducing anxiety.

Classroom Example 2: A kindergarten teacher notices a child hesitating to engage in addition tasks. The teacher sets up a small problem with Dienes blocks: "We have seven units and add three more. Can you show me?" The child physically moves three cubes to join the seven, counts the resulting ten, and experiences success. The tactile, reversible nature of the blocks normalizes error and fosters a sense of mastery. Over repeated interactions, the child begins to approach symbolic addition with reduced apprehension, illustrating the phenomenological principle that embodiment mediates affective and cognitive alignment.

Empirical support for this approach has grown in recent years. McKinnon McQuarrie et al. (2014) demonstrated that first-grade children exhibiting heightened physiological stress responses—elevated heart-rate and cortisol levels—during mathematics tasks performed significantly worse on numerical assessments. Their findings indicate that mathematics anxiety manifests not only as a psychological state but also as a measurable neurobiological reaction. Likewise, Carbonneau et al. (2020) demonstrated that manipulative-based interventions improve numerical fluency while fostering positive emotional engagement, particularly when activities encourage reflection and peer interaction.

Such findings resonate with phenomenological accounts of learning, which view knowledge as emerging through embodied interaction with the world. From a Husserlian perspective, the child's perceptual engagement with concrete materials constitutes a *lifeworld* of meaning in which mathematical structures are first intuited. Likewise, Merleau-Ponty's notion of the body as the primary site of knowing underscores that number, order, and relation are not abstract entities detached from experience, but forms that arise within motor and perceptual intentionality. Integrating manipulatives into early mathematical activity thus becomes not merely a pedagogical technique but a phenomenological act: reconnecting the learner's bodily presence to the lived experience of quantity and form. In this way, embodied play may both mitigate anxiety and reestablish the coherence between feeling, action, and thought that underlies mathematical understanding. Zagorianakos (2019b) further elaborates how phenomenologically-informed observation can reveal the subtle shifts in children's affective states during manipulative interactions. In his studies, children exhibit increased gaze focus, sustained manipulation, and verbalized reasoning when exploring mathematical structures with physical materials. These behaviors indicate alignment of pre-reflective bodily intentionality with conscious understanding, suggesting that Dienes blocks function as both cognitive and affective scaffolds.

2.3 Pre-Reflective Bodily Intentionality, Constructivism, and Embodied Cognition

Merleau-Ponty's (1962/2012) notion of pre-reflective bodily intentionality underscores the idea that cognition is grounded in bodily engagement even before conscious reflection. For young children, the act of stacking, grouping, and exchanging Dienes blocks constitutes a pre-reflective enactment of mathematical concepts. Before articulating "I am making ten," the child's body has already explored, recognized, and internalized the grouping. This pre-reflective engagement provides the foundation for later symbolic reasoning and formal arithmetic understanding.

Constructivist theories reinforce this perspective. Piaget (1936/1952) and Bruner (1966) emphasize that children actively construct knowledge through interaction with the environment. Dienes (1971) operationalized these principles by designing blocks that enable enactive exploration, rule discovery, and progressive formalization. Children can build, dismantle, and reorganize blocks, gradually moving from concrete, hands-on engagement to abstract representation, all within a developmentally appropriate progression.

Classroom Example 3: In a first-grade classroom, children are tasked with representing the number 23 using units, tens, and flats. One child arranges two ten-rods and three units, while another experiments with alternative decompositions. The teacher encourages discussion: "How else could you make 23?" The children verbalize their reasoning, comparing structures. This guided reflection links pre-reflective bodily experience to conscious understanding, illustrating a seamless transition from enactive manipulation to symbolic cognition.

Embodied cognition research supports these pedagogical strategies. Barsalou (2008) and Glenberg (2010) argue that conceptual knowledge is grounded in sensory-motor experience; mental representations are inseparable from the perceptual and motor systems that initially scaffold understanding. In early mathematics, this implies that the conceptual grasp of addition, subtraction, or place value is enriched by physically interacting with Dienes blocks. Recent studies (McKinnon McQuarrie et al 2014) show that children engaging in manipulative-rich environments demonstrate improved working memory, spatial reasoning, and numerical fluency compared to symbolic-only instruction.

2.4 Summary of Theoretical Contributions

Combining phenomenology, constructivism, and embodied cognition provides a robust and comprehensive framework for early mathematics pedagogy, particularly when employing Dienes blocks. This integration foregrounds the child's lived experience, recognizing that mathematical understanding emerges through active engagement, bodily interaction, and reflective thought. The use of manipulatives such as Dienes blocks allows children to experience number, quantity, and arithmetic as concrete phenomena rather than abstract symbols, supporting both cognitive development and emotional resilience.

Several interrelated principles underpin this approach, guiding both the design of learning experiences and the teacher's facilitation of meaningful exploration.

Concrete Manipulation Before Abstraction. Physical interaction with Dienes blocks enables children to internalize numerical relationships and operational principles through enactive engagement. When children group ten unit cubes into a ten-rod, or construct a flat from ten rods, they gain an intuitive understanding of base-ten structures before formal symbolic instruction. This process exemplifies Husserl's principle of intentionality: the child's consciousness is directed toward the blocks as meaningful objects, where perception, touch, and spatial awareness coalesce to produce cognitive insight (Husserl, 1931/1970). Merleau-Ponty (1962/2012) reinforces this by emphasizing the body as the locus of cognition; the manipulation of blocks is an embodied act through which understanding emerges. Through repeated engagement, children develop a tactile sense of numerical magnitude, equivalence, and decomposition, establishing a foundation for subsequent symbolic reasoning. Recent research supports this approach: studies by Saccardo et al. (2024) indicate that manipulative-rich, play-based learning promotes not only procedural skill acquisition but also positive emotional experiences, especially for children prone to math anxiety.

Reflective Dialogue. Linking pre-reflective actions with conscious reasoning strengthens understanding and metacognition. Teachers facilitate reflective dialogue by prompting children to verbalize strategies, compare solutions, and articulate generalizations. For example, after constructing a tower of ten unit cubes and exchanging it for a ten-rod, a teacher might ask: "How did this trade change the tower? Can you find another way to make ten?" Such prompts transform concrete manipulation into a shared, reflective process, consistent with the phenomenological insights of Zagorianakos (2016, 2019) on the role of intuition in constituting mathematical meaning. Through dialogue, children recognize relationships, identify patterns, and explore multiple solution pathways, connecting bodily experience to symbolic representation. This approach ensures that understanding is not merely procedural but deeply conceptual, grounded in both perception and reflection.

Affective Safety. Emotional security is inseparable from cognitive engagement in early mathematics. Error positivity, low-stakes exploration, and playful interaction reduce anxiety and encourage persistence, curiosity, and resilience. Phenomenologically, affect shapes the child's experience of meaning: joy, surprise, and even confusion modulate attention, memory, and the construction of knowledge (Zagorianakos, 2022). Dienes blocks, by their tangible and manipulable nature, provide a safe environment for experimentation. Children can build, trade, decompose, and reconstruct numerical configurations, experiencing control over the mathematical world rather than passivity before abstract symbols. Research indicates that these affective benefits are particularly significant for learners with early signs of math anxiety, offering a scaffolded, emotionally supportive context in which competence and confidence co-develop (Maloney & Beilock, 2012; Saccardo et al., 2024).

Collaborative Learning. Peer interaction magnifies both conceptual and affective gains. When children work together to solve arithmetic problems, construct patterns, or explore multiplicative relationships, they negotiate strategies, articulate reasoning, and co-construct meaning. Phenomenologically, shared experiences influence perception and understanding; children observing each other's manipulations gain new insights into number relationships and alternative solution pathways. For example, in a classroom activity, one child may trade ten units for a rod while another constructs the same total using a different combination of units and rods. Through discussion and comparison, children internalize flexible strategies, reinforcing cognitive schemas while simultaneously developing social competence, patience, and collaborative skills (Siegler & Ramani, 2008; Zagorianakos, 2019a). Such engagement also exemplifies the Husserlian notion that meaning is not passively received but actively constituted within intentional acts that are socially and contextually situated.

Cross-Curricular Integration. Embedding Dienes block activities within broader contexts enhances meaning-making and supports the generalization of mathematical concepts. For instance, during a math-literacy integration task, children might construct towers of Dienes blocks corresponding to the number of letters in words, compare structures, count units, and graph totals. In a science-based activity, blocks can represent quantities of seeds planted in experiments, enabling children to visualize numerical patterns, measure growth, and predict outcomes. Art projects can incorporate block-based symmetry and patterning exercises. Such integrative approaches situate mathematics in real-world contexts, connecting embodied cognition with cognitive abstraction, and fostering engagement, motivation, and transfer of learning (Dowker et al., 2016; Zagorianakos, 2019b; Saccardo et al., 2024;).

Phenomenological Analysis of Error and Discovery. A key insight from Zagorianakos' work is that pre-reflective, embodied interaction with mathematical objects is inseparable from the child's affective and cognitive experience (Zagorianakos, 2016, 2019, 2022). Mistakes are not mere failures; they are informative phenomena through which children discover alternative structures, patterns, and strategies. When a child misaligns rods in building a base-ten flat, the subsequent correction is a lived experience that integrates perception, touch, reasoning, and emotion. The intentionality of the act—the directed awareness of quantity and relationship—is heightened by affective engagement. Teachers can scaffold these moments by prompting reflection: "What did you notice when the rods didn't fit as expected? How could we adjust them?" In this way, phenomenology illuminates how error functions as a generative mechanism for knowledge construction.

Expanded Classroom Examples. In one extended vignette, preschoolers are asked to model addition by combining two separate towers of unit cubes. They observe the resulting total, compare alternative combinations, and then exchange units for rods to simplify counting. The teacher facilitates reflective dialogue, prompting children to verbalize strategies and explore multiple representations. In a parallel activity, children explore subtraction by physically removing blocks from a structure and observing the remaining quantity. Through these guided, embodied experiences, students consolidate the link between action, reflection, and abstract understanding. Zagorianakos (2019, 2022) emphasizes that such observation of pre-reflective engagement is critical: teachers who notice subtle gestures, hesitations, or affective cues can tailor support to align with each child's developmental trajectory, enhancing both cognitive and emotional learning outcomes.

Recent empirical evidence underscores the efficacy of this integrated approach. Saccardo et al. (2024) found that children exposed to manipulative-rich, play-based learning exhibited higher engagement, greater resilience, and more positive attitudes toward mathematics, even among initially math-anxious learners. Zagorianakos (2016, 2019, 2022) further highlights that phenomenologically-informed observation enables educators to design experiences that synchronize bodily manipulation, reflective reasoning, and affective support, fostering an environment where early mathematical competence and confidence emerge simultaneously.

SECTION 3. PRACTICAL INTEGRATION AND PEDAGOGICAL APPLICATION OF DIENES BLOCKS IN EARLY CHILDHOOD MATHEMATICS

Integrating Dienes blocks into early childhood mathematics pedagogy requires a careful balance between theory and practice, one that honors the lived experience of the child while fostering deep cognitive, social, and emotional engagement. Drawing on phenomenology, embodied cognition, and constructivist principles, this section outlines a comprehensive framework for the effective use of Dienes blocks in classrooms, emphasizing intentionality, pre-reflective bodily engagement, affective support, and reflective reasoning (Husserl, 1931/1970; Merleau-Ponty, 1962/2012; Zagorianakos, 2016, 2019, 2022).

3.1 Embodied Manipulation and Concrete Foundations

The use of Dienes blocks in early mathematics instruction begins with concrete manipulation, grounded in the principle that cognition is deeply intertwined with bodily experience (Merleau-Ponty, 1962/2012). Children engage in hands-on exploration, physically grouping units into rods and flats, trading ten units for a ten-rod, or constructing hundreds from smaller components. This enactive engagement allows children to perceive numerical relationships in space, internalize the structure of base ten, and experience arithmetic operations in tangible form. From a phenomenological perspective, these manipulations are intentional acts of consciousness: each grasp, movement, or arrangement directs the child's awareness toward the mathematical object, fostering a meaningful relationship between perception, action, and understanding (Husserl, 1931/1970; Zagorianakos, 2016, 2019a).

In practice, teachers can design tasks that progress from free exploration to structured problem-solving. For instance, a teacher might provide a set of unit cubes and encourage children to build towers of varying lengths, observing patterns and counting aloud. Subsequent tasks might involve combining towers, exchanging units for rods, and decomposing rods back into units. This progressive formalization, first described by Dienes (1960, 1971), allows children to develop an intuitive sense of place value and numerical equivalence before introducing symbolic notation. Observational research supports this approach: when children physically manipulate numerical structures, they not only develop conceptual understanding but also experience greater confidence and agency, reducing early mathematics anxiety (Sowell, 1989; Carbonneau et al., 2013).

3.2 Reflective Dialogue and Metacognitive Scaffolding

While pre-reflective bodily engagement establishes foundational understanding, reflection enables transfer from action to abstraction. Teachers can scaffold reflective thinking through dialogic questioning, encouraging children to articulate their strategies, compare solutions, and generalize concepts across contexts (Bruner, 1966; Piaget, 1952). For example, after constructing a tower of ten units and exchanging them for a rod, the teacher might ask: "How did trading ten units for a rod make counting easier?" or "Can you find another way to make ten?" Such prompts cultivate metacognitive awareness, allowing children to link embodied action with symbolic reasoning.

Zagorianakos (2019b) emphasizes that reflection is not merely verbalization; it involves integrating pre-reflective bodily experience with conscious cognitive appraisal. In phenomenological terms, reflection bridges the lived experience of doing mathematics with conceptual understanding, creating coherence between perception, action, and symbolic representation. Classroom observations demonstrate that children engaged in structured reflection show increased flexibility in problem-solving, a more robust understanding of numerical relationships, and enhanced resilience in the face of challenging tasks (Saccardo et al., 2024; Zagorianakos, 2022).

3.3 Emotional Safety and Affective Engagement

A crucial dimension of Dienes block pedagogy is affective support. Early mathematics anxiety emerges when children perceive tasks as threatening or disconnected from their lived experience (Maloney & Beilock, 2012). Dienes blocks mitigate these risks by creating low-stakes, reversible learning environments. Children can make errors, experiment with different configurations, and explore solutions collaboratively without fear of failure. This aligns with phenomenological interpretations of anxiety as a disruption in the coherence of experience (Heidegger, 1927/1962): by grounding numerical operations in embodied action, manipulatives restore intentional coherence, allowing children to inhabit mathematical relationships confidently.

Classroom Example 1: In a preschool setting, children are asked to build towers representing numbers 1–10. When one child miscounts a tower, peers collaboratively discuss the discrepancy and rebuild the structure together. The teacher encourages dialogue about alternative configurations and validates all attempts, emphasizing exploration over correctness. Such error-positive environments foster emotional regulation, persistence, and a positive disposition toward mathematics (Beilock et al., 2010; Zagorianakos, 2022).

3.4 Collaborative and Socially Situated Learning

Social interaction enhances both cognitive and affective development. Peer collaboration allows children to model strategies, negotiate solutions, and verbalize reasoning. Phenomenologically, shared manipulation of Dienes blocks creates a space where multiple intentionalities converge: each child experiences the object, interprets relationships, and contributes to joint problem-solving. Teachers can facilitate structured collaborative tasks, such as group construction challenges or number composition games, which simultaneously reinforce arithmetic concepts and social competencies (Siegler & Ramani, 2008; Zagorianakos, 2016).

Classroom Example 2: Children work in pairs to represent numbers from 1 to 50 using units, rods, and flats. One child suggests decomposing a flat into rods, while the other proposes combining rods to form larger totals. Together, they discover multiple pathways to achieve the same number, discussing strategies and reasoning aloud. This co-constructed learning promotes both mathematical understanding and socio-emotional skills, including negotiation, empathy, and confidence.

3.5 Cross-Curricular Integration

Dienes blocks can be seamlessly integrated into interdisciplinary learning, linking mathematics with literacy, science, and art. Cross-curricular tasks situate numerical concepts within meaningful, context-rich activities, fostering transfer of learning and deep engagement (Dowker et al., 2016).

Classroom Example 3: During a literacy-math integration, children construct towers representing the number of letters in words from a storybook. They count units, trade for rods, and graph totals on a chart. This activity embeds numerical reasoning in a linguistic context, simultaneously developing spatial, counting, and representational skills. Children later discuss patterns and compare graphs, linking sensorimotor experience with analytical thinking.

Classroom Example 4: In a science-themed activity, children use Dienes blocks to model quantities of seeds, water droplets, or leaves. Through physical manipulation and collaborative discussion, they explore measurement, estimation, and grouping, reinforcing mathematical reasoning in a tangible, meaningful context.

3.6 Gradual Transition from Concrete to Symbolic Representation

A critical pedagogical principle is progressive formalization, which guides the transition from concrete manipulation to abstract representation (Dienes, 1960; Bruner, 1966). Initially, children engage fully with blocks, constructing, trading, and decomposing physical structures. Over time, these experiences are linked explicitly to numerals and symbolic operations. Teachers can scaffold this transition through reflective prompts, notation exercises, and verbal explanation, ensuring that the embodied foundation informs symbolic understanding.

Classroom Example 5: After several sessions manipulating rods and flats, children are introduced to numerals representing quantities they have constructed. They write "10" to represent a ten-rod and "100" for a flat, linking tactile experience with symbolic knowledge. Teachers encourage children to explain in their own words how rods and flats relate to units, reinforcing the phenomenological integration of body, perception, and cognition (Merleau-Ponty, 1962/2012; Zagorianakos, 2016).

3.7 Incorporating Technology Without Disrupting Embodiment

While Dienes blocks are inherently physical, digital technologies can complement hands-on experiences if used thoughtfully. Interactive tablets, digital simulations, or augmented reality overlays can enhance visualizations, provide adaptive challenges, and document student learning, without replacing the embodied experience. The key is maintaining sensorimotor engagement while leveraging technology to scaffold abstraction, reflection, and data analysis (Fischer et al., 2017; Zagorianakos, 2019).

Classroom Example 6: After constructing numbers with blocks, children photograph their arrangements and use a tablet app to create digital graphs, comparing totals across different constructions. Teachers facilitate discussion about similarities, differences, and patterns, linking physical and digital representations.

3.8 Teacher Role: Phenomenological Observation and Responsive Scaffolding

Teachers play a central role in this pedagogical framework, acting as phenomenologically informed guides. They observe children's pre-reflective actions, identify emergent understanding, and provide responsive scaffolds tailored to cognitive, social, and emotional needs (Zagorianakos, 2016, 2019, 2022). For example, noticing a child struggling to conceptualize "ten" as a unit of place value, a teacher might design targeted manipulative activities, prompt reflective discussion, or facilitate peer-assisted construction. Phenomenological observation enables educators to capture the rich lived experience of learning and intervene in ways that preserve agency, curiosity, and affective well-being.

3.9 Supporting Diverse Learners and Inclusive Practice

Dienes blocks are particularly valuable for differentiated instruction and inclusive classrooms. Children with diverse learning profiles—including working memory limitations, language delays, or heightened math anxiety—benefit from the multimodal, tactile, and visual nature of block-based activities. By providing multiple entry points into mathematical reasoning, teachers can scaffold learning at each child's level, allowing equitable participation, competence, and confidence-building (Carbonneau et al., 2013; Saccardo et al., 2024; Zagorianakos, 2019).

Classroom Example 7: A small group of children with varied abilities works together to represent numbers up to 50. Some children use unit cubes, others rely on rods or flats, and each child explains their reasoning in their own words. The teacher documents strategies and rotates materials to ensure everyone engages meaningfully, promoting cognitive accessibility and affective safety.

3.10 Summary

In sum, the practical integration of Dienes blocks in early mathematics classrooms exemplifies the convergence of phenomenology, constructivism, and embodied cognition. By prioritizing concrete manipulation, reflective dialogue, affective safety, collaborative engagement, and cross-curricular integration, educators create rich, developmentally appropriate experiences that foster both conceptual understanding and emotional resilience. Children's pre-reflective bodily interactions with blocks form the substrate for abstract reasoning, while reflective discussion, teacher scaffolding, and peer collaboration deepen understanding and social-emotional competence. When combined with carefully integrated technology, intentional scaffolding, and inclusive practice, Dienes blocks emerge as a powerful, multifaceted tool that supports early numeracy, reduces anxiety, and cultivates curiosity, persistence, and confidence in young learners.

SECTION 4. PEDAGOGICAL APPLICATIONS OF DIENES BLOCKS IN EARLY CHILDHOOD MATHEMATICS

4.1 Introduction

Bringing theory into pedagogical action requires translating abstract principles into tangible experiences that resonate with children's developmental and affective worlds. Dienes blocks—structured manipulatives representing base-ten relationships—offer a medium through which foundational mathematical ideas can emerge experientially rather than didactically. Their power lies not only in their physical composition but in their phenomenological potential: they enable learners to *live* mathematical relations through embodied interaction, reflection, and shared meaning-making.

Building on the theoretical synthesis of phenomenology, constructivism, and embodied cognition developed in the previous chapters, this section turns to practice. It explores how these frameworks converge within classroom environments that employ Dienes blocks to cultivate understanding, autonomy, and emotional security. Pedagogy here becomes an *intentional encounter*: a lived event where child and material co-constitute mathematical meaning.

The chapter demonstrates how educators can design environments and sequences that foster intuitive grasp, reflective reasoning, and affective balance. Each pedagogical dimension—from classroom setup to assessment—reflects a single guiding principle: that mathematical cognition emerges through intentional, embodied, and socially mediated action.

4.2 Designing Developmentally Appropriate Learning Environments

A pedagogical space that supports phenomenologically informed learning must embody openness, flexibility, and sensory accessibility. The arrangement of materials and the structuring of activities are not neutral choices; they constitute the very horizon through which the child perceives and enacts mathematics (Husserl, 1931/1970; Merleau-Ponty, 1962/2012).

A classroom that privileges exploratory engagement with Dienes blocks invites curiosity and collaborative discovery. Materials should be accessible—placed at child height, organized by color and size, and presented without prescriptive instruction. Such spatial design encourages the *intentional arc* of perception and action: children see, reach for, and manipulate objects according to self-generated hypotheses. As Zagorianakos (2019a) notes, the phenomenological horizon of learning is defined not by the transmission of content but by the structure of experience in which content appears as meaningful.

Teachers thus serve as *architects of possibility*. They shape an atmosphere that balances freedom and subtle guidance, ensuring cognitive challenge within emotional safety. Affective security—what Dienes called *playful mathematics*—allows learners to take risks, embrace reversibility of thought, and tolerate ambiguity. As recent work by Dowker et al. (2016) and Saccardo et al. (2024) confirms, such conditions reduce anxiety and heighten persistence in early numerical reasoning.

A practical example: In a reception classroom, materials are organized into zones—"build," "compare," and "record." Children choose their activity, constructing structures or patterns using Dienes blocks. The teacher circulates, posing phenomenological prompts ("What do you notice as you change this?") that draw awareness from pre-reflective manipulation to reflective articulation. This transition mirrors the movement from lived experience toward conceptual insight—a process central to both Husserl's intentionality and Vygotsky's perezhivanie as reframed by Zagorianakos (2022).

4.3 Concrete Manipulation and Progressive Formalization

Phenomenological pedagogy honors the body as the first site of knowing. In Dienes-based instruction, this principle aligns with Bruner's enactive-iconic-symbolic model, which charts a developmental path from action to representation to abstraction (Bruner, 1966).

When children handle Dienes blocks, they enact the *constitution of number*. The grouping of ten unit cubes into a rod or the decomposition of a flat into smaller parts are not mechanical tasks but acts of intentional synthesis. Meaning arises through doing: the child's perception of part–whole relations, weight, and spatial configuration coalesce into an intuitive sense of quantity.

From a phenomenological stance, each manipulation is a lived event through which the essence of numerical structure is intuited (Zagorianakos, 2016). The blocks thus become *intentional objects*—media through which mathematical essence is grasped pre-reflectively before being symbolized.

Progressive formalization involves guiding children from these sensorimotor intuitions toward explicit reasoning. Teachers facilitate this by encouraging pattern recognition ("What happens every time we have ten?") and by introducing symbolic representations only once they have emerged experientially (Zagorianakos, 2019a).

For instance, in a small-group activity, children trade ten unit cubes for a ten-rod, verbalizing what they observe: "It's still ten, but now it's together." Later, they record the transformation using drawn symbols or number sentences. This enactment of *eidetic variation*—seeing one phenomenon (ten) across changing appearances—reflects Husserl's (1931/1970) method of uncovering essential invariants.

Recent research supports such embodied-to-symbolic trajectories. Sarama and Clements (2019) show that manipulatives like Dienes blocks are most effective when children are prompted to connect physical configurations to conceptual structures, bridging enactive and symbolic cognition.

4.4 Integrating Reflection and Dialogue

Phenomenological pedagogy depends on cultivating reflection—not as afterthought but as co-moment of action. Reflection transforms manipulation into meaning by enabling learners to articulate and reinterpret their lived experiences (Zagorianakos, 2019b).

Teachers can foster reflective dialogue through open-ended questioning, encouraging children to describe processes rather than products: "What did you notice when you changed that?" "How is this tower different from the one before?" Such questions engage the *reflective intentionality* that follows pre-reflective doing.

Peer dialogue further deepens understanding by externalizing thought. When two children compare constructions—say, towers of eight and ten—they co-constitute mathematical relations intersubjectively. This shared intentionality (Husserl, 1950/1973) transforms solitary intuition into communicable concept.

An illustrative sequence: After free building, the teacher gathers children to observe two models—one made of a ten-rod, one of ten cubes. "Are these the same?" she asks. As children debate, they move between perceptual evidence and conceptual reasoning, arriving at equivalence through collaborative discourse. Such transitions from *Erlebnis* (immediate experience) to *Erfahrung* (conceptualized understanding) form the phenomenological backbone of mathematical reflection.

4.5 Fostering Affective Safety and Reducing Math Anxiety

Mathematical understanding in early childhood is inseparable from emotion. Saccardo et al. (2024) have shown that early negative experiences with number tasks can entrench math anxiety, limiting working-memory resources and suppressing exploratory motivation. Phenomenologically, anxiety constricts the horizon of possibility—it narrows what can appear as meaningful.

Creating an *affectively safe* classroom thus becomes a central pedagogical act. Dienes blocks support this by offering tactile feedback, visible reversibility, and collaborative play—conditions that restore agency and reduce evaluative pressure.

For example, during an addition game, children collectively build "number towers." Errors are not corrected but explored: "What happens if we add one more block?" Such framing reframes error as discovery. The physicality of Dienes blocks renders mistakes reversible—an embodied metaphor for conceptual flexibility.

Zagorianakos (2022) interprets this affective openness through Vygotsky's *perezhivanie*: the integration of emotional and cognitive dimensions in learning. Each successful manipulation carries an affective charge of achievement, anchoring abstract insight in lived joy.

4.6 Collaborative and Social Learning

Social interaction magnifies learning by transforming private intuition into shared understanding. Phenomenologically, this occurs through *intersubjectivity*—the recognition of others as co-constitutors of meaning (Husserl, 1931/1970).

Collaborative Dienes activities invite negotiation, dialogue, and mutual correction. When children collectively construct a "city" using tens, hundreds, and units, they must coordinate perspectives: agreeing on scale, comparing quantities, and resolving discrepancies. These processes mirror mathematical reasoning itself—systematic, relational, and communicative.

Zagorianakos (2019b) argues that such intersubjective exchanges constitute a phenomenological laboratory of consciousness: through the other's gaze and discourse, one becomes aware of one's own reasoning. Social play with Dienes blocks thus nurtures both cognitive and metacognitive awareness.

Siegler and Ramani (2008) found that structured peer interaction in early numerical games significantly enhanced number sense and symbolic fluency, supporting the pedagogical emphasis on collaborative construction.

4.7 Cross-Curricular Integration and Interdisciplinary Approaches

Embedding mathematical meaning in real-world contexts enriches conceptual transfer and motivation. Phenomenology insists that meaning arises within lived experience; thus, mathematics must appear as an aspect of life, not an isolated code.

Cross-curricular integration enables this synthesis. In a literacy–math activity, children build Dienes towers corresponding to the number of letters in their names, then compare heights and record results. The exercise connects numerical reasoning to identity, language, and physical embodiment.

In science, blocks can model atomic structures, ecosystems, or balance; in art, they form patterns and mosaics exploring symmetry and proportion. Each domain re-situates mathematics within experiential horizons, confirming Dowker et al. (2016) and Sarama and Clements (2019) on the benefits of contextualized learning.

Such integration transforms the classroom into a *lifeworld* (Lebenswelt) of mathematics, where numerical relations intertwine with linguistic, aesthetic, and ethical dimensions—a notion resonant with Zagorianakos's (2015, 2022, 2019b) exploration of phenomenological depth in educational experience.

4.8 Assessment, Observation, and Responsive Scaffolding

Phenomenologically informed assessment prioritizes *observation over measurement*. The teacher becomes a reflective participant, attending to children's gestures, hesitations, and affective cues as expressions of understanding.

Rather than relying solely on written tests, educators document the *process* of engagement with Dienes blocks—photographs of constructions, transcripts of dialogue, and reflective notes. These data reveal the evolving intentional structures of learning.

Zagorianakos (2019b) emphasizes that assessment should capture both the *objectification* of mathematical meaning and the *subjective horizon* of experience through which it unfolds. Teachers thus engage in what he calls *phenomenological attunement*: a receptive stance that aligns instructional scaffolding with learners' lived trajectories.

Example: A child persistently organizes blocks by color rather than value. Instead of correcting, the teacher observes and asks, "What does this pattern help you see?" Gradually, value and color merge in the child's awareness—a micro-phenomenon of conceptual transformation.

4.9 Digital Augmentation and Blended Approaches

While the essence of Dienes pedagogy is tactile, digital tools can extend opportunities for visualization and replay. The challenge is to preserve embodied intentionality while leveraging technology's flexibility.

Augmented-reality (AR) applications and tablet-based virtual blocks allow children to manipulate representations of Dienes sets, experiment with regrouping, and visualize equivalence dynamically. Recent studies (e.g., Kim & Lee, 2023; Nguyen et al., 2022) show that blended manipulatives enhance spatial reasoning and symbolic transition when paired with physical exploration.

From a phenomenological viewpoint, digital augmentation should not replace the tactile encounter but extend its horizon. Virtual environments can replay lived actions, enabling children to reflect on prior gestures—an echo of Husserl's *retention and protention* structure of time-consciousness.

Teachers can design hybrid tasks: children build with real blocks, capture the configuration on tablets, then annotate patterns or narrate reasoning. This integration maintains the corporeal root of cognition while fostering reflective abstraction.

4.10 Conclusion

The pedagogical application of Dienes blocks represents more than a methodological choice; it exemplifies a philosophy of learning grounded in embodiment, intentionality, and intersubjectivity. Through phenomenological insight, the manipulative transcends its material form, becoming a *medium of revelation*—a means through which mathematical essences appear to the child's consciousness.

Constructivism provides the developmental scaffolding, ensuring that action leads to abstraction, while embodied cognition anchors learning in perception and movement. Together, these perspectives yield a pedagogy that is cognitively rigorous, emotionally sustaining, and ontologically grounded in lived experience.

Teachers, as reflective practitioners, assume a dual role: they design conditions for discovery while observing the unfolding of meaning in real time. Their practice becomes phenomenological research—an ongoing inquiry into how number, structure, and relation are constituted through experience.

Ultimately, classrooms enriched with Dienes blocks cultivate not only numeracy but a sense of agency, curiosity, and aesthetic appreciation for mathematical form. As Zagorianakos (2016, 2019b, 2022) affirms, such experiences transform learners' horizons: mathematics ceases to be an external code to decode and becomes a lived mode of being-in-the-world.

SECTION 5. CHALLENGES, LIMITATIONS, AND RESEARCH PERSPECTIVES

5.1 Introduction: Re-examining the Limits of Phenomenological Pedagogy

While the pedagogical integration of Dienes blocks within phenomenological and constructivist frameworks has demonstrated significant potential, such approaches also face methodological, conceptual, and practical limitations. These challenges stem from the inherent tension between phenomenology's philosophical depth and the procedural demands of empirical educational research (Zagorianakos, 2019a). Translating phenomenological insight into classroom praxis—particularly in early mathematics education—requires confronting epistemological ambiguities: how can the lived experience of number, quantity, or relation be systematically observed, analyzed, and cultivated without reducing it to measurable behavior?

Phenomenology seeks to describe the *intentional constitution of meaning*, not to quantify it. Yet, educational systems often privilege measurable outcomes and standardized assessment. This mismatch between phenomenological intentionality and empirical validation represents a central limitation. As Zagorianakos (2016) emphasizes, the intuitive grasp (*Anschauung*) of mathematical essence cannot be fully operationalized without distorting its qualitative richness. Nevertheless, researchers and educators must strive to navigate this tension—developing hybrid methodologies that preserve the fidelity of lived experience while satisfying the evidentiary rigor expected in contemporary research.

5.2 Epistemological and Methodological Challenges

Phenomenological inquiry in mathematics education prioritizes *Erlebnis*—the lived, pre-reflective experience of the learner—as the origin of understanding. However, capturing this dimension empirically presents profound methodological difficulties. Observation alone cannot access the subjective intentional horizon in which a child constitutes numerical meaning. Even sophisticated qualitative methods, such as micro-ethnography or stimulated recall, can only approximate the lived experience retrospectively (Zagorianakos, 2019a).

This challenge is magnified when Dienes blocks are used with very young learners who may not yet possess the linguistic capacity to articulate their reasoning. Researchers must therefore rely on triangulated data—gesture, gaze, material configuration, and affective expression—as proxies for intentional meaning. Yet such data remain interpretive rather than definitive, demanding hermeneutic sensitivity rather than statistical certainty.

Zagorianakos (2015, 2019a) proposes a *phenomenological methodology of observation*, where the researcher brackets (in the Husserlian sense of *epoché*) preconceptions about correctness and instead attends to the learner's *mode of being with the material*. This reflective stance transforms observation from evaluation into *attunement*, aligning with the notion that knowledge arises from intersubjective resonance rather than external verification. Nonetheless, adopting such a stance in formal research contexts—dominated by performance metrics and accountability—poses institutional and philosophical challenges.

Another limitation concerns the phenomenological reduction itself. While powerful as a philosophical method, the *reduction* (the suspension of the natural attitude to examine experience as experience) may be impractical for teachers under real classroom conditions. Teachers rarely have the temporal or reflective space to perform reduction while managing 20 children simultaneously engaged in manipulative play. Developing professional-development models that train educators in "micro-phenomenological attention" (Petitmengin et al., 2019) may offer a pragmatic compromise, allowing teachers to cultivate reflective sensitivity without the full philosophical procedure.

5.3 Material and Contextual Limitations of Dienes Blocks

Although Dienes blocks offer powerful affordances for embodied learning, their physical design also introduces constraints. As fixed geometric units reflecting base-ten structure, they may inadvertently reinforce a rigid conception of number if not supplemented by open-ended exploration (Sarama & Clements, 2019). The phenomenological richness of the experience depends not on the material itself but on how it is *lived*. Without teacher mediation, children may focus on superficial aspects—color, size, or stacking—rather than the underlying mathematical essence.

Moreover, cross-cultural studies reveal that the conceptual resonance of Dienes blocks varies with linguistic and curricular contexts. In educational systems emphasizing rote counting, the blocks may be perceived as secondary "toys," not epistemic mediators (Nguyen et al., 2022). A phenomenologically informed pedagogy must therefore attend to the *lifeworld* (*Lebenswelt*) of each educational setting, ensuring that materials are embedded in meaningful social and linguistic practices.

Another challenge concerns the transition from tactile to abstract reasoning. While embodied engagement grounds early understanding, it can also create dependency on the concrete. Some children struggle to detach from physical manipulatives and generalize to symbolic representations (Mix et al., 2020). From a Husserlian perspective, this indicates an incomplete *eidetic reduction*—the learner has not yet grasped the invariant essence underlying varying appearances. Effective pedagogy must therefore facilitate "progressive de-embodiment," leading the learner from the perceptual to the conceptual without rupturing continuity (Zagorianakos, 2016).

Finally, logistical constraints—cost, storage, time, and teacher training—limit the widespread implementation of phenomenological manipulative-based instruction. As Saccardo et al. (2024) note, while manipulative-rich environments enhance engagement, they require sustained professional support to be pedagogically effective.

5.4 The Challenge of Phenomenological Generalization

A persistent critique of phenomenological approaches concerns their perceived lack of generalizability. Because phenomenology privileges the *particularity of lived experience*, its findings are often dismissed as anecdotal or idiosyncratic. Yet, as Husserl (1931/1970) insisted, *eidetic* knowledge—knowledge of essences—is general precisely because it transcends empirical contingency. The task, then, is not to generalize statistically but *phenomenologically*: to identify invariant structures of experience across different subjects.

Zagorianakos (2019b) operationalizes this in mathematics education by analyzing *learning episodes* to discern the essential structure of insight. In his studies of prospective teachers, the process of objectification—where intuition crystallizes into explicit concept—revealed consistent phases: perceptual engagement, imaginative variation, affective dissonance, and eventual synthesis. Similar patterns appear in children's interactions with Dienes blocks: manipulation, exploration of alternatives, momentary confusion, and the "aha" of realization. Future research can build on such micro-phenomenological frameworks to articulate generalizable phenomenological patterns without resorting to psychometric reductionism.

To strengthen validity, mixed-method designs can combine phenomenological description with process-tracing, eye-tracking, or gesture analysis, capturing how perceptual–motor activity corresponds to moments of insight. Such triangulation does not betray phenomenology; rather, it enriches its descriptive precision, bringing the *invisible intentional arc* into observable form.

5.5 Affective and Sociocultural Dimensions

Recent studies underscore that affect is not peripheral to cognition but constitutive of it (Immordino-Yang & Damasio, 2007). In phenomenological terms, every act of consciousness is affectively "colored." However, capturing this affective dimension in empirical work is notoriously difficult. Emotional states fluctuate rapidly, intertwining with task engagement, social context, and self-concept.

Zagorianakos (2022) reinterprets Vygotsky's *perezhivanie* as *radical Erlebnis*—a phenomenological unification of cognition and emotion within lived experience. Applied to Dienes pedagogy, this suggests that each manipulative encounter carries an affective tone that either expands or contracts the learner's horizon of meaning. Yet most classroom research isolates affect as an external variable (e.g., "math anxiety") rather than as an intrinsic structure of experience.

Future research must therefore develop methodologies that attend to affect phenomenologically. Video micro-analysis combined with teacher self-reflection could trace the affective rhythms of engagement—moments of frustration, surprise, delight—as indicators of learning dynamics. Similarly, participatory inquiry with children, using art or storytelling, can externalize emotional meanings embedded in manipulative play (Saccardo et al., 2024).

Socioculturally, implementing phenomenologically informed manipulative pedagogy requires reconfiguring classroom hierarchies. The teacher must shift from transmitter to co-experiencer, engaging children as epistemic partners. However, this egalitarian stance may conflict with institutional expectations for control, pacing, and curriculum coverage. Creating spaces for "slow pedagogy" (Clark, 2020)—where exploration unfolds at the child's temporal rhythm—is essential but politically challenging in high-stakes educational systems.

5.6 Digital Transformation and the Risk of Disembodiment

Digital technologies offer new possibilities for extending Dienes-based learning—through augmented reality, haptic feedback, and interactive simulations—but they also introduce risks of disembodiment. If poorly designed, digital manipulatives can sever the perceptual–motor loop that anchors phenomenological experience (Kim & Lee, 2023).

A critical research direction involves exploring *hybrid embodiment*: integrating physical and virtual manipulation while preserving intentional coherence. Zagorianakos's (2019) notion of *reflective mediation* provides a conceptual lens: technology should mediate, not replace, lived contact with materiality. Mixed-reality environments where children manipulate physical blocks while receiving real-time digital feedback exemplify this synergy, maintaining bodily intentionality while expanding representational depth.

However, ethical and accessibility considerations remain. Digital inequities can exacerbate educational disparities, and the data-intensive nature of emerging technologies raises privacy concerns. Phenomenological pedagogy must therefore align technological innovation with the ethical imperative to safeguard the learner's dignity and autonomy—a theme resonant with Husserl's later reflections on the *Crisis of the European sciences* (1936/1970).

5.7 Future Research Directions

To address these challenges, future inquiry should pursue the following complementary trajectories:

1. **Phenomenological Microgenesis:** Detailed analyses of children's moment-to-moment interactions with Dienes blocks, using slow-motion video and phenomenological transcription, could reveal the microstructure of mathematical insight—how gesture, perception, and affect intertwine in the genesis of number sense (Zagorianakos, 2015, 2019).
2. **Teacher Phenomenology:** Research should focus on the teacher's *lived experience of facilitation*—how educators perceive, interpret, and respond to children's emerging meanings. Such studies could inform professional development grounded in *phenomenological attunement*, complementing constructivist training.
3. **Comparative Embodiment Studies:** Longitudinal, cross-cultural comparisons could explore how different manipulatives (Dienes blocks, pattern blocks, digital hybrids) elicit distinct phenomenological structures of understanding. This

would bridge phenomenology and design-based research, uniting philosophical depth with pedagogical pragmatism.

Each trajectory must balance fidelity to lived experience with methodological innovation—an endeavor that reflects Husserl's enduring call for a "rigorous science of the lifeworld."

6. CONCLUSION

The challenges and limitations of phenomenologically informed pedagogy are not deficiencies but invitations to refinement. They compel educators and researchers to re-examine what counts as knowledge, evidence, and success in early mathematics education. When viewed through this lens, the use of Dienes blocks in early childhood classrooms transcends their typical instructional function and becomes a way of disclosing how children constitute mathematical meaning through embodied, affective, and intersubjective engagement. In doing so, such pedagogy shifts the focus of mathematics education from the transmission of pre-existing knowledge to the lived encounter between child and phenomenon — an encounter through which mathematical sense emerges not as something taught but as something experienced and co-constructed.

To see pedagogy phenomenologically is to acknowledge that mathematics is not merely an abstract system of symbols and operations but a human mode of being, rooted in perception, gesture, language, and relation. Children do not receive mathematical meaning ready-made; they constitute it through their bodily and social activity. Dienes blocks, as tangible and visual representations of quantity, structure, and relation, act as mediating artifacts in this process. Their value lies not simply in helping children "understand" mathematical concepts but in allowing them to enter into a relationship with mathematical phenomena. In handling, grouping, stacking, and rearranging these blocks, children are not following instructions; they are engaging in acts of inquiry. They feel the rhythm of pattern, they notice the harmony of structure, they sense correspondence between movement and number. Through this embodied and exploratory engagement, they begin to disclose mathematics as something belonging to their lived world rather than as an alien symbolic domain imposed from outside.

Such a stance transforms our notion of teaching. The teacher is no longer a transmitter of truths but a facilitator of encounters. Teaching becomes the art of arranging situations in which mathematical phenomena can show themselves to the child. It involves creating a space where children are invited to play, explore, and articulate their discoveries, while the teacher listens, observes, and gently guides reflection.

In this view, the pedagogical task is less about control and more about care — care for how meaning arises, how confidence grows, how curiosity unfolds. The use of Dienes blocks provides a particularly powerful medium for this kind of teaching because the blocks invite action, dialogue, and interpretation. They allow the teacher to see learning happening in real time: in gestures, in pauses, in shared laughter, in moments of confusion and resolution. Mathematics becomes a conversation rather than an evaluation, a lived process rather than a fixed product.

Phenomenologically informed pedagogy, however, does not offer an easy or straightforward path. It resists the simplifications of standardized instruction and demands a different kind of attentiveness from educators. Its first challenge is methodological ambiguity. Traditional pedagogies, grounded in behaviorist or constructivist paradigms, lend themselves easily to measurement: the teacher introduces a concept, the child performs a task, and success is measured by correct answers. Phenomenological pedagogy, by contrast, asks what it is like for the child to engage with a phenomenon, what inner movements and meanings accompany their actions, what kind of world is opened in that engagement. These questions do not yield easily to quantification, yet they are essential to understanding learning as lived experience. The ambiguity is not a weakness but an invitation to look more closely, to describe with precision the unfolding of meaning in children's interactions with materials, peers, and teachers. It calls for new kinds of documentation: detailed observation, narrative description, video analysis, reflection on gesture, and attention to the temporal flow of understanding.

The second invitation arises from the affective and embodied nuance of such pedagogy. When children manipulate Dienes blocks, they do so not only cognitively but emotionally and bodily. They experience delight, frustration, curiosity, satisfaction, hesitation. Their hands learn as much as their minds. A phenomenological stance requires teachers to notice these subtleties — the way a child's shoulders tense when uncertain, the moment their eyes light up when they perceive a pattern, the rhythm of their movements as they group or separate blocks. These micro-events are part of mathematical learning. They show how understanding is born in the interplay between body, material, and meaning. Yet, in most classrooms, such subtle dimensions are often overlooked in favor of overt cognitive outcomes. The challenge, then, is to cultivate pedagogical patience — to value the slow rhythms of discovery, to see uncertainty as productive, to resist the impulse to correct too quickly. By doing so, teachers honor the child's process of sense-making and allow confidence to grow organically rather than through external validation.

A related complexity concerns the transition from concrete to abstract understanding. One of the central insights of both Dienes' theory and phenomenological pedagogy is that abstraction must emerge from concrete experience. Children first meet mathematics through perception and action, not through symbols. However, the transition from handling Dienes blocks to manipulating numbers on paper must be managed carefully. If this movement is too abrupt, children may lose the sense of meaning that grounded their learning and anxiety may reappear. The teacher's role here is to weave continuity between the tactile and the symbolic — to help children recognize that the relationships they built with blocks persist in numerical form. This requires deliberate scaffolding, dialogue, and reflection: inviting children to describe what they did with the blocks, to draw it, to represent it with numerals, and to see the correspondences between these representations. The process cannot be rushed; it must respect the child's readiness to internalize the concrete experience as abstract understanding. This attention to pacing and continuity exemplifies the phenomenological commitment to remaining faithful to the child's experience rather than to external curricular demands.

The social and intersubjective dimensions of phenomenological pedagogy add another layer of invitation. Learning mathematics through Dienes blocks is seldom a solitary act; it unfolds in interaction with peers and teachers. The classroom becomes a small community where meaning is negotiated and shared. When two children manipulate blocks together, they co-constitute understanding through dialogue, imitation, and collaboration. Yet, these same interactions can also produce tension, competition, or withdrawal. Some children may dominate, others may hesitate to speak. The teacher's challenge is to cultivate intersubjectivity that supports rather than hinders sense-making — to facilitate conversations where each child's contribution is heard and valued, where curiosity is collective, and where mistakes are seen as opportunities for communal reflection. This requires skillful orchestration, sensitivity to group dynamics, and a commitment to relational pedagogy. The classroom becomes a site not just of cognitive growth but of ethical and emotional formation, where children learn to listen, to negotiate meaning, to care for each other's understanding.

Beyond the classroom, phenomenologically informed pedagogy raises questions about evidence, assessment, and accountability. In educational systems dominated by standardized metrics, it may appear difficult to justify approaches that privilege lived experience over measurable outcomes. Yet, to reduce learning to test scores is to betray its human depth. The phenomenological perspective insists that genuine learning includes changes in perception, attitude, and relationship — dimensions not easily captured by conventional assessments. The invitation here is to redefine what counts as evidence. Teachers might use observational notes, transcripts of dialogue, children's drawings, video recordings, and reflective journals to capture the evolving texture of learning. Assessment becomes descriptive rather than judgmental; it tells the story of how understanding grows rather than merely scoring its endpoint. In this way, evidence becomes a record of transformation, documenting not only what children know but how they come to know, how they move from fear to confidence, from confusion to clarity.

Scaling and sustainability pose further challenges. Phenomenological pedagogy, with its emphasis on attentiveness, flexibility, and dialogue, may seem ill-suited to large class sizes, rigid curricula, or resource-limited contexts. Providing Dienes blocks for every classroom, training teachers to observe and reflect phenomenologically, and allowing time for open exploration may appear impractical. Yet these obstacles are themselves calls for innovation. Schools and policymakers must rethink priorities, acknowledging that depth of learning cannot be achieved without attention to experience. Teacher education programs must include opportunities for prospective teachers to engage with manipulatives phenomenologically — to explore how meaning arises in their own embodied experience, to reflect on their affective relationship with mathematics, to learn to notice children's gestures and emotions. Professional development should emphasize reflective practice, collaborative inquiry, and documentation as forms of research. Equity, too, must be central: all children, regardless of linguistic background, cognitive profile, or socioeconomic status, deserve access to rich, embodied mathematical experiences. Manipulatives like Dienes blocks democratize mathematical access by reducing reliance on verbal or symbolic fluency and inviting multiple modes of understanding.

Through all these challenges, phenomenologically informed pedagogy demonstrates that education can be both empirically credible and existentially true. Empirically credible, because research has consistently shown that manipulatives enhance conceptual understanding and reduce anxiety; existentially true, because such pedagogy honors the child's lived experience of learning. When children manipulate Dienes blocks, they engage mathematics not as an external demand but as a phenomenon that belongs to their world. They see, touch, and move mathematical relationships; they feel the satisfaction of discovery; they share understanding with peers. The result is not only cognitive development but the formation of a mathematical identity — a sense of belonging in the world of number and pattern.

For the researcher, this convergence of the empirical and the existential opens new methodological possibilities. It calls for approaches that capture both the observable and the lived: mixed-methods studies that combine video analysis, gesture tracking, and affective observation with standardized measures of learning and anxiety. Longitudinal studies could explore whether early phenomenological experiences with manipulatives have lasting effects on mathematical confidence, identity, and achievement. Qualitative research could delve into teachers' own phenomenological awareness: how they perceive children's engagement, how their beliefs about mathematics evolve through embodied practice, and how their emotional presence influences classroom climate. In this way, research itself becomes a form of pedagogy — a process of learning from the lived world of the classroom, not imposing abstractions upon it.

What emerges from this synthesis is a renewed vision of mathematics education. Mathematics is no longer a detached body of knowledge to be mastered but a lived domain to be inhabited. The child does not merely learn mathematics but becomes mathematical — perceiving, acting, and communicating in ways that reveal structure and relation. Dienes blocks, within this vision, are more than teaching aids; they are bridges between worlds. They connect the child's lifeworld of touch, movement, and perception with the formal world of numbers and symbols. They allow abstraction to grow organically out of concrete experience, linking body and mind, feeling and thought. This reconceptualization restores to mathematics its human dimension. It reminds us that at its core, mathematics is an act of meaning-making, a way of orienting oneself in the world, a form of wonder.

The implications are profound. If educators accept this view, early childhood mathematics can become a domain not of fear but of joy. Anxiety, which so often shadows children's encounters with mathematics, can be transformed into curiosity through experiences of agency and success. When children see that mathematics is something they can touch and play with, something that responds to their actions, they learn to trust their own reasoning. They come to associate mathematics with discovery rather than judgment. Over time, this affective foundation may prove more important than any specific content learned, because it shapes lifelong attitudes toward problem-solving and learning itself.

To realize this vision, however, the educational system must be willing to embrace complexity. Phenomenological pedagogy cannot be reduced to simple formulas or quick interventions. It requires time, reflection, and commitment. Teachers must learn to observe before they instruct, to listen before they explain, to follow the child's line of inquiry before imposing their own. They must design spaces that invite exploration, tolerate ambiguity, and value process as much as product. Administrators must recognize that meaningful learning cannot always be accelerated or standardized. Policymakers must appreciate that qualitative growth — confidence, curiosity, agency — is as vital an outcome as quantitative achievement. Only through such systemic openness can phenomenologically informed pedagogy flourish.

The limitations of this approach, therefore, are the very sources of its vitality. Its methodological ambiguity challenges us to develop richer ways of knowing. Its affective nuance reminds us that learning is emotional as well as intellectual. Its demand for embodiment restores the body to education. Its insistence on intersubjectivity grounds knowledge in community. Its apparent impracticality calls forth creativity and innovation. Each limitation is an invitation — to refine theory, to redesign practice, to re-imagine what teaching and learning can mean.

Ultimately, to teach phenomenologically with Dienes blocks is to engage in an act of faith: faith that meaning arises in encounter, that understanding grows from lived experience, that the child's world is worthy of philosophical attention. As Zagorianakos (2016, 2019, 2022) has argued, genuine understanding arises not from external imposition but from the child's intentional meeting with phenomena. The researcher's and teacher's task is to honor that meeting, to describe without distorting the fragile emergence of meaning in the lived world of the learner. To do so is to participate in a pedagogy that is both scientific and poetic, one that measures without reducing, guides without constraining, teaches without silencing.

By embracing the complexity of this task — its methodological openness, its affective richness, its technological and material mediation — the field moves toward a pedagogy and a science of mathematics education that are both empirically credible and existentially true. Such a pedagogy recognizes that mathematics anxiety is not an inevitable feature of childhood but a symptom of alienation, of a disconnect between abstract symbol and lived experience. Through phenomenological engagement and the thoughtful use of tools like Dienes blocks, that alienation can be healed. Mathematics can become a space of belonging, where children encounter the beauty of structure, the play of pattern, and the joy of understanding.

The conclusion, then, is not closure but continuation. Phenomenologically informed pedagogy remains an unfinished project, constantly renewed in each classroom, each gesture, each act of discovery. It asks educators and researchers to see teaching not as the delivery of knowledge but as the co-creation of meaning, not as the management of anxiety but as the cultivation of confidence. Its limitations are its lifeblood, its challenges the conditions of its truth. To teach phenomenologically is to believe that every child's encounter with mathematics holds the possibility of revelation — that within the simple movement of a hand placing a Dienes block upon another lies the profound act of making sense of the world.

REFERENCES

Barsalou, L. W. (2008). Grounded cognition. *Annual Review of Psychology*, *59*(1), 617–645. DOI: 10.1146/annurev.psych.59.103006.093639 PMID: 17705682

Beilock, S. L., Gunderson, E. A., Ramirez, G., & Levine, S. C. (2010). Female teachers' math anxiety affects girls' math achievement. *Proceedings of the National Academy of Sciences of the United States of America*, *107*(5), 1860–1863. DOI: 10.1073/pnas.0910967107 PMID: 20133834

Bruner, J. S. (1966). *Toward a theory of instruction*. Harvard University Press.

Carbonneau, K. J., Marley, S. C., & Selig, J. P. (2013). A meta-analysis of the efficacy of teaching mathematics with concrete manipulatives. *Journal of Educational Psychology*, *105*(2), 380–400. DOI: 10.1037/a0031084

Clark, A. (2020). *Slow pedagogy: Learning in the rhythm of time*. Routledge.

Dienes, Z. P. (1971). *Building up mathematics* (4th ed.). Hutchinson Educational.

Dowker, A., Sarkar, A., & Looi, C. Y. (2016). Mathematics anxiety: What have we learned in 60 years? *Frontiers in Psychology*, *7*, 508. DOI: 10.3389/fpsyg.2016.00508 PMID: 27199789

Glenberg, A. M. (2010). Embodiment as a unifying perspective for psychology. *Wiley Interdisciplinary Reviews: Cognitive Science*, *1*(4), 586–596. DOI: 10.1002/wcs.55 PMID: 26271505

Heidegger, M. (1927/1962). *Being and time* (Macquarrie, J., & Robinson, E., Trans.). Harper & Row.

Husserl, E. (1931/1970). *Cartesian meditations: An introduction to phenomenology* (D. Cairns, Trans.). Martinus Nijhoff.

Husserl, E. (1936/1970). *The crisis of European sciences and transcendental phenomenology: An introduction to phenomenological philosophy* (Carr, D., Trans.). Northwestern University Press.

Immordino-Yang, M. H., & Damasio, A. (2007). We feel, therefore we learn: The relevance of affective and social neuroscience to education. *Mind, Brain and Education : the Official Journal of the International Mind, Brain, and Education Society*, *1*(1), 3–10. DOI: 10.1111/j.1751-228X.2007.00004.x

Kim, J., & Lee, H. (2023). Digital manipulatives and augmented reality in early mathematics education: Effects on spatial reasoning. *Journal of Educational Technology & Society*, *26*(2), 45–60.

Maloney, E. A., & Beilock, S. L. (2012). Math anxiety: Who has it, why it develops, and how to guard against it. *Trends in Cognitive Sciences*, *16*(8), 404–406. DOI: 10.1016/j.tics.2012.06.008 PMID: 22784928

McKinnon McQuarrie, M. A., Siegel, L. S., Perry, N. E., & Weinberg, J. (2014). Reactivity to stress and the cognitive components of math disability in Grade 1 children. *Journal of Learning Disabilities*, *47*(4), 349–365. DOI: 10.1177/0022219412463436 PMID: 23124381

Merleau-Ponty, M. (1962/2012). *Phenomenology of perception* (Smith, C., Trans.). Routledge.

Mix, K. S., Smith, L. B., & Ni, Y. (2020). The transition from concrete to abstract in early mathematics learning. *Developmental Review*, *57*, 100922. DOI: 10.1016/j.dr.2020.100922

Nguyen, T., Lee, J., & Wong, P. (2022). Cross-cultural perspectives on manipulatives in early mathematics classrooms. *International Journal of Science and Mathematics Education*, *20*, 1125–1144. DOI: 10.1007/s10763-021-10242-3

Petitmengin, C., Van Beek, M., Bitbol, M., Nissou, J. M., & Roepstorff, A. (2019). Studying the experience of meditation through micro-phenomenology. *Current Opinion in Psychology*, *28*, 54–59. DOI: 10.1016/j.copsyc.2018.10.009 PMID: 30502663

Piaget, J. (1936/1952). *The origins of intelligence in children* (Cook, M., Trans.). International Universities Press.

Saccardo, S., Clements, D., & Sarama, J. (2024). Manipulative-rich environments in early mathematics: Emotional and cognitive outcomes. *Early Childhood Research Quarterly*, *65*, 1–15. DOI: 10.1016/j.ecresq.2024.102044

Sarama, J., & Clements, D. H. (2019). *Hands-on, minds-on: Learning mathematics through manipulatives*. Routledge.

Siegler, R. S., & Ramani, G. B. (2008). Playing linear numerical board games promotes low-income children's numerical development. *Developmental Science*, *11*(5), 655–661. DOI: 10.1111/j.1467-7687.2008.00714.x PMID: 18801120

Zagorianakos, A. (2016). The study of the intuition of essence of a prospective teacher of mathematics from a phenomenological perspective. *Mediterranean Journal for Research in Mathematics Education*, *15*, 69–94.

Zagorianakos, A. (2019a, February). *A phenomenological methodology based on Husserl's work in the service of mathematics education research.* Paper presented at the Eleventh Congress of the European Society for Research in Mathematics Education (CERME 11), Utrecht University, Utrecht, Netherlands. https://hal.archives-ouvertes.fr/hal-02417428

Zagorianakos, A. (2019b). A phenomenological approach to the mathematical lived experience: Towards a radical change of attitude to students' (mis)conceptions. In Shvarts, A. (Ed.), *Proceedings of the PME and Yandex Russian Conference: Technology and Psychology for Mathematics Education* (pp. xxx–xxx). Moscow, Russia: HSE Publishing House.

Zagorianakos, A. (2022). The capturing of Vygotskyan perezhivanie as radical Erlebnis, through the analysis of a prospective teacher's learning episode. In C. Derouet, A. Nechache, P. R. Richard, L. Vivier, I. M. Gómez-Chacón, A. Kuzniak, M. Maschietto, & E. Montoya Delgadillo (Eds.), *Actes du septième symposium d'Étude sur le Travail Mathématique* (pp. 417–430). IREM de Strasbourg.

Zagorianakos, A., & Shvarts, A. (2015). The role of intuition in the process of objectification of mathematical phenomena from a Husserlian perspective: A case study. *Educational Studies in Mathematics*, *88*(1), 137–157. DOI: 10.1007/s10649-014-9576-9

Chapter 8
Equations of Stress: Visual Math and Well-Being in Primary Education With Cuisenaire Rods

Andonis Zagorianakos
http://orcid.org/0009-0006-3002-6609
National and Kapodistrian University, Greece

ABSTRACT

Primary mathematics education offers both opportunities and challenges, as stress and anxiety often arise from early experiences emphasizing rote learning and fear of mistakes. Mathematics anxiety in young learners stems from rigid, abstract instruction. Hands-on tools like Cuisenaire rods help children visualize concepts, reduce cognitive load, and build confidence. Activities involving addition, subtraction, multiplication, division, and fractions enhance understanding through play and collaboration. Storytelling and creative exploration make math meaningful and support emotional well-being. Low-pressure games and formative assessment foster differentiation and reduce stress. Inclusive, manipulative-based learning promotes equity and participation. Integrating visual, tactile, and reflective activities nurtures cognitive growth, emotional resilience, and a lifelong positive relationship with mathematics.

1. INTRODUCTION

Primary mathematics education represents a unique domain in which young learners encounter both remarkable opportunities for cognitive growth and significant challenges that may induce stress, frustration, and anxiety. Numerous studies

DOI: 10.4018/979-8-2600-3085-1.ch008

have documented that mathematics anxiety, characterized by feelings of tension, worry, and apprehension during numerical problem-solving, can emerge even in early childhood (Ashcraft & Moore, 2009; Dowker, Sarkar, & Looi, 2016). While anxiety can impede both learning and performance, early interventions using hands-on, visual, and creative pedagogical strategies have shown promise in reducing stress and fostering resilience. The present chapter explores how tactile and visual tools, particularly Cuisenaire rods, can be employed to facilitate both cognitive understanding and emotional regulation in primary classrooms.

Traditional mathematics instruction, which often emphasizes rote memorization, procedural fluency, and timed assessments, can exacerbate stress, particularly for children who benefit from concrete, kinesthetic, and visual representations (Boaler, 2016). By contrast, manipulative-based pedagogy allows learners to externalize abstract concepts, construct meaning, and explore relationships between quantities in a tangible way (Fosnot & Dolk, 2001). Cuisenaire rods, which vary in length and color, serve as ideal instruments for these purposes, providing a multi-sensory bridge between concrete experience and abstract reasoning. The rods can be used to model addition, subtraction, multiplication, division, and fractions, while simultaneously engaging students in play, collaboration, and reflection (Sarama & Clements, 2009).

Beyond cognitive development, mathematics learning is intricately linked to affective dimensions, including self-efficacy, confidence, and emotional well-being (Carey, Hill, Devine, & Szűcs, 2016). Hands-on visual mathematics allows learners to experience agency and mastery, mitigating the fear of mistakes that often underpins mathematics anxiety. Furthermore, embedding creative and collaborative activities within these lessons promotes social resilience, as children develop communication skills, negotiate strategies, and celebrate collective achievements. Reflective practices, such as journaling, drawing, or verbalizing problem-solving steps, provide opportunities for learners to articulate emotional responses to challenges, thereby cultivating self-awareness and adaptive coping strategies.

Research has consistently highlighted the role of early visual and tactile experiences in supporting numerical cognition and mathematical reasoning. Sarama and Clements (2009) emphasized that manipulatives provide children with concrete referents for abstract symbols, facilitating deeper conceptual understanding. Similarly, Kamii and Lewis (1993) argued that young learners often "reinvent arithmetic" through hands-on exploration, highlighting the importance of play and active construction of knowledge. These theoretical perspectives align with contemporary views on socio-emotional learning, suggesting that cognition and emotion are deeply intertwined in early mathematics education (Mix, Levine, Cheng, Young, Hambrick, & Konstantopoulos, 2016).

The present chapter advances this body of work by integrating a phenomenological perspective, drawing on Husserl's (1901/1970) conceptualization of intentionality and Merleau-Ponty's (1945/2002) account of embodied perception. By considering mathematics learning as an experience grounded in perception, action, and embodiment, the chapter emphasizes how learners' engagement with physical manipulatives fosters both cognitive and emotional understanding. In doing so, the chapter argues for a re-conceptualization of primary mathematics classrooms as environments in which well-being, conceptual development, and social collaboration are mutually reinforcing.

This chapter is organized as follows: Section 2 presents the theoretical framework, situating the study within Husserlian and Merleau-Pontian phenomenology and articulating principles of embodied learning. Section 3 elaborates on pedagogical applications, detailing how Cuisenaire rods can be employed in classroom settings to foster conceptual understanding, emotional regulation, and resilience. Section 4 discusses implications for inclusive and digital mathematics pedagogy, integrating phenomenological principles with contemporary instructional strategies. Finally, Section 5 (to be written later) provides concluding reflections on how a phenomenologically informed, hands-on approach can transform early mathematics education.

2. THEORETICAL FRAMEWORK: PHENOMENOLOGY, EMBODIMENT, AND MATHEMATICS LEARNING

2.1 Husserl's Phenomenology of Intentionality and Primary Mathematics

Edmund Husserl's phenomenology, particularly his foundational work on intentionality, provides a compelling framework for understanding early mathematics learning (Husserl, 1901/1970). Intentionality refers to the notion that consciousness is always directed toward something; mental acts are inherently relational, directed at objects, events, or experiences. In the context of mathematics education, this perspective underscores that learners' engagement with numbers, operations, and spatial relations is not a mere mechanical activity but a directed act of meaning-making.

For young children, abstract symbols such as numerals or operational signs initially lack intrinsic significance. They must be experienced, manipulated, and integrated into the child's perceptual world. Here, Cuisenaire rods act as intentional objects: their colors, lengths, and tactile qualities become focal points for directed attention, allowing learners to explore numerical relationships actively. For instance, combining a red rod (length 2) and a light green rod (length 3) to create a yellow rod (length 5) constitutes a lived experience of addition, in which the abstract operation is anchored in perception and action. Husserl's emphasis on the constitutive process—the ways in which consciousness constitutes meaning from experience—illuminates why such hands-on engagement is cognitively and emotionally potent.

Furthermore, Husserl's phenomenology highlights the temporal structure of experience: learning unfolds in the flow of consciousness, with retention, protention, and present awareness shaping understanding. In classroom practice, this implies that sequencing activities from concrete manipulation to symbolic representation, while providing opportunities for reflection and anticipatory reasoning, aligns with learners' temporal experience of understanding. Cognitive load is mitigated because learners can anchor complex mathematical relations in concrete, temporally coherent activities, rather than grappling prematurely with abstract symbols.

2.2 Merleau-Ponty's Embodied Perception and Learning

Maurice Merleau-Ponty (1945/2002) extends Husserl's phenomenology by emphasizing embodiment: perception, cognition, and action are inseparably intertwined. For Merleau-Ponty, knowledge is not purely abstract; it emerges from bodily engagement with the world. In primary mathematics education, this insight has direct pedagogical implications. Learners' understanding of numbers, spatial relations, and operations is scaffolded by sensory-motor interactions, gestures, and manipulation of physical objects.

The use of Cuisenaire rods exemplifies this principle. When a child constructs a tower of rods to represent the number 10, the act is not only a cognitive abstraction but an embodied negotiation of length, proportion, and balance. Gestures, visual alignment, and haptic feedback co-constitute understanding. The rod becomes an extension of the learner's perceptual field, linking touch, vision, and proprioception to conceptual reasoning. As Merleau-Ponty (1945/2002) emphasizes, perception is always already structured by the body, meaning that mathematics learning can be profoundly shaped by embodied activity rather than solely symbolic instruction.

Moreover, Merleau-Ponty's notion of the lived body implies that mathematics learning is affectively and socially situated. Manipulating rods in collaboration with peers fosters shared perception and intersubjective meaning-making. Learners communicate strategies through gestures, jointly negotiate solutions, and witness multiple perspectives on the same problem. Such experiences cultivate not only cognitive understanding but also social and emotional skills, including resilience, patience, and cooperative problem-solving.

2.3 Implications for Embodied and Multisensory Learning

Phenomenological insights suggest that primary mathematics instruction should prioritize multisensory, embodied experiences that foreground learner agency.

Cuisenaire rods are ideal in this regard because they allow children to engage simultaneously visually, tactilely, and kinesthetically. Learning activities can be sequenced to progress from direct manipulation, to discussion of strategies, to symbolic representation, thereby leveraging perception, action, and reflection in tandem.

In addition, phenomenology supports attentiveness to lived experience, including affective and emotional dimensions of learning. Mathematics anxiety can be understood not merely as a cognitive deficit but as a disruption in the learner's lived intentional engagement with numbers. By fostering meaningful, hands-on experiences where success and exploration are emphasized, teachers can help children reconstruct mathematics as an accessible, playful, and emotionally safe domain (Ashcraft & Moore, 2009; Boaler, 2016).

3. PEDAGOGICAL APPLICATIONS: EMBODIED EXPLORATION WITH CUISENAIRE RODS

3.1 The Perceptual Ground of Abstraction

A key challenge in early mathematics education is bridging the gap between concrete perception and abstract reasoning. Phenomenology offers a framework for understanding this process: abstraction is not detached from experience but emerges through structured, intentional engagement with perceptible phenomena (Husserl, 1901/1970; Merleau-Ponty, 1945/2002). Cuisenaire rods serve as ideal tools for this bridge, allowing learners to see, touch, and manipulate numerical and spatial relationships, making mathematical ideas tangible.

For instance, when a child combines a red rod of length 2 with a light green rod of length 3 to create a yellow rod of length 5, the act is simultaneously cognitive, perceptual, and motor. The learner anticipates the outcome (Husserl's protention), experiences the act of combining the rods (the present), and retains the visual and tactile feedback in memory (retention). This embodied process situates abstract operations such as addition in a tangible, lived experience, enhancing comprehension and reducing cognitive overload.

Teachers can further scaffold this learning by posing predictive challenges. For example, before combining rods, learners can be asked to guess the resulting length or to arrange multiple combinations that sum to the same total. This encourages reflection on relationships between numbers, comparison, and pattern recognition, aligning with phenomenological principles of intentionality and consciousness directed toward meaningful goals.

3.2 Supporting Arithmetic and Early Algebra

Beyond basic arithmetic, Cuisenaire rods provide a platform for exploring early algebraic reasoning. Through hands-on manipulation, learners can model unknown quantities, identify equivalencies, and experiment with relational thinking. For example, presenting two rods of different lengths and asking which combination equals a third rod introduces the child to an embodied experience of equations, such as $2+x=5$.

By physically manipulating rods, children can "solve" for x through trial, observation, and reflection, experiencing the equality concept concretely. This contrasts with traditional symbolic instruction, which may present numbers and letters in isolation, often increasing anxiety in learners with limited prior exposure.

Furthermore, arranging rods in repeated patterns fosters early understanding of multiplication and proportionality. A learner can physically place three red rods (length 2) alongside three green rods (length 3) and observe the total length as a product or combined sum. This tangible interaction grounds abstract arithmetic in perceptual experience, embodying Merleau-Ponty's (1945/2002) principle that cognition is inseparable from bodily engagement. By actively exploring these relationships, children develop a sense of agency and ownership over their mathematical reasoning.

3.3 Fractions, Ratios, and Partitioning

Fractions, ratios, and division often present particular challenges to early learners, as these concepts require reasoning about part-whole relationships. Cuisenaire rods can make these relationships perceptible and manipulable. For instance, if a rod of length 8 is subdivided by rods of length 2, children can physically see that four smaller rods constitute the larger rod, concretely illustrating the concept of 1/4 (one quarter). Similarly, ratios can be explored by arranging rods of different colors and lengths, prompting learners to notice patterns of equivalence and proportion.

Such embodied experiences foster conceptual clarity that purely symbolic instruction may struggle to achieve. Children can experiment, make mistakes safely, and adjust their reasoning, experiencing the temporal and intentional structure of understanding emphasized by Husserl. They are not simply memorizing rules; they are constituting meaning from action and perception, which is fundamental to resilient learning.

3.4 Integrating Play, Creativity, and Social Collaboration

A central principle of phenomenologically informed pedagogy is the integration of play and creativity into learning. When children use rods to create narratives, construct shapes, or design patterns, mathematics becomes a meaningful and emotionally engaging activity rather than a high-stakes evaluation. For example, children might be asked to represent a "mathematical story" using rods, arranging lengths to depict characters or actions while simultaneously performing calculations.

Collaborative work enhances this further. Group-based rod activities promote peer-to-peer learning, social negotiation, and intersubjective meaning-making, aligning with Merleau-Ponty's emphasis on perception as a shared and socially situated experience. Learners articulate strategies, resolve conflicts, and celebrate collective achievements, reinforcing emotional resilience, confidence, and persistence in problem-solving.

3.5 Reflection, Metacognition, and Emotional Regulation

Reflection is a crucial component of embodied mathematics learning. Phenomenology suggests that awareness of lived experience deepens understanding. Teachers can incorporate structured reflection activities, such as drawing or photographing rod arrangements and explaining their reasoning, writing brief journals about the steps taken to solve problems, and discussing alternative strategies with peers.

Such reflective practices allow learners to externalize their cognitive processes, link action to abstract reasoning, and recognize emotional responses to challenges. Reflection helps children develop metacognitive skills, fostering an understanding that mistakes are part of the learning process, and thus reducing anxiety. Over time, learners build emotional resilience, learning to approach mathematics as a domain for exploration rather than judgment.

3.6 Classroom Implementation: Structuring Rod Activities

Practical classroom strategies can integrate Cuisenaire rods systematically. Examples include:

- **Stations or centers:** Different manipulatives, including rods, allow learners to rotate among activities targeting addition, subtraction, multiplication, fractions, and pattern recognition.
- **Problem-solving tasks:** Present challenges such as constructing all combinations of rods that sum to a target length, prompting reasoning, creativity, and collaboration.
- **Game-based exploration:** Incorporate rods into simple math games, encouraging speed-independent play that reinforces conceptual understanding.

Teachers can scaffold these activities through prompts, questioning, and observation, always attending to learners' embodied engagement and emotional state. The combination of structured exploration and freedom to experiment embodies phenomenological principles, supporting both cognitive development and emotional well-being.

3.7 Extending Rod Use to Early Algebra and Pattern Recognition

As learners progress in their mathematical understanding, Cuisenaire rods can be used to introduce and explore early algebraic concepts through embodied and visual reasoning, thus developing a visually and kinesthetically grounded sense of algebra. When children manipulate rods to model simple equations, they physically represent relationships of balance, equivalence, and transformation. These tactile experiences allow them to perceive algebra not as a set of abstract symbols but as a dynamic system of relationships grounded in action and perception. By arranging rods into sequences or patterns, learners begin to recognize patterns, such as regularities, symmetries, and proportional relationships that mirror algebraic structures. This process cultivates an intuitive grasp of generalization and variable thinking, which are foundational to algebraic reasoning. Because the exploration engages both body and mind, it transforms potentially intimidating symbolic ideas into approachable and meaningful experiences. In doing so, it strengthens learners' confidence, nurtures flexible thinking, and fosters a deeper appreciation of mathematical structure as a coherent, discoverable system.

3.8 Summary of Pedagogical Principles

The use of Cuisenaire rods in primary education exemplifies several core principles grounded in phenomenological theory and constructivist pedagogy. At its foundation lies the principle of embodiment, emphasizing that learning emerges through perception, action, and bodily engagement with the world (Merleau-Ponty, 1945/2002). When children manipulate rods, they do not merely handle physical objects; they enact a process of meaning-making through sensory experience and movement. This embodied interaction transforms abstract mathematical relationships—such as equivalence, proportion, and number composition—into tangible, perceivable patterns that can be explored and discussed.

Closely related is the notion of intentionality, as described by Husserl (1901/1970), which posits that consciousness is always directed toward something meaningful. In the classroom, this means that learners focus their attention on specific tasks, outcomes, or relationships, constructing understanding through intentional interaction with materials and peers. Reflection deepens this process, as learners become aware of their own cognitive and emotional responses, linking perception to self-regulation and resilience. Through guided reflection, children learn to recognize strategies, manage frustration, and celebrate discovery.

Play and collaboration further enrich the phenomenological learning experience by situating mathematical exploration within a social and creative context. Through shared problem-solving, learners co-construct understanding, develop communicative competence, and experience mathematics as an inclusive, participatory practice. The gradual transition from concrete manipulation to abstract reasoning consolidates this process, as learners internalize mathematical structures once rooted in embodied activity. Ultimately, systematic engagement with Cuisenaire rods fosters not only conceptual understanding but also confidence, curiosity, and agency—qualities that sustain meaningful and lifelong mathematical learning.

4. IMPLICATIONS FOR INCLUSIVE AND DIGITAL MATHEMATICS PEDAGOGY

4.1 Phenomenology and Inclusive Mathematics Learning

Phenomenology, with its focus on lived experience, intentionality, and embodiment, offers a powerful framework for rethinking inclusive mathematics pedagogy. From a Husserlian perspective, cognition is grounded in conscious experience, while Merleau-Ponty emphasizes the inseparability of perception, body, and environment (Husserl, 1901/1970; Merleau-Ponty, 1945/2002). In the context of primary mathematics education, these insights highlight the importance of designing learning environments where all students, regardless of ability or background, can actively engage with mathematical concepts through perception and action.

Inclusive mathematics education involves ensuring that diverse learners—including those with neurodiverse profiles, learning difficulties, or limited early numeracy experience—can access, manipulate, and internalize mathematical structures meaningfully. Tools such as Cuisenaire rods provide a multisensory bridge between concrete experience and abstract reasoning, supporting learners who might struggle with symbolic notation or procedural instruction. By physically manipulating rods, learners embody mathematical relationships, fostering understanding through lived experience rather than relying solely on symbolic representation, which can often be exclusionary (Sarama & Clements, 2009).

4.2 Reducing Mathematics Anxiety and Promoting Resilience

Inclusive pedagogy also necessitates attention to emotional and psychological factors in learning. Mathematics anxiety is prevalent even in early primary education and disproportionately affects children from under-resourced or marginalized backgrounds (Devine et al., 2012; Dowker et al., 2016). Phenomenological principles suggest that anxiety is experienced through the body and perceptual engagement: tense posture, avoidance of eye contact, or withdrawal from manipulatives signal a learner's stress response.

Classroom interventions grounded in embodied mathematics can mitigate these effects. For example, arranging Cuisenaire rods collaboratively in small groups allows learners to approach problem-solving playfully, socially, and without fear of error. Reflection activities—such as drawing rod-based solutions or explaining reasoning orally—foster metacognition and self-awareness, helping children regulate emotional responses and recognize learning as a process rather than a high-stakes performance (Liljedahl, 2020). This approach aligns with Merleau-Ponty's understanding that perception and cognition are situated, embodied, and relational, meaning that inclusive strategies must account for the holistic lived experience of the learner.

4.3 Digital Tools as Embodied Extensions

Digital technology offers further avenues to implement inclusive and phenomenologically informed pedagogy. Interactive apps, virtual manipulatives, and augmented reality can replicate the tactile and visual affordances of Cuisenaire rods while providing adaptive support for individual learners. For instance, digital platforms can allow children to experiment with combining rods, exploring patterns, or modeling fractions in a low-pressure, manipulable environment. The interactive, responsive nature of digital tools supports intentional action and feedback loops central to phenomenological learning: learners perceive, act, and adjust their understanding in real time (Benson et al., 2022).

Digital tools also facilitate differentiation, enabling teachers to scaffold challenges according to learners' developmental level. Visual cues, dynamic feedback, and adjustable difficulty levels help students explore multiple representations—from concrete to abstract—while maintaining agency over their learning. Moreover, digital collaboration platforms allow learners to share rod-based constructions, exchange strategies, and reflect collectively, reinforcing the intersubjective dimensions of learning emphasized by Merleau-Ponty.

4.4 Equity and Accessibility Considerations

Implementing inclusive and digital pedagogy requires attention to equity and access. Learners from socioeconomically disadvantaged contexts may lack prior exposure to manipulatives, digital devices, or enriched home numeracy experiences (Devine et al., 2012). Educators must therefore provide readily available, high-quality resources, ensuring that both physical manipulatives and digital tools are integrated meaningfully in the classroom.

Inclusive practices also entail culturally responsive pedagogy. Rod-based activities can be contextualized in narratives, examples, and problem-solving tasks relevant to learners' experiences, supporting meaning-making and engagement. Digital environments, when designed inclusively, can allow multilingual support, visual scaffolds, and flexible pacing, helping students overcome barriers that traditional instruction may inadvertently reinforce.

4.5 Integration of Play, Reflection, and Digital Creativity

Phenomenological pedagogy emphasizes the dynamic interplay between action, perception, and reflection. Digital and physical manipulatives together offer a spectrum of embodied learning experiences. Children might first explore addition through Cuisenaire rods, then use a tablet application to visualize and animate rod combinations, followed by group reflection on patterns and strategies. Such integration promotes conceptual understanding, engagement, and emotional confidence simultaneously.

Creativity and exploration are essential. Learners can design rod-based "mathematical stories" in both physical and digital media, fostering imagination, collaboration, and agency. Reflection on these activities—through discussions, journaling, or digital portfolios—helps students recognize their cognitive and emotional growth, consolidating knowledge and reinforcing self-efficacy. By situating mathematics within playful, embodied, and socially meaningful contexts, learners develop resilience and a positive, enduring relationship with mathematics.

4.6 Teacher Practices and Scaffolding

Teachers play a pivotal role in shaping inclusive and digital pedagogy, serving as mediators between learners, tools, and the broader sociocultural environment. From a phenomenological perspective, learning emerges through embodied interaction with the environment and through intersubjective engagement with others. In this view, knowledge is not a static entity transmitted from teacher to student, but a dynamic process of meaning-making grounded in lived experience. The teacher, therefore, becomes both observer and participant, guiding students' sense-making through intentional scaffolding and reflective dialogue. By attending to how children perceive, manipulate, and interpret materials such as Cuisenaire rods or digital equivalents, educators can foster a more authentic connection between mathematical structures and children's experiential world.

In inclusive mathematics pedagogy, this phenomenological stance requires educators to design environments where all learners can access, explore, and express mathematical ideas through multiple modes of engagement. Teachers model strategies not only verbally but also physically, demonstrating manipulations of rods and visual representations in ways that highlight spatial, relational, and proportional reasoning. Such modeling bridges the gap between abstract concepts and sensory experience, allowing children with diverse learning profiles to anchor understanding in perceptual and kinesthetic activity. The verbal explanation accompanying the demonstration serves to link action with conceptual language, reinforcing both communication and comprehension.

Moreover, the encouragement of peer explanation and collaborative problem-solving deepens intersubjectivity—the mutual recognition of others as co-constructors of meaning. When children articulate their reasoning and listen to peers, they externalize thought processes that can then be negotiated, challenged, or extended within the group. This dialogic interaction supports the development of metacognitive awareness and empathy, as learners come to appreciate different perspectives and strategies. For children with special educational needs, such collaborative practices foster belonging and agency, ensuring that their voices contribute to the shared construction of knowledge.

Within digital contexts, teachers translate these embodied and social principles into technologically mediated experiences. Structured yet flexible digital challenges that mirror hands-on tasks enable continuity between physical and virtual learning. Interactive simulations, for example, can replicate the tactile manipulation of rods while offering adaptive feedback and accessibility features. Teachers curate these experiences to ensure that digital tools do not replace embodiment but extend it, maintaining the centrality of perception, action, and reflection in learning.

Finally, reflective prompts—whether delivered verbally, through journaling, or via digital platforms—invite learners to articulate not only what they learned but also how they felt during the process. This integration of cognitive and emotional reflection aligns with contemporary views of mathematics as an affective as well as intellectual domain. By foregrounding emotional awareness, teachers help students build resilience and a positive relationship with mathematics.

Through this multifaceted role, educators enact a pedagogy that unites inclusion, digital innovation, and phenomenological insight. They transform mathematics learning into an accessible, engaging, and deeply human experience, one that respects each child's individuality while nurturing collective understanding and equitable participation.

4.7 Summary

The integration of inclusive and digital strategies in mathematics education can be enriched through a phenomenological lens. Embodied tools like Cuisenaire rods, combined with interactive digital technologies, allow learners to perceive, act, and reflect on mathematical structures meaningfully. Attention to emotional well-being, equity, and social interaction ensures that all children can access and internalize mathematical concepts while developing resilience and confidence. Phenomenologically informed pedagogy thus transforms classrooms into spaces of intentional, embodied, and inclusive learning, bridging the gap between concrete perception and abstract reasoning, and fostering holistic development.

5. IMPLICATIONS FOR INCLUSIVE AND DIGITAL MATHEMATICS PEDAGOGY

Mathematics education stands at a crossroads between abstraction and lived experience. As classrooms become increasingly technologized and diverse, the challenge for educators is not merely to transmit mathematical knowledge but to cultivate a *felt understanding* of mathematics as part of the child's being-in-the-world. Through a phenomenological lens, learning mathematics becomes an inquiry into *how meaning arises* from embodied, perceptual, and social experience. This chapter has argued that phenomenology—grounded in Husserl's (1901/1970) account of intentionality and Merleau-Ponty's (1945/2002) notion of embodied perception—provides a transformative framework for inclusive and emotionally grounded mathematics pedagogy.

The journey from stress and anxiety to well-being and agency in mathematical learning begins with a shift in the teacher's gaze: from viewing mathematics as an external structure to be mastered, toward viewing it as a *phenomenon to be lived.* In Husserlian terms, the teacher practices a form of *epoché*, suspending preconceived notions of ability and progress to encounter mathematics as it manifests in the learner's consciousness. Every act of counting, arranging, or manipulating Cuisenaire rods becomes an expression of *intentional life*—a directedness of consciousness toward number, relation, and pattern. By attending to these acts phenomenologically, the teacher encounters mathematics as the child's own project of world-constitution.

5.1 Phenomenological Foundations for Inclusive Learning

Inclusive mathematics pedagogy demands attention not only to cognitive accessibility but also to the lived experience of learners, encompassing both emotional and perceptual dimensions. Phenomenology provides a conceptual framework for understanding how learners experience mathematical concepts through their intentional consciousness (Husserl, 1901/1970) and through embodied perception (Merleau-Ponty, 1945/2002). Husserl emphasizes that all cognitive acts are grounded in experience, suggesting that mathematical understanding emerges not solely from abstract symbols, but from the meaningful interplay between perception, action, and reflection. Merleau-Ponty extends this perspective by asserting that the body is the primary site of knowing, mediating the learner's engagement with objects and concepts in the world.

Within inclusive classrooms, these phenomenological insights translate into concrete strategies that enable all learners to perceive, manipulate, and internalize mathematical structures. Cuisenaire rods, as tangible manipulatives, exemplify this principle: they provide visual, tactile, and spatial experiences of addition, subtraction, multiplication, division, and fractions, allowing learners with diverse abilities to interact with mathematics directly and meaningfully (Sarama & Clements, 2009). By engaging the senses, learners are able to form embodied representations of abstract relationships, enhancing conceptual understanding while reducing cognitive load and mitigating anxiety.

5.2 Addressing Mathematics Anxiety through Embodied and Digital Practices

Mathematics anxiety is a significant barrier in primary education, particularly for learners from under-resourced backgrounds or with limited prior exposure to numerical reasoning (Devine et al., 2012; Dowker et al., 2016). Phenomenology suggests that anxiety is not only a cognitive phenomenon but a bodily experience: tense posture, avoidance behaviors, or hesitation during problem-solving signal the learner's stress response. By creating environments in which learners can explore mathematics physically and socially, educators can reduce these stress responses.

Hands-on manipulatives, such as Cuisenaire rods, facilitate low-pressure experimentation, allowing children to explore relationships among numbers, shapes, and patterns without fear of error. Incorporating digital extensions, including interactive virtual rods or gamified arithmetic tasks, provides additional opportunities for learners to engage with concepts repeatedly and adaptively, reinforcing mastery and confidence. Digital environments can offer immediate feedback, adjustable challenge levels, and multimodal representation, which support learners in perceiving and correcting errors in real time, in line with Merleau-Ponty's view of perception as active, adaptive, and situated (Merleau-Ponty, 1945/2002).

5.3 Multimodal Representation and Differentiation

Inclusive pedagogy requires attention to diverse learning modalities. While some learners grasp mathematical relationships most effectively through visual cues, others rely on tactile, auditory, or kinesthetic experiences. Combining physical manipulatives with digital tools allows educators to offer multimodal representations that cater to varied learner needs. For instance, learners may first manipulate rods to model a fraction visually, then engage a digital application to animate rod combinations, and finally use reflective journaling to articulate reasoning. This tri-modal approach promotes deep understanding, self-reflection, and metacognition (Benson et al., 2022).

Digital platforms also facilitate adaptive differentiation, adjusting tasks according to learner readiness. Interactive visualizations of rod arrangements, for example, allow students to explore relationships between sums and differences at their own pace. Incorporating scaffolded challenges, such as stepwise exploration of multiplication arrays or fraction equivalence, ensures that learners of different abilities can engage meaningfully, while also cultivating executive functioning skills, including planning, inhibition, and cognitive flexibility (Carey et al., 2016).

5.4 Collaborative Learning and Social Inclusion

Phenomenology highlights that learning is inherently intersubjective: knowledge emerges not solely from individual experience but through engagement with others in a shared world (Merleau-Ponty, 1945/2002). Inclusive mathematics pedagogy can harness this principle through collaborative exploration. Small-group tasks with Cuisenaire rods encourage learners to share strategies, articulate reasoning, and negotiate solutions, fostering both cognitive and socio-emotional development.

Digital environments extend collaborative possibilities: learners can construct shared virtual rod models, annotate problem-solving steps, and provide peer feedback in real time. These social practices support inclusive engagement, allowing learners who might otherwise struggle with verbal explanation or symbolic reasoning to participate meaningfully and contribute to group problem-solving. This approach not only strengthens mathematical understanding but also builds social resilience, empathy, and communication skills (Liljedahl, 2020).

5.5 Designing Culturally Responsive and Equitable Learning Environments

Equity considerations are central to inclusive pedagogy. Learners from diverse linguistic, cultural, and socio-economic backgrounds may face structural barriers to mathematics learning (Devine et al., 2012). By integrating embodied and digital strategies, educators can mitigate these inequities. Physical manipulatives are inexpensive, reusable, and immediately accessible, providing concrete experiences for learners with limited prior exposure. Digital tools, when used thoughtfully, offer multilingual support, adjustable difficulty, and alternative representation modes, broadening access.

Culturally responsive pedagogy further enhances inclusion. Educators can contextualize rod-based activities within learners' lived experiences, linking numerical exploration to familiar stories, games, or community contexts. Such practices help learners perceive mathematics not as abstract rules but as meaningful and relevant, reinforcing both engagement and self-efficacy. Phenomenologically, this approach acknowledges that experience is situated, and mathematical understanding emerges from interaction with the social and physical environment (Husserl, 1901/1970; Merleau-Ponty, 1945/2002).

5.6 Reflective and Metacognitive Practices

Reflection is a cornerstone of inclusive pedagogy. Learners who can articulate their thought processes, strategies, and challenges develop both conceptual understanding and emotional regulation. Activities such as drawing rod-based solutions, maintaining digital portfolios, or narrating problem-solving journeys encourage metacognition and self-awareness. Phenomenology emphasizes that reflection is an intentional act, connecting perception, action, and understanding (Husserl, 1901/1970). When learners reflect on their embodied manipulations, they consolidate abstract reasoning in a manner that is experiential and personally meaningful.

Teachers can scaffold reflection through guiding questions, peer discussion, and digital annotation tools. For example, a learner may construct a fraction equivalence model using rods, then use a tablet to simulate multiple configurations, finally reflecting in a journal how different combinations maintain equivalence. Such practices reinforce both cognitive and affective engagement, making mathematics accessible, enjoyable, and inclusive.

5.7 Integration of Physical and Digital Tools for Holistic Development

The combination of embodied and digital approaches provides a spectrum of learning experiences that supports cognitive, emotional, and social development simultaneously. Physical manipulation of rods grounds abstract concepts in perception and action. Digital simulations extend these manipulations by offering adaptive feedback, collaborative opportunities, and multimodal representation. Learners navigate between concrete, virtual, and reflective spaces, developing flexible problem-solving skills while strengthening their self-concept and resilience.

Inclusive mathematics pedagogy, therefore, requires intentional integration of physical manipulatives, digital technologies, and reflective practices. By embedding these strategies within a phenomenological framework, educators create environments in which all learners—regardless of prior experience, ability, or background—can engage deeply, explore creatively, and achieve meaningful understanding.

5.8 Teacher Roles and Scaffolding in Inclusive Digital Environments

Educators are central to the successful integration of phenomenological, inclusive, and digital approaches to mathematics learning. From a phenomenological standpoint, teaching is not a neutral act of delivering content but an intentional process of perceiving, interpreting, and responding to learners' lived experiences. Guided intentionality—a key concept in phenomenology—underscores that teachers must remain attuned to how children experience mathematical phenomena through their bodies, senses, and social interactions. Learning, in this view, arises from the dynamic interplay between perception and action, and it is through these encounters that understanding takes shape. The teacher's role, therefore, is to create conditions that allow such embodied inquiry to unfold meaningfully for all learners, ensuring that mathematics remains both accessible and experientially rich.

In practice, educators achieve this by demonstrating and modeling manipulations of Cuisenaire rods while simultaneously verbalizing their reasoning. This dual mode of communication—physical and linguistic—connects movement to meaning and supports the formation of conceptual bridges between concrete experiences and abstract relationships. When teachers encourage collaborative dialogue and peer scaffolding, they promote intersubjective learning, where ideas are shared, contested, and refined through interaction. Such exchanges help children develop not only mathematical reasoning but also social awareness, empathy, and confidence. In inclusive settings, this peer-oriented dynamic is particularly powerful, as it affirms the value of every contribution and nurtures a sense of collective agency.

Digital environments further extend these pedagogical intentions. When educators integrate digital tasks that replicate embodied experiences—such as manipulating virtual rods or constructing patterns in interactive applications—they provide learners with multimodal opportunities to explore mathematical structures. The continuity between physical and virtual experience reinforces the unity of perception, thought, and action, enabling diverse learners to engage with content in personally meaningful ways. Teachers can then offer reflection prompts that invite students to consider both cognitive and emotional aspects of learning, fostering self-awareness and metacognition.

By continually adjusting challenges to accommodate different abilities and developmental stages, educators ensure that every learner experiences success and agency. This responsive and situated pedagogy embodies Merleau-Ponty's (1945/2002) insight that cognition is not detached or purely mental but relational, embodied, and embedded in the world. Through these interwoven practices, teachers cultivate classrooms where exploration, error, and discovery are integral to mathematical understanding, sustaining an inclusive learning culture that values process over performance and growth over correctness.

5.9 Conclusion

In conclusion, inclusive and digital mathematics pedagogy benefits profoundly from a phenomenological framework. Ultimately, the phenomenological reframing of mathematics pedagogy transforms the question from "How can we teach mathematical content?" to "How can learners come to see mathematical structure in the world they inhabit?" The answer lies in cultivating perception, reflection, and dialogue—dimensions embodied in every Cuisenaire rod placed, every relation perceived, every meaning shared. Such education, rooted in the lived body and open to difference, constitutes not only inclusive mathematics but a pedagogy of humanity itself. By integrating Cuisenaire rods, digital tools, collaborative strategies, and reflective practices, educators create learning environments where perception, action, and understanding are interconnected. These approaches reduce mathematics anxiety, support diverse learning needs, and cultivate both cognitive competence and emotional resilience. Phenomenologically informed pedagogy ensures that mathematics is experiential, meaningful, and inclusive, bridging the gap between concrete and abstract reasoning, and promoting holistic development for all learners.

6. CHALLENGES, LIMITATIONS, AND RESEARCH PERSPECTIVES

Despite the substantial pedagogical promise of integrating Cuisenaire rods and digital tools within phenomenologically grounded mathematics education, several challenges and limitations must be acknowledged. These pertain to practical constraints in classroom implementation, variability in teacher expertise, technological infrastructure, learner differences, and the broader research landscape. Addressing these challenges is critical for advancing both inclusive practice and theoretical understanding.

6.1 Practical and Logistical Constraints

One of the most salient challenges relates to the practical realities of classroom management. While Cuisenaire rods provide an accessible, concrete representation of mathematical concepts, their effective use requires careful planning, sufficient quantities, and organized storage systems. Large primary classrooms may face limitations in distributing manipulatives equitably, resulting in potential inequities in participation (Sarama & Clements, 2009). Furthermore, transitions between whole-class instruction, small-group activities, and individual exploration can be time-consuming and require explicit routines. Phenomenologically, these logistical considerations intersect with learners' lived experience: disruptions or delays in hands-on activity can diminish engagement and interfere with the embodied perception-action loops that are central to learning (Merleau-Ponty, 1945/2002).

Digital integration compounds these challenges. While interactive applications and virtual manipulatives offer significant affordances for exploration, not all classrooms possess the necessary technological infrastructure, such as tablets, high-speed internet, or adaptive input devices. Even where technology is available, technical issues, device maintenance, and software compatibility can disrupt the flow of learning. Teachers must therefore develop contingency strategies that maintain pedagogical continuity while ensuring that all learners can participate meaningfully.

6.2 Teacher Expertise and Professional Development

The effectiveness of embodied and digital pedagogy is closely linked to teacher knowledge and pedagogical skill. Research consistently shows that teachers' beliefs, familiarity with manipulatives, and comfort with digital tools influence the quality of implementation and student outcomes (Boaler, 2016; Benson et al., 2022). In phenomenological terms, the teacher's presence mediates the students' perception and engagement; the ability to guide attention, scaffold exploration, and articulate connections between concrete and abstract concepts is essential (Husserl, 1901/1970).

Professional development programs that focus exclusively on content knowledge without addressing experiential, embodied, and reflective aspects of mathematics learning may inadequately prepare teachers for this pedagogical approach. In addition, integrating inclusive and culturally responsive practices requires nuanced understanding of learner diversity, socio-emotional factors, and equity issues. Teacher training must therefore encompass not only technical proficiency with Cuisenaire rods and digital tools but also phenomenologically informed strategies that foreground lived experience, intersubjectivity, and embodied reasoning.

6.3 Learner Variability and Cognitive Differences

While Cuisenaire rods and digital manipulatives support multisensory learning, learners differ in cognitive, perceptual, and emotional profiles, which can impact engagement and efficacy. For example, children with fine motor challenges may struggle to manipulate rods effectively, while others may encounter difficulties in mapping spatial representations onto symbolic mathematics. Students with high mathematics anxiety or low self-efficacy may require additional scaffolding and emotional support to benefit fully from open-ended explorations (Ashcraft & Moore, 2009; Dowker et al., 2016).

Phenomenologically, each learner's experience of mathematics is uniquely situated, shaped by prior experiences, perceptual tendencies, and social interactions (Merleau-Ponty, 1945/2002). Inclusive pedagogy demands adaptive strategies that respect these differences. Teachers must observe and respond to subtle cues—gestures, facial expressions, engagement patterns—to maintain a supportive environment that fosters competence and resilience. This attention to lived experience is especially critical in digital contexts, where screen-mediated interaction can reduce opportunities for embodied and intersubjective engagement.

6.4 Equity and Access Considerations

Equity remains a persistent challenge in both physical and digital implementations. Students from under-resourced schools may lack access to sufficient manipulatives, devices, or high-quality instructional support, exacerbating existing disparities in mathematics achievement (Devine et al., 2012). Digital tools, while offering potential for personalization and scaffolding, may inadvertently privilege students with greater technological familiarity or home access to devices and internet connectivity. Phenomenologically, inequitable access alters the nature of learners' lived experience of mathematics, potentially restricting the embodiment of concepts and limiting opportunities for meaningful exploration.

Strategies to address these disparities include pooling resources, integrating low-cost or recycled materials, leveraging shared devices, and designing lessons that allow alternating physical and digital engagement. Additionally, culturally responsive pedagogy can enhance relevance and motivation, ensuring that learners' experiences, values, and contexts are recognized in the design of mathematical problems.

6.5 Assessment Challenges

Assessment within phenomenologically informed, hands-on mathematics pedagogy presents its own set of complexities. Traditional summative assessments often emphasize symbolic computation, speed, and procedural correctness, which may not capture the depth of understanding achieved through embodied, exploratory learning (Fosnot & Dolk, 2001). Formative assessment, including observation, reflective journals, collaborative discussions, and digital activity logs, aligns more closely with phenomenological principles by attending to learners' processes, strategies, and embodied engagement.

However, implementing formative assessment effectively requires substantial teacher expertise, time, and interpretive skill. Teachers must analyze multiple dimensions of performance—conceptual understanding, problem-solving approaches, collaboration, and emotional engagement—while providing timely and constructive feedback. Digital platforms can support assessment through data tracking, visualization of student interactions, and immediate feedback, yet careful design is needed to ensure that these tools augment rather than replace human judgment and teacher presence.

6.6 Research Gaps and Future Directions

Despite promising evidence for the effectiveness of Cuisenaire rods and digital manipulatives, several research gaps persist. Longitudinal studies examining the sustained impact of embodied and phenomenologically informed interventions on mathematical understanding, problem-solving flexibility, and socio-emotional outcomes are limited. Most studies focus on short-term gains, leaving questions about retention, transfer, and the development of higher-order reasoning unanswered.

Moreover, phenomenological research in mathematics education remains relatively underdeveloped. While studies highlight the importance of embodiment, perception, and intersubjectivity, few provide systematic frameworks for investigating these dimensions empirically. Mixed-methods designs, combining qualitative phenomenological approaches with quantitative measures of achievement, engagement, and affect, offer a promising avenue for capturing the richness of students' lived experiences.

Another priority is the exploration of hybrid learning environments that integrate physical and digital manipulatives. Research should investigate optimal blends of tactile and virtual engagement, the role of teacher scaffolding, and strategies for maintaining inclusivity and equity. Comparative studies across socio-cultural contexts could elucidate how learners' perceptions, motivations, and embodied experiences vary, informing the design of adaptable and context-sensitive interventions.

6.7 Concluding Reflections

Phenomenology re-centers mathematics education on lived experience. By foregrounding the body as the locus of intentionality, it dissolves the dichotomy between concrete and abstract, sensory and intellectual, individual and collective. Cuisenaire rods exemplify this synthesis: they mediate a dynamic interplay between perception, action, and reflection through which mathematical forms are constituted.

For inclusive education, the implications are profound. A phenomenological classroom honors the multiplicity of ways in which learners inhabit the world. Differences in sensory orientation are not deficits but variations in access to meaning. The educator's role becomes one of creating perceptual constellations where each learner's experience contributes to the communal articulation of mathematical sense. Through such practice, phenomenology unites the ethical and epistemic dimensions of education: to teach mathematics is to invite others into shared perception of order, proportion, and possibility.

In conclusion, while the integration of Cuisenaire rods and digital tools within phenomenologically informed mathematics pedagogy offers considerable promise, it is not without challenges. Practical constraints, teacher expertise, learner variability, equity concerns, and assessment complexities must be addressed systematically. Phenomenology provides a guiding framework, emphasizing the inseparability of cognition, perception, and embodiment, and highlighting the centrality of lived experience in learning. Future research and professional development must focus on operationalizing these principles in ways that are sustainable, inclusive, and responsive to the diverse realities of contemporary classrooms. Only through such deliberate, evidence-informed, and reflective practice can the transformative potential of embodied mathematics learning be fully realized.

7. SYNTHESIS AND EXTENDED CONCLUSION: A PHENOMENOLOGICAL PEDAGOGY FOR THE 21ST CENTURY

The preceding sections of this chapter have explored the interplay among embodied cognition, hands-on tools such as Cuisenaire rods, digital technologies, and phenomenologically informed teaching practices in primary mathematics education. Drawing from Husserl's (1901/1970) and Merleau-Ponty's (1945/2002) foundational insights, alongside contemporary research on mathematics anxiety, manipulatives, and inclusive pedagogy, we now synthesize these findings into a cohesive vision for phenomenologically grounded mathematics pedagogy for the 21st century.

Central to this vision is the recognition that mathematics learning is fundamentally an embodied and hands-on experience. Husserl's (1901/1970) exploration of intentionality and the structures of consciousness illuminates how learners' awareness of mathematical objects is inseparable from their perceptual and bodily engagement. Children do not merely encounter numbers or symbols abstractly; their understanding emerges through active manipulation, construction, and exploration. Hands-on tools like Cuisenaire rods transform abstract concepts into perceptually and physically accessible forms, enabling learners to visualize quantities, compare lengths, explore arithmetic relationships, and construct equations concretely (Sarama & Clements, 2009; Fosnot & Dolk, 2001). By physically manipulating rods to represent addition, subtraction, multiplication, division, and fractions, learners enact mathematical reasoning, internalize relationships, and gain a sense of mastery that reduces anxiety and builds confidence.

Merleau-Ponty's (1945/2002) phenomenology of perception further emphasizes the inseparability of body, perception, and environment in knowledge acquisition. Learning is not a passive reception of pre-formed knowledge; rather, it is an active, situated, and hands-on process. Aligning bodily actions with perceptual feedback—such as stacking rods, arranging them into patterns, or subdividing lengths—allows children to engage in sensorimotor problem-solving that bridges concrete experience and abstract understanding. This hands-on engagement provides immediate feedback, supports error detection, and encourages experimentation, transforming mistakes into learning opportunities and fostering resilience (Ashcraft & Moore, 2009; Dowker et al., 2016). By physically enacting mathematical relationships, learners cultivate both conceptual knowledge and embodied confidence.

Digital technologies complement this hands-on approach, offering dynamic visualization and interactive experimentation. Virtual manipulatives can simulate mathematical operations at scales or complexities not feasible in the physical classroom, while touch-based interfaces preserve sensorimotor engagement. When integrated with physical manipulatives, digital tools enhance hands-on exploration, allowing learners to manipulate numerical and geometric representations, rotate shapes, scale patterns, and receive immediate adaptive feedback. A phenomenological perspective emphasizes that even in digital spaces, learning remains embodied: learners' gestures, visual attention, and exploratory actions mediate understanding, and technology must be designed to maintain this active, perceptually grounded engagement (Benson et al., 2022).

Social and collaborative dimensions of hands-on learning are also critical. Intersubjective engagement, as emphasized by Husserl, positions peer interaction as central to mathematical development (Husserl, 1901/1970). Collaborative construction with Cuisenaire rods encourages dialogue, joint problem-solving and shared reflection. Learners articulate reasoning, negotiate strategies, and co-construct understanding. Group tasks with manipulatives promote inclusion, as children with varying abilities, experiences, and learning styles participate equitably. Peer modeling, observation of hands-on strategies, and discussion reinforce embodied understanding and social learning simultaneously (Devine et al., 2012; Boaler, 2016).

Hands-on pedagogy also supports learners' socio-emotional development. Mathematics anxiety, often intensified by rigid, high-stakes instruction, can be mitigated by providing manipulatives and activities that normalize trial and error. Safe, playful, and exploratory tasks with rods enable children to experiment without fear of failure, strengthening self-efficacy and persistence. Integrating reflective practices, such as journals or drawings of manipulative-based problem-solving, fosters metacognition and emotional awareness, promoting resilience and positive attitudes toward mathematics (Liljedahl, 2020; Carey et al., 2016).

Teacher intentionality and scaffolding remain central. Educators observe how learners physically and perceptually engage with manipulatives, adapt tasks based on embodied cues, and scaffold understanding without over-directing. Hands-on activities become both assessment tools and learning experiences, revealing conceptual and emotional states, informing differentiation, and guiding pedagogical decisions (Fosnot & Dolk, 2001; Sarama & Clements, 2009). Teachers may provide structured challenges, collaborative problem sets, or open-ended explorations, always attending to students' bodily and perceptual engagement while fostering autonomy. Phenomenological reflection prompts educators to consider not only what learners know but how they experience mathematics through perception, action, and emotion. For instance, noticing how a child pauses, reorients, or compares rods can inform the teacher about the child's understanding and affective state, prompting subtle interventions that guide learning without diminishing agency.

Moreover, hands-on pedagogy encourages iterative and reflective learning cycles, where perception, action, and reflection converge. Children may model a problem with rods, observe patterns, verbalize reasoning, adjust constructions, and reflect on emerging understanding. This cyclical engagement embodies both Husserlian intentionality and Merleau-Ponty's notion of perceptual openness, reinforcing the intertwined nature of cognition, perception, and action. In practice, classrooms might feature stations with manipulatives, small-group problem-solving rotations, or project-based tasks, allowing learners to explore concepts in multiple ways while fostering autonomy, collaboration, and critical thinking.

Finally, this extended conclusion emphasizes that a 21st-century phenomenological pedagogy is multimodal, hands-on, socially mediated, digitally enriched, and reflective. Cuisenaire rods, other manipulatives, and complementary digital tools provide embodied pathways to understanding, facilitate conceptual abstraction, reduce mathematics anxiety, and promote resilience. By attending to perception, embodiment, intersubjectivity, and affective experience, educators can design inclusive learning environments where mathematics is engaging, meaningful, and emotionally supportive. Through active, hands-on, and reflective practices, primary mathematics classrooms transform into spaces where cognition, emotion, and action converge, producing not only competent mathematicians but confident, resilient, and curious learners. In this vision, phenomenology and hands-on pedagogy are inseparable: each action, perception, and reflection contributes to a holistic learning experience in which mathematical concepts are lived, explored, and internalized in their full complexity.

This perspective underscores that the future of mathematics education depends not solely on content mastery but on fostering experiential understanding and the embodied engagement of learners. The phenomenologically informed, hands-on approach cultivates deep, lasting comprehension, nurtures socio-emotional well-being, and equips learners with the tools to navigate increasingly complex mathematical landscapes with confidence, curiosity, and resilience.

REFERENCES

Ashcraft, M. H., & Moore, A. M. (2009). Mathematics anxiety and the affective drop in performance. *Journal of Psychoeducational Assessment*, *27*(3), 197–205. DOI: 10.1177/0734282908330580

Benson, I., Marriott, N., & McCandliss, B. D. (2022). Dynamic visualizations and embodied cognition in early mathematics learning: A systematic review of the Cuisenaire–Gattegno approach. *Frontiers in Education*, *7*, 902899. DOI: 10.3389/feduc.2022.902899

Boaler, J. (2016). *Mathematical mindsets: Unleashing students' potential through creative math, inspiring messages, and innovative teaching*. Jossey-Bass.

Carey, E., Hill, F., Devine, A., & Szűcs, D. (2016). The chicken or the egg? The direction of the relationship between mathematics anxiety and mathematics performance. *Frontiers in Psychology*, *6*, 1987. DOI: 10.3389/fpsyg.2015.01987 PMID: 26779093

Devine, A., Fawcett, K., Szűcs, D., & Dowker, A. (2012). Gender differences in mathematics anxiety and the relation to mathematics performance while controlling for test anxiety. *Behavioral and Brain Functions : BBF*, *8*(1), 33. DOI: 10.1186/1744-9081-8-33 PMID: 22769743

Dowker, A., Sarkar, A., & Looi, C. Y. (2016). Mathematics anxiety: What have we learned in 60 years? *Frontiers in Psychology*, *7*, 508. DOI: 10.3389/fpsyg.2016.00508 PMID: 27199789

Fosnot, C. T., & Dolk, M. (2001). *Young mathematicians at work: Constructing number sense, addition, and subtraction*. Heinemann.

Husserl, E. (1970). *Logical investigations* (Findlay, J. N., Trans.). Routledge. (Original work published 1901)

Kamii, C., & Lewis, B. A. (1993). *Young children reinvent arithmetic: Implications of Piaget's theory*. Teachers College Press.

Liljedahl, P. (2020). *Building thinking classrooms in mathematics, grades K–12: 14 teaching practices for enhancing learning*. Corwin.

Merleau-Ponty, M. (2002). *Phenomenology of perception* (Smith, C., Trans.). Routledge Classics. (Original work published 1945) DOI: 10.4324/9780203994610

Mix, K. S., Levine, S. C., Cheng, Y.-L., Young, C., Hambrick, D. Z., & Konstantopoulos, S. (2016). Separate but correlated: The latent structure of space and mathematics across development. *Journal of Experimental Psychology. General*, *145*(10), 1364–1384. DOI: 10.1037/xge0000182 PMID: 27560854

Sarama, J., & Clements, D. H. (2009). Building blocks and cognitive building blocks: Playing to know the world mathematically. *American Journal of Play*, *1*(3), 313–337.

Compilation of References

Abokhashabah, T., Jamoussi, B., Summan, A. S., Abdelfattah, E., & Ahmad, I. (2021). Effects of Heat Stress Exposure and Climate Change on Health and Safety of Outdoor Workers. *Current World Environment*, *16*(3), 836–847. DOI: 10.12944/CWE.16.3.15

Aburn, G., Gott, M., & Hoare, K. (2016). What is resilience? An integrative review of the empirical literature. *Journal of Advanced Nursing*, *72*(5), 980–1000. DOI: 10.1111/jan.12888 PMID: 26748456

Agochukwu, N. Q., Skolarus, T. A., & Wittmann, D. (2018). Telemedicine and prostate cancer survivorship: A narrative review. *mHealth*, *4*(0), 45–45. DOI: 10.21037/mhealth.2018.09.08 PMID: 30505843

Ainsworth, M. D. (1985). Patterns of infant-mother attachments: Antecedents and effects on development. *Bulletin of the New York Academy of Medicine*, *61*(9), 771. PMID: 3864510

Alanzi, T. M. (2021). Gig health vs ehealth: Future prospects in saudi arabian health-care system. *Journal of Multidisciplinary Healthcare*, *14*, 1945–1953. DOI: 10.2147/JMDH.S304690 PMID: 34326645

Andersson, N., & Ledogar, R. J. (2008). The CIET Aboriginal Youth Resilience Studies: 14 Years of Capacity Building and Methods Development in Canada. *Pimatisiwin*, *6*(2), 65–88. PMID: 20862230

Anisman, H., Doubad, D., Asokumar, A., & Matheson, K. (2024). Psychosocial and neurobiological aspects of the worldwide refugee crisis: From vulnerability to resilience. *Neuroscience and Biobehavioral Reviews*, *165*, 105859. DOI: 10.1016/j.neubiorev.2024.105859 PMID: 39159733

Anwar, M. A., & Graham, M. (2021). Between a rock and a hard place: Freedom, flexibility, precarity and vulnerability in the gig economy in Africa. *Competition & Change*, *25*(2), 237–258. DOI: 10.1177/1024529420914473

Applebaum, K. M., Graham, J., Gray, G. M., LaPuma, P., McCormick, S. A., Northcross, A., & Perry, M. J. (2016). An Overview of Occupational Risks From Climate Change. *Current Environmental Health Reports*, *3*(1), 13–22. DOI: 10.1007/s40572-016-0081-4 PMID: 26842343

Ashcraft, M. H., & Moore, A. M. (2009). Mathematics anxiety and the affective drop in performance. *Journal of Psychoeducational Assessment*, *27*(3), 197–205. DOI: 10.1177/0734282908330580

Ayentimi, D. T., Abadi, H. A., & Burgess, J. (2023). Decent gig work in Sub Sahara Africa? *The Journal of Industrial Relations*, *65*(1), 112–125. DOI: 10.1177/00221856221111693

Azahra, A. S., Pirdaus, D. I., & Prabowo, A. (2024). Digital Health Literacy and Telemedicine in the Information Age: A Comprehensive Review and Future Prospects. *International Journal of Linguistics. Communication & Broadcasting*, *2*(1), 13–19. DOI: 10.46336/ijlcb.v2i1.89

Αθανασέκου, Μ. (2020). επιμ. και συγγραφή, Γιατί με αφορά η τέχνη. Οι πολλές της διαστάσεις και πως αξιοποιούνται στη ζωή μας», Ηδυέπεια.

Αθανασέκου, Μ. (2021). *Η σχέση της τέχνης με την ψυχολογία - Η πρόσληψη της νοητικής υστέρησης και η απεικόνισή της στη ζωγραφική από τον 15ο έως τον 19ο αιώνα, στο βιβλίο Αργυριάδης, Α., Λόγος, αναπηρία, θεραπευτικές και εκπαιδευτικές παρεμβάσεις –Νέα δεδομένα και τάσεις στην Ειδική Αγωγή, σελ.* Εκδόσεις Ηδυέπεια.

Bajwa, U., Gastaldo, D., Di Ruggiero, E., & Knorr, L. (2018). The health of workers in the global gig economy. *Globalization and Health*, *14*(1), 1–4. DOI: 10.1186/s12992-018-0444-8 PMID: 30563539

Bakker, D., Kazantzis, N., Rickwood, D., & Rickard, N. (2016). Mental health smartphone apps: Review and evidence-based recommendations for future developments. *JMIR Mental Health*, *3*(1), e7. DOI: 10.2196/mental.4984 PMID: 26932350

Bandura, A. (1997). *Self-efficacy: The exercise of control*. W. H. Freeman.

Barrita, A. M., & Wong-Padoongpatt, G. (2023). Ethnic identity and resilience: A moderated mediation analysis of protective factors for self-blame and racial microaggressions. *Frontiers in Psychology*, *14*, 1198375. DOI: 10.3389/fpsyg.2023.1198375 PMID: 37457064

Barsalou, L. W. (2008). Grounded cognition. *Annual Review of Psychology*, *59*(1), 617–645. DOI: 10.1146/annurev.psych.59.103006.093639 PMID: 17705682

Bauer, M., Glenn, T., Monteith, S., Bauer, R., Whybrow, P. C., & Geddes, J. (2017). Ethical perspectives on recommending digital technology for patients with mental illness. *International Journal of Bipolar Disorders*, *5*(1), 6. DOI: 10.1186/s40345-017-0073-9 PMID: 28155206

Beaty, R. E., Benedek, M., Kaufman, S. B., & Silvia, P. J. (2016). Default and executive network coupling supports creative idea production. *Scientific Reports*, *5*(1), 10964. DOI: 10.1038/srep10964

Beauchamp, T. L., & Childress, J. F. (2019). *Principles of biomedical ethics* (8th ed.). Oxford University Press.

Beilock, S. L., Gunderson, E. A., Ramirez, G., & Levine, S. C. (2010). Female teachers' math anxiety affects girls' math achievement. *Proceedings of the National Academy of Sciences of the United States of America*, *107*(5), 1860–1863. DOI: 10.1073/pnas.0910967107 PMID: 20133834

Benson, I., Marriott, N., & McCandliss, B. D. (2022). Dynamic visualizations and embodied cognition in early mathematics learning: A systematic review of the Cuisenaire–Gattegno approach. *Frontiers in Education*, *7*, 902899. DOI: 10.3389/feduc.2022.902899

Berreman, G. D. (1972). Race, caste, and other invidious distinctions in social stratification. *Race*, *13*(4), 385–414. DOI: 10.1177/030639687201300401

Bhardwaj, A., Sharma, S., & Singh, R. (2021). Ethical implications of digital mental health interventions: A review. *Indian Journal of Psychological Medicine*, *43*(4), 333–340. DOI: 10.1177/02537176211008583

Boaler, J. (2016). *Mathematical mindsets: Unleashing students' potential through creative math, inspiring messages, and innovative teaching*. Jossey-Bass.

Bogaerts, A., Claes, L., Raymaekers, K., Buelens, T., Bastiaens, T., & Luyckx, K. (2023). Trajectories of adaptive and disturbed identity dimensions in adolescence: Developmental associations with self-esteem, resilience, symptoms of depression, and borderline personality disorder features. *Frontiers in Psychiatry*, *14*, 1125812. DOI: 10.3389/fpsyt.2023.1125812 PMID: 37168080

Bolier, L., Haverman, M., Westerhof, G. J., Riper, H., Smit, F., & Bohlmeijer, E. (2013). Positive psychology interventions: A meta-analysis of randomized controlled studies. *BMC Public Health*, *13*(1), 119. DOI: 10.1186/1471-2458-13-119 PMID: 23390882

Bolwerk, A., Mack-Andrick, J., Lang, F. R., Dörfler, A., & Maihöfner, C. (2014). How art changes your brain: Differential effects of visual art production and cognitive art evaluation on functional brain connectivity. *PLoS One*, *9*(7), e101035. DOI: 10.1371/journal.pone.0101035 PMID: 24983951

Bonanno, G. A., Romero, S. A., & Klein, S. I. (2015). The temporal elements of psychological resilience: An integrative framework for the study of individuals, families, and communities. *Psychological Inquiry*, *26*(2), 139–169. DOI: 10.1080/1047840X.2015.992677

Bowlby, J. (1944). Forty-four juvenile thieves: Their characters and home-life. *The International Journal of Psycho-Analysis*, *25*, 19.

Bradt, J., & Dileo, C. (2014). Music interventions for mechanically ventilated patients. *Cochrane Database of Systematic Reviews*, *12*(12), CD006902. Advance online publication. DOI: 10.1002/14651858.CD006902.pub3 PMID: 25490233

Bretherton, I. & American Psychological Association, Inc. (1992). The Origins of Attachment Theory: John Bowlby and Mary Ainsworth. In Developmental Psychology (Vol. 28, Issue 5, pp. 759–775). American Psychological Association, Inc. https://psychology.psy.sunysb.edu/attachment/online/inge_origins%20DP1992.pdf

Brown, D. D., & Kulig, J. C. (1996). The concepts of resiliency: Theoretical lessons from community research.

Brown, T. (2008). Design thinking. *Harvard Business Review*, *86*(6), 84–92. PMID: 18605031

Bruner, J. S. (1966). *Toward a theory of instruction*. Harvard University Press.

Burnaford, G., Brown, S., Doherty, J., & McLaughlin, H. J. (2007). *Arts integration frameworks, research and practice: A literature review*. Arts Education Partnership.

Camic, P. M. (2010). Participatory art for older adults: A review of benefits and mechanisms. *Perspectives in Public Health*, *130*(6), 277–283. DOI: 10.1177/1757913910386206 PMID: 21213564

Camic, P. M., Baker, E. L., & Tischler, V. (2014). Theorizing how art gallery interventions impact people with dementia. *The Gerontologist*, *54*(6), 912–921. DOI: 10.1093/geront/gnt103 PMID: 25063936

Camic, P. M., & Chatterjee, H. J. (2013). Museums and art galleries as partners for public health interventions. *Perspectives in Public Health*, *133*(1), 66–71. DOI: 10.1177/1757913912468523

Carbonneau, K. J., Marley, S. C., & Selig, J. P. (2013). A meta-analysis of the efficacy of teaching mathematics with concrete manipulatives. *Journal of Educational Psychology, 105*(2), 380–400. DOI: 10.1037/a0031084

Carey, E., Hill, F., Devine, A., & Szűcs, D. (2016). The chicken or the egg? The direction of the relationship between mathematics anxiety and mathematics performance. *Frontiers in Psychology, 6*, 1987. DOI: 10.3389/fpsyg.2015.01987 PMID: 26779093

Case, C., & Dalley, T. (2014). *The handbook of art therapy* (3rd ed.). Routledge. DOI: 10.4324/9781315779799

CASEL. (2020). *SEL framework.* Collaborative for Academic, Social, and Emotional Learning. https://casel.org/sel-framework/

Cassidy, J., Jones, J. D., & Shaver, P. R. (2013). Contributions of attachment theory and research: A framework for future research, translation, and policy. *Development and Psychopathology, 25*(4pt2), 1415–1434. DOI: 10.1017/S0954579413000692 PMID: 24342848

CAST. (2018). *Universal design for learning guidelines version 2.2.* http://udlguidelines.cast.org

Catterall, J. S., Dumais, S. A., & Hampden-Thompson, G. (2012). *The arts and achievement in at-risk youth: Findings from four longitudinal studies.* National Endowment for the Arts.

Chanda, M. L., & Levitin, D. J. (2013). The neurochemistry of music. *Trends in Cognitive Sciences, 17*(4), 179–193. DOI: 10.1016/j.tics.2013.02.007 PMID: 23541122

Chandel, A. S. (2025). Traffic congestion in Shimla: A smart city in the Himalayan mountain landscape—analyzing socioeconomic impacts from the perspectives of drivers and passengers. *Urban, Planning and Transport Research, 13*(1), 2502000. Advance online publication. DOI: 10.1080/21650020.2025.2502000

Chang, R., Barrita, A. M., & Wong-Padoongpatt, G. (2007). Race (racism). *The Blackwell Encyclopedia of Sociology*, 1-3.

Chatterjee, A. (2014). Neuroaesthetics: Brain at the intersection of art and science. *Perspectives on Psychological Science, 9*(2), 113–117. DOI: 10.1177/1745691613513468

Chatterjee, A., & Vartanian, O. (2014). Neuroaesthetics. *Trends in Cognitive Sciences, 18*(7), 370–375. DOI: 10.1016/j.tics.2014.03.003

Chen, T., Song, W., Song, J., Ren, Y., Dong, Y., Yang, J., & Zhang, S. (2022). Measuring Well-Being of Migrant Gig Workers: Exampled as Hangzhou City in China. *Behavioral Sciences (Basel, Switzerland)*, *12*(10), 365. DOI: 10.3390/bs12100365 PMID: 36285934

Choi, N. G., & Dinitto, D. M. (2013). The digital divide among low-income homebound older adults: Internet use patterns, eHealth literacy, and attitudes toward computer/Internet use. *Journal of Medical Internet Research*, *15*(5), e93. DOI: 10.2196/jmir.2645 PMID: 23639979

Cianconi, P., Hanife, B., Hirsch, D., & Janiri, L. (2023). Is climate change affecting mental health of urban populations? In *Current Opinion in Psychiatry* (Vol. 36, Issue 3, pp. 213–218). Curr Opin Psychiatry. DOI: 10.1097/YCO.0000000000000859

Clark, A. (2020). *Slow pedagogy: Learning in the rhythm of time*. Routledge.

Clayton, S. (2020). Climate anxiety: Psychological responses to climate change. *Journal of Anxiety Disorders*, *74*, 102263. DOI: 10.1016/j.janxdis.2020.102263

Clift, S., & Camic, P. (2016). *Oxford textbook of creative arts, health, and wellbeing: International perspectives on practice, policy, and research*. Oxford University Press.

Clift, S., & Morrison, I. (2011). Group singing fosters mental health and wellbeing: Findings from the East Kent "singing for health" network project. *Mental Health and Social Inclusion*, *15*(2), 88–97. DOI: 10.1108/20428301111140930

Cocking, C. (2013). The role of "zero-responders" during 7/7: Implications for the emergency services. *International Journal of Emergency Services*, *2*(2), 79–93. DOI: 10.1108/IJES-08-2012-0035

Cohen-Yatziv, L., & Regev, D. (2019). The effectiveness of art therapy with children: A review of the empirical literature. *Frontiers in Psychology*, *10*, 2375. DOI: 10.3389/fpsyg.2019.02375

Coholic, D., & Eys, M. (2016). Benefits of an arts-based mindfulness group intervention for vulnerable children. *Child & Adolescent Social Work Journal*, *33*(1), 1–13. DOI: 10.1007/s10560-015-0431-3

Colpitts, E., & Gahagan, J. (2016). The utility of resilience as a conceptual framework for understanding and measuring LGBTQ health. *International Journal for Equity in Health*, *15*(1), 60. DOI: 10.1186/s12939-016-0349-1 PMID: 27048319

Comlek, S., & Ordu, A. (2021). Interventional pain management during sars-cov-2 pandemic. *Signa Vitae*, *17*(4), 178–184. DOI: 10.22514/sv.2021.008

Corbett, B. A., Gunther, J. R., Comins, D., Price, J., Ryan, N., Simon, D., Jenson, A., & Rios, T. (2014). Brief report: Theatre as therapy for children with autism spectrum disorder. *Journal of Autism and Developmental Disorders*, *44*(2), 466–472. DOI: 10.1007/s10803-013-1883-0

Cox, J. A., Read, G. J. M., Butler, G. L., & Salmon, P. M. (2024). Examining gender differences in gig worker safety. *Human Factors and Ergonomics in Manufacturing*, *34*(1), 3–15. DOI: 10.1002/hfm.21007

Cox, M. (2005). *The pictorial world of the child*. Cambridge University Press.

Crane, K., Li, L., Subramanian, P., Rovit, E., & Liu, J. (2022). Climate Change and Mental Health: A Review of Empirical Evidence, Mechanisms and Implications. In *Atmosphere* (Vol. 13, Issue 12). Atmosphere (Basel). DOI: 10.3390/atmos13122096

Creswell, J. D., Lindsay, E. K., & Moyers, T. B. (2015). How does mindfulness training affect health? A mindfulness stress buffering account. *Current Directions in Psychological Science*, *24*(6), 401–407. DOI: 10.1177/0963721414547415

Creswell, J. W., & Plano Clark, V. L. (2017). *Designing and conducting mixed methods research* (3rd ed.). SAGE Publications.

Cropanzano, R., Keplinger, K., Lambert, B. K., Caza, B., & Ashford, S. J. (2022). The Organizational Psychology of Gig Work: An Integrative Conceptual Review. *The Journal of Applied Psychology*, *108*(3), 492–519. DOI: 10.1037/apl0001029 PMID: 36222635

Czamanski-Cohen, J., & Weihs, K. L. (2023). The role of emotion processing in art therapy (REPAT) intervention protocol. *Frontiers in Psychology, 14*, 1208901. https://doi.org/, G. L. (1977). The need for a new medical model: A challenge for biomedicine. *Science, 196*(4286), 129–136. https://doi.org/DOI: 10.3389/fpsyg.2023.1208901Engel

Deasy, R. J. (Ed.). (2002). *Critical links: Learning in the arts and student academic and social development*. Arts Education Partnership.

Deriglazov, D., Halamová, J., & Kernová, L. (2025). Burnout, Compassion Fatigue, and Compassion Satisfaction Interventions via Mobile Applications: A Systematic Review and a Meta-Analysis. *Worldviews on Evidence-Based Nursing*, *22*(3), e70033. DOI: 10.1111/wvn.70033 PMID: 40361274

Devine, A., Fawcett, K., Szűcs, D., & Dowker, A. (2012). Gender differences in mathematics anxiety and the relation to mathematics performance while controlling for test anxiety. *Behavioral and Brain Functions : BBF*, *8*(1), 33. DOI: 10.1186/1744-9081-8-33 PMID: 22769743

Diamond, A. (2013). Executive functions. *Annual Review of Psychology*, *64*(1), 135–168. DOI: 10.1146/annurev-psych-113011-143750

Diamond, A., & Lee, K. (2011). Interventions shown to aid executive function development in children 4 to 12 years old. *Science*, *333*(6045), 959–964. DOI: 10.1126/science.1204529

Diener, E., & Chan, M. Y. (2011). Happy people live longer: Subjective well-being contributes to health and longevity. *Applied Psychology. Health and Well-Being*, *3*(1), 1–43. DOI: 10.1111/j.1758-0854.2010.01045.x PMID: 26286968

Dienes, Z. P. (1971). *Building up mathematics* (4th ed.). Hutchinson Educational.

Dowker, A., Sarkar, A., & Looi, C. Y. (2016). Mathematics anxiety: What have we learned in 60 years? *Frontiers in Psychology*, *7*, 508. DOI: 10.3389/fpsyg.2016.00508 PMID: 27199789

Drury, J., Carter, H., Cocking, C., Ntontis, E., Tekin Guven, S., & Amlôt, R. (2019). Facilitating Collective Psychosocial Resilience in the Public in Emergencies: Twelve Recommendations Based on the Social Identity Approach. *Frontiers in Public Health*, *7*, 429165. DOI: 10.3389/fpubh.2019.00141 PMID: 31214561

Durojaiye, O. C., Jibril, I., & Kritsotakis, E. I. (2022). Effectiveness of telemedicine in outpatient parenteral antimicrobial therapy (Tele-OPAT): A systematic review. In *Journal of Telemedicine and Telecare*. SAGE PublicationsSage UK: London, England. DOI: 10.1177/1357633X221131842

Du, Y., Zhou, Q., Cheng, W., Zhang, Z., Hoelzer, S., Liang, Y., Xue, H., Ma, X., Sylvia, S., Tian, J., & Tang, W. (2022). Factors Influencing Adoption and Use of Telemedicine Services in Rural Areas of China: Mixed Methods Study. *JMIR Public Health and Surveillance*, *8*(12), e40771. DOI: 10.2196/40771 PMID: 36563026

Ecclestone, K., & Hayes, D. (2009). *The dangerous rise of therapeutic education*. Routledge. DOI: 10.4324/9780203870563

Eggenberger, S. K., Meiers, S. J., Krumwiede, N., Bliesmer, M., & Earle, P. (2011). Reintegration within families in the context of chronic illness: A family health promoting process. *Journal of Nursing and Healthcare of Chronic Illness*, *3*(3), 283–292. DOI: 10.1111/j.1752-9824.2011.01101.x

Eisenberg, N., Spinrad, T. L., & Eggum, N. D. (2010). Emotion-related self-regulation and its relation to children's maladjustment. *Annual Review of Clinical Psychology*, *6*(1), 495–525. DOI: 10.1146/annurev.clinpsy.121208.131208

Eisner, E. W. (2002). *The arts and the creation of mind*. Yale University Press.

Elliott, T. R., Perrin, P. B., Powers, M. B., Duffeck, D., & Warren, A. M. (2023). Resilience and distress among individuals with chronic health conditions during the initial wave of the COVID-19 pandemic. *Journal of Affective Disorders Reports, 15*, 100710. DOI: 10.1016/j.jadr.2023.100710

Emami, S. G., Lorenzoni, V., & Turchetti, G. (2024). Towards Resilient Healthcare Systems: A Framework for Crisis Management. *International Journal of Environmental Research and Public Health, 21*(3), 286. DOI: 10.3390/ijerph21030286 PMID: 38541286

Engel, G. L. (1977). The need for a new medical model: A challenge for biomedicine. *Science, 196*(4286), 129–136. DOI: 10.1126/science.847460 PMID: 847460

Erikson, E. H. (1963). *Childhood and society* (2nd ed.). Norton.

Estrada-Moreno, I. S., Palma-Garcia, M. D. L. O., Gomez Jacinto, L., & Hombrados-Mendieta, M. I. (2025). Resilience in immigrants: A facilitating resource for their social integration. *Journal of Ethnic & Cultural Diversity in Social Work*, •••, 1–16.

Fancourt, D., Aufegger, L., & Williamon, A. (2019). Low-stress and high-stress singing have contrasting effects on glucocorticoid response. *Frontiers in Psychology, 10*, 1–13. DOI: 10.3389/fpsyg.2019.00005 PMID: 26388794

Fan, Y., & Lyu, X. (2021). Exploring Two Decades of Research in Community Resilience: A Content Analysis Across the International Literature. *Psychology Research and Behavior Management, 14*, 1643–1654. DOI: 10.2147/PRBM.S329829 PMID: 34675704

Ferbežar, N., Kopinič, A., & Gavriloski Tretjak, M. (2025). Elements of minority stress and resilience in LGBTQ+ students' experience of education. *Journal of Homosexuality, 72*(3), 520–543. DOI: 10.1080/00918369.2024.2326473 PMID: 38470515

Firth, J., Torous, J., Nicholas, J., Carney, R., Pratap, A., Rosenbaum, S., & Sarris, J. (2019). The efficacy of smartphone-based mental health interventions for depressive symptoms: A meta-analysis. *World Psychiatry; Official Journal of the World Psychiatric Association (WPA), 18*(3), 325–336. DOI: 10.1002/wps.20673 PMID: 31496095

Firth, J., Torous, J., Nicholas, J., Carney, R., Rosenbaum, S., & Sarris, J. (2017). Can smartphone mental health interventions reduce symptoms of anxiety? A meta-analysis of randomized controlled trials. *Journal of Affective Disorders, 218*, 15–22. DOI: 10.1016/j.jad.2017.04.046 PMID: 28456072

Fitzpatrick, P. J. (2023). Improving health literacy using the power of digital communications to achieve better health outcomes for patients and practitioners. In *Frontiers in Digital Health* (Vol. 5, p. 1264780). Frontiers Media SA. DOI: 10.3389/fdgth.2023.1264780

Fleming, J., & Ledogar, R. J. (2008). Resilience, an Evolving Concept: A Review of Literature Relevant to Aboriginal Research. *Pimatisiwin*, *6*(2), 7–23. PMID: 20963184

Fletcher, D., & Sarkar, M. (2013). Psychological resilience. *European Psychologist*, *18*(1), 12–23. DOI: 10.1027/1016-9040/a000124

Flouris, A. D., Dinas, P. C., Ioannou, L. G., Nybo, L., Havenith, G., Kenny, G. P., & Kjellstrom, T. (2018). Workers' health and productivity under occupational heat strain: A systematic review and meta-analysis. *The Lancet. Planetary Health*, *2*(12), e521–e531. DOI: 10.1016/S2542-5196(18)30237-7 PMID: 30526938

Ford, J. H. II, Jolles, S. A., Heller, D., Langenstroer, M., & Crnich, C. (2022). There and back again: The shape of telemedicine in U.S. nursing homes following COVID-19. *BMC Geriatrics*, *22*(1), 1–12. DOI: 10.1186/s12877-022-03046-y PMID: 35436869

Forgeard, M. J. C., & Elstein, J. G. (2014). Advancing the clinical science of creativity. *Frontiers in Psychology*, *5*, 613. DOI: 10.3389/fpsyg.2014.00613 PMID: 24994990

Fosnot, C. T., & Dolk, M. (2001). *Young mathematicians at work: Constructing number sense, addition, and subtraction*. Heinemann.

Frank, A. W., & Frank, J. (1991). *At the will of the body: Reflections on illness*. Houghton Mifflin.

Frankl, V. E. (1963). *Man's search for meaning: An introduction to logotherapy*. Beacon Press.

Fuchs, T. (2018). *Ecology of the brain: The phenomenology and biology of the embodied mind*. Oxford University Press., DOI: 10.1093/oso/9780199646883.001.0001

Fullerton, D. J., Zhang, L. M., & Kleitman, S. (2021). An integrative process model of resilience in an academic context: Resilience resources, coping strategies, and positive adaptation. *PLoS One*, *16*(2), e0246000. DOI: 10.1371/journal.pone.0246000 PMID: 33529232

Garvis, S., & Pendergast, D. (2011). An investigation of early childhood teacher self-efficacy beliefs in the teaching of arts education. *International Journal of Education & the Arts*, *12*(9), 1–15. DOI: 10.59236/ijea12n9

Geretsegger, M., Elefant, C., Mössler, K. A., & Gold, C. (2014). Music therapy for people with autism spectrum disorder. *The Cochrane Library*, *6*(3), CD004381. Advance online publication. DOI: 10.1002/14651858.CD004381.pub3

Geue, K., Goetze, H., Buttstaedt, M., Kleinert, E., Richter, D., & Singer, S. (2010). An overview of art therapy interventions for cancer patients and the results of research. *Complementary Therapies in Medicine*, *18*(3–4), 160–170. DOI: 10.1016/j.ctim.2010.04.001 PMID: 20688262

Ghanei Gheshlagh, R., Sayehmiri, K., Ebadi, A., Dalvandi, A., Dalvand, S., & Nourozi Tabrizi, K. (2016). Resilience of Patients With Chronic Physical Diseases: A Systematic Review and Meta-Analysis. *Iranian Red Crescent Medical Journal*, *18*(7), e38562. DOI: 10.5812/ircmj.38562 PMID: 27703800

Ghosh, A., & Deb, A. (2017). Positive psychology interventions for chronic physical illnesses: A systematic review. *Psychological Studies*, *62*(4), 354–362. DOI: 10.1007/s12646-017-0421-y

Gibb, K., Beckman, S., Vergara, X. P., Heinzerling, A., & Harrison, R. (2024). Extreme Heat and Occupational Health Risks. *Annual Review of Public Health*, *45*(1), 315–335. DOI: 10.1146/annurev-publhealth-060222-034715 PMID: 38166501

Gleiss, A., & Lewandowski, S. (2022). Removing barriers for digital health through organizing ambidexterity in hospitals. *Journal of Public Health (Berlin)*, *30*(1), 21–35. DOI: 10.1007/s10389-021-01532-y

Glenberg, A. M. (2010). Embodiment as a unifying perspective for psychology. *Wiley Interdisciplinary Reviews: Cognitive Science*, *1*(4), 586–596. DOI: 10.1002/wcs.55 PMID: 26271505

Gonzalez Garcia, M., Fatehi, F., Bashi, N., Varnfield, M., Iyngkaran, P., Driscoll, A., Neil, C., Hare, D. L., & Oldenburg, B. (2019). A Review of Randomized Controlled Trials Utilizing Telemedicine for Improving Heart Failure Readmission: Can a Realist Approach Bridge the Translational Divide? *Clinical Medicine Insights. Cardiology*, *13*, 1179546819861396. Advance online publication. DOI: 10.1177/1179546819861396 PMID: 31316270

Goudet, J. M., Arif, F. B., Owais, H., Ahmed, H. U., & Ridde, V. (2024). Climate change and women's mental health in two vulnerable communities of Bangladesh: An ethnographic study. *PLOS Global Public Health, 4*(6 June), e0002080. DOI: 10.1371/journal.pgph.0002080

Goudet, J.-M., Arif, F. B., Owais, H., Ahmed, H. U., & Ridde, V. (2023). Intersecting Vulnerabilities: Unraveling the Complex Relationship between Women, Climate Change, and Mental Health in Bangladeshi Communities. In medRxiv (p. 2023.06.06.23290721). Cold Spring Harbor Laboratory Press. DOI: 10.1101/2023.06.06.23290721

Grady, C. (2015). Enduring and emerging challenges of informed consent. *The New England Journal of Medicine*, *372*(9), 855–862. DOI: 10.1056/NEJMra1411250 PMID: 25714163

Graham, A. L., Cobb, N. K., Raymond, L., Sill, S., & Young, J. (2011). Effectiveness of an internet-based worksite smoking cessation intervention at 12 months. *Journal of Occupational and Environmental Medicine*, *53*(7), 821–828. DOI: 10.1097/JOM.0b013e318220c5b3 PMID: 17693778

Grande, D., Luna Marti, X., Feuerstein-Simon, R., Merchant, R. M., Asch, D. A., Lewson, A., & Cannuscio, C. C. (2020). Health Policy and Privacy Challenges Associated with Digital Technology. *JAMA Network Open*, *3*(7), e208285–e208285. DOI: 10.1001/jamanetworkopen.2020.8285 PMID: 32644138

Gregory, K. (2021). 'My Life Is More Valuable Than This': Understanding Risk among On-Demand Food Couriers in Edinburgh. *Work, Employment and Society*, *35*(2), 316–331. DOI: 10.1177/0950017020969593

Gunasiri, H., Wang, Y., Watkins, E. M., Capetola, T., Henderson-Wilson, C., & Patrick, R. (2022). Hope, Coping and Eco-Anxiety: Young People's Mental Health in a Climate-Impacted Australia. *International Journal of Environmental Research and Public Health*, *19*(9), 5528. Advance online publication. DOI: 10.3390/ijerph19095528 PMID: 35564923

Gussek, L., Schned, L., & Wiesche, M. (2021). Obsolescence in IT Work: Causes, Consequences and Counter-Measures. *Lecture Notes in Information Systems and Organisation, 48 LNISO*, 572–586. DOI: 10.1007/978-3-030-86800-0_40

Hadi, A. A. W. K., & Pratono, A. H. (2024). Ethical predicaments of gig economy: Bibliometric approach. *Optimum: Jurnal Ekonomi Dan Pembangunan*, *14*(1), 40–48. DOI: 10.12928/optimum.v14i1.9316

Haeyen, S., van Hooren, S., van der Veld, W., & Hutschemaekers, G. (2015). Perceived effects of art therapy in the treatment of personality disorders, cluster B/C: A qualitative study. *The Arts in Psychotherapy*, *45*(3), 1–9. DOI: 10.1016/j.aip.2015.04.005

Haleem, A., Javaid, M., Singh, R. P., & Suman, R. (2021). Telemedicine for healthcare: Capabilities, features, barriers, and applications. In *Sensors International.* DOI: 10.1016/j.sintl.2021.100117

Hallam, S. (2010). The power of music: Its impact on the intellectual, social and personal development of children and young people. *International Journal of Music Education, 28*(3), 269–289. https://doi.org/. https://doi.org/DOI: 10.1177/0255761413490659

Hallam, S. (2010). The power of music: Its impact on the intellectual, social and personal development of children and young people. *International Journal of Music Education, 28*(3), 269–289. DOI: 10.1177/0255761410370658

Halprin, D. (2003). *The expressive body in life, art, and therapy: Working with movement, metaphor, and meaning*. Jessica Kingsley Publishers.Malchiodi, C. A. (2020). *Creative interventions with traumatized children.* Guilford Press.

Hardiman, M. (2016). *The brain-targeted teaching model for 21st-century schools.* Corwin Press.

Harpur, P., & Blanck, P. (2020). Gig Workers with Disabilities: Opportunities, Challenges, and Regulatory Response. *Journal of Occupational Rehabilitation, 30*(4), 511–520. DOI: 10.1007/s10926-020-09937-4 PMID: 33146784

Hart, A., Romney, D., Sarin, R., Mechanic, O., Hertelendy, A. J., Larson, D., Rhone, K., Sidel, K., Voskanyan, A., & Ciottone, G. R. (2022). Developing Telemedicine Curriculum Competencies for Graduate Medical Education: Outcomes of a Modified Delphi Process. *Academic Medicine, 97*(4), 577–585. DOI: 10.1097/ACM.0000000000004463 PMID: 34670239

Heidegger, M. (1927/1962). *Being and time* (Macquarrie, J., & Robinson, E., Trans.). Harper & Row.

Hjelm, N. M. (2005). Benefits and drawbacks of telemedicine. In *Journal of Telemedicine and Telecare* (Vol. 11, Issue 2, pp. 60–70). SAGE PublicationsSage UK: London, England. DOI: 10.1258/1357633053499886

Hollis, C., Falconer, C. J., Martin, J. L., Whittington, C., Stockton, S., Glazebrook, C., & Davies, E. B. (2017). Annual research review: Digital health interventions for children and young people with mental health problems–a systematic and meta-review. *Journal of Child Psychology and Psychiatry, and Allied Disciplines, 58*(4), 474–503. DOI: 10.1111/jcpp.12663 PMID: 27943285

Horne, R., Bell, K., Marin, D., & Weinman, J. (2015). Understanding patients' adherence-related beliefs about medicines prescribed for long-term conditions: A meta-analytic review. *Annals of Behavioral Medicine*, *49*(1), 1–15. DOI: 10.1007/s12160-014-9649-2 PMID: 24841509

Horvath, A. O., Del Re, A. C., Flückiger, C., & Symonds, D. (2011). Alliance in individual psychotherapy. *Psychotherapy (Chicago, Ill.)*, *48*(1), 9–16. DOI: 10.1037/a0022186 PMID: 21401269

Hosseini, S. M., Boushehri, S. A., & Alimohammadzadeh, K. (2024). Challenges and solutions for implementing telemedicine in Iran from health policymakers' perspective. *BMC Health Services Research*, *24*(1), 1–11. DOI: 10.1186/s12913-023-10488-6 PMID: 38200535

Howard, A. H., Roberts, M., Mitchell, T., & Wilke, N. G. (2023). The Relationship Between Spirituality and Resilience and Well-being: A Study of 529 Care Leavers from 11 Nations. *Adversity and Resilience Science*, *4*(2), 177–190. DOI: 10.1007/s42844-023-00088-y PMID: 36816809

Hui, C. Y., Abdulla, A., Ahmed, Z., Goel, H., Habib, G. M. M., Hock, T. T., Khandakr, P., Mahmood, H., Nautiyal, A., Nurmansyah, M., Panwar, S., Patil, R., Rinawan, F. R., Salim, H., Satav, A., Shah, J. N., Shukla, A., Tanim, C. Z. H., Balharry, D., & Pinnock, H. (2022). Mapping national information and communication technology (ICT) infrastructure to the requirements of potential digital health interventions in low and middle-income countries. *Journal of Global Health*, *12*, 04094. DOI: 10.7189/jogh.12.04094 PMID: 36579436

Huppert, F. A., & So, T. T. (2013). Flourishing across Europe: Application of a new conceptual framework for defining well-being. *Social Indicators Research*, *110*(3), 837–861. DOI: 10.1007/s11205-011-9966-7 PMID: 23329863

Husserl, E. (1931/1970). *Cartesian meditations: An introduction to phenomenology* (D. Cairns, Trans.). Martinus Nijhoff.

Husserl, E. (1936/1970). *The crisis of European sciences and transcendental phenomenology: An introduction to phenomenological philosophy* (Carr, D., Trans.). Northwestern University Press.

Husserl, E. (1970). *Logical investigations* (Findlay, J. N., Trans.). Routledge. (Original work published 1901)

Hwong, A. R., Wang, M., Khan, H., Chagwedera, D. N., Grzenda, A., Doty, B., Benton, T., Alpert, J., Clarke, D., & Compton, W. M. (2022). Climate change and mental health research methods, gaps, and priorities: a scoping review. In *The Lancet Planetary Health* (Vol. 6, Issue 3, pp. e281–e291). Lancet Planet Health. DOI: 10.1016/S2542-5196(22)00012-2

Illingworth, P. (2024). Will Including Health at COP28 Mean Transformation of Global Mental Health Action? And will Mental Health Professionals transform to help achieve it? *Mental Health: Global Challenges*, *7*(1), 50–54. DOI: 10.56508/mhgcj.v7i1.187

Immordino-Yang, M. H. (2016). *Emotions, learning, and the brain: Exploring the educational implications of affective neuroscience*. W. W. Norton.

Immordino-Yang, M. H., Christodoulou, J. A., & Singh, V. (2012). Rest is not idleness: Implications of the brain's default mode for human development and education. *Perspectives on Psychological Science*, *7*(4), 352–364. DOI: 10.1177/1745691612447308

Immordino-Yang, M. H., & Damasio, A. (2007). We feel, therefore we learn: The relevance of affective and social neuroscience to education. *Mind, Brain and Education : the Official Journal of the International Mind, Brain, and Education Society*, *1*(1), 3–10. DOI: 10.1111/j.1751-228X.2007.00004.x

Jacklitsch, B., Williams, W., Musolin, K., Coca, A., Kim, J.-H., & Turner, N. (2016). NIOSH criteria for a recommended standard: occupational exposure to heat and hot environments. *US Department of Health and Human Services*, Publication 2016-106.

Jeanmonod, D., Irick, J., Munday, A. R., Awosika, A. O., & Jeanmonod, R. (2024). Compassion Fatigue in Emergency Medicine: Current Perspectives. *Open Access Emergency Medicine : OAEM*, *16*, 167–181. DOI: 10.2147/OAEM.S418935 PMID: 39045605

Jelinek, R., Pandita, D., Linzer, M., Engoang, J. B. B. N., & Rodin, H. (2022). An Evidence-Based Roadmap for the Provision of More Equitable Telemedicine. *Applied Clinical Informatics*, *13*(3), 612–620. DOI: 10.1055/s-0042-1749597 PMID: 35675839

Jiang, L., Wang, J., Castaño-Rosa, R., Zhong, C., & Cao, S. (2024). Heat exposure and coping strategies for food delivery riders under urban heat extremes. *Energy and Building*, *322*, 114693. DOI: 10.1016/j.enbuild.2024.114693

Jiaojiao, L., & Lifei, M. (2023). The Dilemma and Thinking of Gig Workers in the Digital Organization Environment. *Information Systems and Economics*, *4*(6). Advance online publication. DOI: 10.23977/infse.2023.040606

Johnson, C. V., Mimiaga, M. J., & Bradford, J. (2008). Health care issues among lesbian, gay, bisexual, transgender and intersex (LGBTI) populations in the United States: Introduction. *Journal of Homosexuality*, *54*(3), 213–224. DOI: 10.1080/00918360801982025 PMID: 18825859

Joyce, S., Shand, F., Tighe, J., Laurent, S. J., Bryant, R. A., & Harvey, S. B. (2018). Road to resilience: A systematic review and meta-analysis of resilience training programmes and interventions. *BMJ Open*, *8*(6), e017858. DOI: 10.1136/bmjopen-2017-017858 PMID: 29903782

Junge, M. B., & Linesch, D. (1993). Our own voices: New paradigms for art therapy research. *Art Therapy: Journal of the American Art Therapy Association*, *10*(1), 3–11. DOI: 10.1080/07421656.1993.10758986

Jung, H. H., Emlet, C. A., Kim, H. J., & Fredriksen-Goldsen, K. (2025). Predictors of Generativity Among SGM Midlife and Older Adults. *The Gerontologist*, *65*(4), gnaf023. DOI: 10.1093/geront/gnaf023 PMID: 39878371

Kaimal, G., Ray, K., & Muniz, J. (2017). Reduction of cortisol levels and participants' responses following art making. *Art Therapy: Journal of the American Art Therapy Association*, *33*(2), 74–80. DOI: 10.1080/07421656.2016.1166832 PMID: 27695158

Kalbalia, P., & Koushik, K. (2025a). Driving Better Health Outcomes for Gig Workers Through Strategic Health Initiatives. In *Immersive Technology for the Gig Economy* (pp. 323–346). IGI Global Scientific Publishing., DOI: 10.4018/979-8-3373-1290-3.ch012

Kalbalia, P., & Koushik, K. (2025b). Health Communication as Capability: Gig Workers' Freedoms Through Sen's Approach. *The Howard Journal of Communications*, •••, 1–13. DOI: 10.1080/10646175.2025.2570753

Kalbalia, P., & Koushik, K. (2025c). Regulating the gig economy: Addressing worker rights in India's quick commerce sector. In *Sustainability and Adaptability of Gig Economies in Global Business* (pp. 85–105). IGI Global., DOI: 10.4018/979-8-3693-9385-7.ch004

Kalbalia, P., Nath, N. J., & Haneefa, K. V. (2024). Utilisation and Accessibility of Healthcare Services Among Gig Workers: A Systematic Review. In *Population, Environment and Disease: Towards Health Geography* (pp. 77–95). Springer., DOI: 10.1007/978-3-031-67624-6_5

Kamii, C., & Lewis, B. A. (1993). *Young children reinvent arithmetic: Implications of Piaget's theory*. Teachers College Press.

Kapitan, L. (2016). *Introduction to art therapy research* (2nd ed.). Routledge.

Katzman, J. G., Tomedi, L. E., Herring, D., Jones, H., Groves, R., Norsworthy, K., Martin, C., Liu, J., Kazhe-Dominguez, B., & Arora, S. (2022). Educating Community Health Professionals About the Health-Related Effects of Climate Change Through ECHO Telementoring. *Journal of Primary Care & Community Health, 13*, 21501319221102033. Advance online publication. DOI: 10.1177/21501319221102033 PMID: 35603993

Kaushik, A. (2024). Comprehensive Impact of On-Demand Platforms: Examining the Gig Economy\'s Influence on Specialized Professionals, Work-Life Balance, and Gig Workers\' Perspectives. *International Journal for Research in Applied Science and Engineering Technology, 12*(1), 552–559. DOI: 10.22214/ijraset.2024.58005

Keyes, C. L. (2002). The mental health continuum: From languishing to flourishing in life. *Journal of Health and Social Behavior, 43*(2), 207–222. DOI: 10.2307/3090197 PMID: 12096700

Khanijahani, A., Akinci, N., & Quitiquit, E. (2022). A Systematic Review of the Role of Telemedicine in Blood Pressure Control: Focus on Patient Engagement. In *Current Hypertension Reports* (Vol. 24, Issue 7, pp. 247–258). Springer. DOI: 10.1007/s11906-022-01186-5

Khreis, H., Warsow, K. M., Verlinghieri, E., Guzman, A., Pellecuer, L., Ferreira, A., Jones, I., Heinen, E., Rojas-Rueda, D., Mueller, N., Schepers, P., Lucas, K., & Nieuwenhuijsen, M. (2016). The health impacts of traffic-related exposures in urban areas: Understanding real effects, underlying driving forces and co-producing future directions. In *Journal of Transport and Health* (Vol. 3, Issue 3, pp. 249–267). Elsevier. DOI: 10.1016/j.jth.2016.07.002

Kim, J., & Lee, H. (2023). Digital manipulatives and augmented reality in early mathematics education: Effects on spatial reasoning. *Journal of Educational Technology & Society, 26*(2), 45–60.

Koch, S. C., & Fuchs, T. (2011). Embodied arts therapies. *Frontiers in Psychology, 2*, 1–12. DOI: 10.3389/fpsyg.2011.00124

Koch, S. C., Kunz, T., Lykou, S., & Cruz, R. (2014). Effects of dance movement therapy and dance on health-related psychological outcomes: A meta-analysis. *The Arts in Psychotherapy, 41*(1), 46–64. DOI: 10.1016/j.aip.2013.10.004

Koelsch, S. (2014). Brain correlates of music-evoked emotions. *Nature Reviews. Neuroscience, 15*(3), 170–180. DOI: 10.1038/nrn3666 PMID: 24552785

Kolb, B., & Gibb, R. (2011). Brain plasticity and behaviour in the developing brain. *Journal of the Canadian Academy of Child and Adolescent Psychiatry = Journal de l'Académie Canadienne de Psychiatrie de l'Enfant et de l'Adolescent, 20*(4), 265–276.

Koutsimpogiorgos, N., van Slageren, J., Herrmann, A., & Frenken, K. (2020). Conceptualizing the Gig Economy and Its Regulatory Problems. *Policy & Internet*. https://doi.org/DOI: 10.31235/OSF.IO/JMQYT

Krebs, P., Prochaska, J. O., & Rossi, J. S. (2010). A meta-analysis of computer-tailored interventions for health behavior change. *Preventive Medicine, 51*(3–4), 214–221. DOI: 10.1016/j.ypmed.2010.06.004 PMID: 20558196

Kruse, C. S., Karem, P., Shifflett, K., Vegi, L., Ravi, K., & Brooks, M. (2018). Evaluating barriers to adopting telemedicine worldwide: A systematic review. In *Journal of Telemedicine and Telecare* (Vol. 24, Issue 1, pp. 4–12). J Telemed Telecare. DOI: 10.1177/1357633X16674087

Lambert, S. J., Haley-Lock, A., & Henly, J. R. (2012). Schedule flexibility in hourly jobs: Unanticipated consequences and promising directions. *Community Work & Family, 15*(3), 293–315. DOI: 10.1080/13668803.2012.662803

Landes, S. D., Ardelt, M., Vaillant, G. E., & Waldinger, R. J. (2014). Childhood adversity, midlife generativity, and later life well-being. *The Journals of Gerontology. Series B, Psychological Sciences and Social Sciences, 69*(6), 942–952. DOI: 10.1093/geronb/gbu055 PMID: 24870028

Landsbergis, P. A., Schnall, P. L., Belkic, K. L., Baker, D., Schwartz, J., & Pickering, T. G. (2001). Work stressors and cardiovascular disease. In *Work* (Vol. 17, Issue 3, pp. 191–208). John Wiley & Sons, Ltd. DOI: 10.3233/WOR-2001-00189

Lattie, E. G., Stiles-Shields, C., & Graham, A. K. (2019). An overview of and recommendations for more accessible digital mental health services. *Nature Reviews Psychology, 1*(2), 87–100. DOI: 10.1038/s44159-021-00003-1 PMID: 38515434

Lauss, J., & Helm, C. (2024). The role of the arts in the classroom: Does integration of the arts promote social relationships in the classroom? *ResearchGate*. https://www.researchgate.net/publication/387452576

Lazarus, R. S., & Folkman, S. (1984). *Stress, appraisal, and coping*. Springer.

Lei, Y. W. (2021). Delivering Solidarity: Platform Architecture and Collective Contention in China's Platform Economy. *American Sociological Review, 86*(2), 279–309. DOI: 10.1177/0003122420979980

Lester, G. V., Brock Baskin, M. E., & Clinton, M. S. (2021). Employer-Sponsored Benefits in the United States: The Past, Present, and Future. *Compensation and Benefits Review*, *53*(1), 24–42. DOI: 10.1177/0886368720947609 PMID: 34955602

Levison, M. M., Butler, A. J., Rebellato, S., Armstrong, B., Whelan, M., & Gardner, C. (2018). Development of a climate change vulnerability assessment using a public health lens to determine local health vulnerabilities: An Ontario health unit experience. *International Journal of Environmental Research and Public Health*, *15*(10), 2237. Advance online publication. DOI: 10.3390/ijerph15102237 PMID: 30322040

Liljedahl, P. (2020). *Building thinking classrooms in mathematics, grades K–12: 14 teaching practices for enhancing learning*. Corwin.

Liyanage, S., Dia, H., Abduljabbar, R., & Bagloee, S. A. (2019). Flexible mobility on-demand: An environmental scan. In *Sustainability (Switzerland)* (Vol. 11, Issue 5, p. 1262). Multidisciplinary Digital Publishing Institute. DOI: 10.3390/su11051262

Lõhmus, M. (2018). Possible biological mechanisms linking mental health and heat—a contemplative review. In *International Journal of Environmental Research and Public Health* (Vol. 15, Issue 7). Int J Environ Res Public Health. DOI: 10.3390/ijerph15071515

Luxton, D. D., Kayl, R. A., & Mishkind, M. C. (2011). mHealth data security: The need for HIPAA-compliant standardization. *Telemedicine Journal and e-Health*, *18*(4), 284–288. DOI: 10.1089/tmj.2011.0180 PMID: 22400974

Luyckx, K., Goossens, L., Soenens, B., Beyers, W., & Vansteenkiste, M. (2005). Identity statuses based on 4 rather than 2 identity dimensions: Extending and refining Marcia's paradigm. *Journal of Youth and Adolescence*, *34*(6), 605–618. DOI: 10.1007/s10964-005-8949-x

Malchiodi, C. A. (2012). *Handbook of art therapy* (2nd ed.). Guilford Press.

Malchiodi, C. A. (2020). *Trauma and expressive arts therapy: Brain, body, and imagination in the healing process*. Guilford Press.

Maloney, E. A., & Beilock, S. L. (2012). Math anxiety: Who has it, why it develops, and how to guard against it. *Trends in Cognitive Sciences*, *16*(8), 404–406. DOI: 10.1016/j.tics.2012.06.008 PMID: 22784928

Manning, L., Ferris, M., Rosario, C. N., Prues, M., & Bouchard, L. (2019). Spiritual resilience: Understanding the protection and promotion of well-being in the later life. *Journal of Religion, Spirituality and Aging*, *31*(2), 168–186. DOI: 10.1080/15528030.2018.1532859 PMID: 33335455

Marks, D. F., Murray, M., Evans, B., & Estacio, E. V. (2018). *Health psychology: Theory, research and practice* (5th ed.). Sage.

Marsh, Z., Nguyen, Y., Teegala, Y., & Cotter, V. T. (2022). Diabetes management among underserved older adults through telemedicine and community health workers. In *Journal of the American Association of Nurse Practitioners* (Vol. 34, Issue 1, pp. 26–31). Lippincott Williams and Wilkins. DOI: 10.1097/JXX.0000000000000595

Marshall, A. I., Lasco, G., Phaiyarom, M., Pangkariya, N., Leuangvilay, P., Sinam, P., Suphanchaimat, R., Julchoo, S., Kunpeuk, W., & Zhang, Y. (2021). Evidence on child nutrition recommendations and challenges in crisis settings: A scoping review. *International Journal of Environmental Research and Public Health*, *18*(12), 6637. DOI: 10.3390/ijerph18126637 PMID: 34203109

Martín Quintana, J. C., Alemán Ramos, P. F., & Morales Almeida, P. (2023). The Influence of Perceived Security in Childhood on Adult Self-Concept: The Mediating Role of Resilience and Self-Esteem. *Healthcare (Basel)*, *11*(17), 2435. DOI: 10.3390/healthcare11172435 PMID: 37685469

Masten, A. S. (2014). Global perspectives on resilience in children and youth. *Child Development*, *85*(1), 6–20. DOI: 10.1111/cdev.12205 PMID: 24341286

Masten, A. S., & Barnes, A. J. (2018). Resilience in Children: Developmental Perspectives. *Children (Basel, Switzerland)*, *5*(7), 98. DOI: 10.3390/children5070098 PMID: 30018217

Mayer, K. H., Bradford, J. B., Makadon, H. J., Stall, R., Goldhammer, H., & Landers, S. (2008). Sexual and gender minority health: What we know and what needs to be done. *American Journal of Public Health*, *98*(6), 989–995. DOI: 10.2105/AJPH.2007.127811 PMID: 18445789

Mayhew, C., & Quinlan, M. (2002). Fordism in the fast food industry: Pervasive management control and occupational health and safety risks for young temporary workers. *Sociology of Health & Illness*, *24*(3), 261–284. DOI: 10.1111/1467-9566.00294

Mayhew, C., & Quinlan, M. (2006). Economic pressure, multi-tiered subcontracting and occupational health and safety in Australian long-haul trucking. *Employee Relations*, *28*(3), 212–229. DOI: 10.1108/01425450610661216

McAllister, M., & McKinnon, J. (2009). The importance of teaching and learning resilience in the health disciplines: A critical review of the literature. *Nurse Education Today*, *29*(4), 371–379. DOI: 10.1016/j.nedt.2008.10.011 PMID: 19056153

McKinnon McQuarrie, M. A., Siegel, L. S., Perry, N. E., & Weinberg, J. (2014). Reactivity to stress and the cognitive components of math disability in Grade 1 children. *Journal of Learning Disabilities*, *47*(4), 349–365. DOI: 10.1177/0022219412463436 PMID: 23124381

Megasari, A. L., Masbahah, , Riatma, D. L., & Fatsena, R. A. (2023). The effect of telemedicine plus application on the covid-19 patients' quality of life. *Journal of Public Health Dentistry*, *21*(2), 56–68. DOI: 10.55131/jphd/2023/210205

Merleau-Ponty, M. (1962/2012). *Phenomenology of perception* (Smith, C., Trans.). Routledge.

Meyer, I. H. (2013). Prejudice, social stress, and mental health in lesbian, gay, and bisexual populations: Conceptual issues and research evidence.

Meyer, I. H. (1995). Minority stress and mental health in gay men. *Journal of Health and Social Behavior*, *36*(1), 38–56. DOI: 10.2307/2137286 PMID: 7738327

Meyer, I. H. (2003). Prejudice, social stress, and mental health in lesbian, gay, and bisexual populations: Conceptual issues and research evidence. *Psychological Bulletin*, *129*(5), 674–697. DOI: 10.1037/0033-2909.129.5.674 PMID: 12956539

Meyer, I. H. (2015). Resilience in the study of minority stress and health of sexual and gender minorities. *Psychology of Sexual Orientation and Gender Diversity*, *2*(3), 209–213. DOI: 10.1037/sgd0000132

Miner, A. S., Milstein, A., Schueller, S., Hegde, R., Mangurian, C., & Linos, E. (2016). Smartphone-based conversational agents and responses to questions about mental health, interpersonal violence, and physical health. *JAMA Internal Medicine*, *176*(5), 619–625. DOI: 10.1001/jamainternmed.2016.0400 PMID: 26974260

Mittelstadt, B. D., Allo, P., Taddeo, M., Wachter, S., & Floridi, L. (2016). The ethics of algorithms: Mapping the debate. *Big Data & Society*, *3*(2), 1–21. DOI: 10.1177/2053951716679679

Mix, K. S., Levine, S. C., Cheng, Y.-L., Young, C., Hambrick, D. Z., & Konstantopoulos, S. (2016). Separate but correlated: The latent structure of space and mathematics across development. *Journal of Experimental Psychology. General*, *145*(10), 1364–1384. DOI: 10.1037/xge0000182 PMID: 27560854

Mix, K. S., Smith, L. B., & Ni, Y. (2020). The transition from concrete to abstract in early mathematics learning. *Developmental Review*, *57*, 100922. DOI: 10.1016/j.dr.2020.100922

Mohr, D. C., Weingardt, K. R., Reddy, M., & Schueller, S. M. (2017). Three problems with current digital mental health research... and three things we can do about them. *Psychiatric Services (Washington, D.C.)*, *68*(5), 427–429. DOI: 10.1176/appi.ps.201600541 PMID: 28412890

Morales, M. J., King, M. D., Hiler, H., Coopwood, M. S., & Wayland, S. (2017). The greater St. Louis LGBT health and human services needs assessment: An examination of the silent and baby boom generations. In *Community-Based Research on LGBT Aging* (pp. 103–128). Routledge.

Mosher, C. E., & DuHamel, K. N. (2006). An examination of distress, physical symptoms, and health behaviors among cancer survivors. *Cancer*, *107*(4), 831–838.

Moula, Z., Powell, J., & Karkou, V. (2020). *A systematic review of child-focused outcomes and experiences in arts therapies.* Edge Hill University. https://research.edgehill.ac.uk/files/23144225/Systematic_review_Final_version.pdf

Musa, S., Ramatu, A., Haliru, L., Abigail, D., & Gumbi, S. (2023). Establishing a paediatric telemedicine centre in a low-resource setting: Experience and challenges from a teaching hospital in Kaduna, Nigeria. *Sri Lanka Journal of Child Health*, *52*(2), 155–160. DOI: 10.4038/sljch.v52i2.10548

Nadeau, C. P., Urban, M. C., & Bridle, J. R. (2017). Climates Past, Present, and Yet-to-Come Shape Climate Change Vulnerabilities. In *Trends in Ecology and Evolution* (Vol. 32, Issue 10, pp. 786–800). Elsevier Ltd. DOI: 10.1016/j.tree.2017.07.012

Narimani, M., Abolghasemi, A., & Ilbeigy Ghalenei, R. (2018). Effect of art therapy (painting) on executive functions and visual motor coordination in dyslexic children. *Middle Eastern Journal of Disability Studies, 8,* 50. https://jdisabilstud.org/article-1-645-en.html

Nebeker, C., Torous, J., & Bartlett Ellis, R. J. (2019). Building the case for actionable ethics in digital health research supported by artificial intelligence. *BMC Medicine*, *17*(1), 137. DOI: 10.1186/s12916-019-1377-7 PMID: 31311535

Nguyen, M. L. T., Garcia, F., Juarez, J., Zeng, B., Khoong, E. C., Nijagal, M. A., Sarkar, U., Su, G., & Lyles, C. R. (2022). Satisfaction can co-exist with hesitation: Qualitative analysis of acceptability of telemedicine among multi-lingual patients in a safety-net healthcare system during the COVID-19 pandemic. *BMC Health Services Research*, *22*(1), 1–9. DOI: 10.1186/s12913-022-07547-9 PMID: 35164746

Nguyen, T., Lee, J., & Wong, P. (2022). Cross-cultural perspectives on manipulatives in early mathematics classrooms. *International Journal of Science and Mathematics Education*, *20*, 1125–1144. DOI: 10.1007/s10763-021-10242-3

Nikulin, D., Wolszczak-Derlacz, J., & Parteka, A. (2022). Working Conditions in Global Value Chains: Evidence for European Employees. *Work, Employment and Society*, *36*(4), 701–721. DOI: 10.1177/0950017020986107

Norman, D. A. (2013). *The design of everyday things: Revised and expanded edition*. Basic Books.

Nutbeam, D., & Lloyd, J. E. (2020). Understanding and Responding to Health Literacy as a Social Determinant of Health. In *Annual Review of Public Health* (Vol. 42, pp. 159–173). Annual Reviews Inc., DOI: 10.1146/annurev-publhealth-090419-102529

Obar, J. A., & Oeldorf-Hirsch, A. (2020). The biggest lie on the internet: Ignoring the privacy policies and terms of service policies of social networking services. *Information Communication and Society*, *23*(1), 128–147. DOI: 10.1080/1369118X.2018.1486870

Ojala, M., Cunsolo, A., Ogunbode, C. A., & Middleton, J. (2021). Anxiety, Worry, and Grief in a Time of Environmental and Climate Crisis: A Narrative Review. In *Annual Review of Environment and Resources* (Vol. 46, Issue Volume 46, 2021, pp. 35–58). Annual Reviews Inc. DOI: 10.1146/annurev-environ-012220-022716

Omaghomi, T. T. (2023). Telemedicine in rural Africa: A review of accessibility and impact. *World Journal of Advanced Research and Reviews*, *21*(2), 421–431. DOI: 10.30574/wjarr.2024.21.2.0475

Ong, A. D., Graham, E. K., Jackson, K., Atherton, O. E., Luo, J., Willroth, E. C., Beck, E. D., Yoneda, T., Cintron, D. W., Mroczek, D. K., & Steptoe, A. (2024). Associations Between Generativity and Social Asymmetry Among Older Adults in Japan. *The Journals of Gerontology. Series B, Psychological Sciences and Social Sciences*, *79*(2), gbad183. Advance online publication. DOI: 10.1093/geronb/gbad183 PMID: 38149998

Onsongo, S., Kamotho, C., Rinke De Wit, T. F., & Lowrie, K. (2023). Experiences on the Utility and Barriers of Telemedicine in Healthcare Delivery in Kenya. *International Journal of Telemedicine and Applications*, *2023*(1), 1487245. DOI: 10.1155/2023/1487245 PMID: 37180825

Orenstein, G. A., & Lewis, L. (2022). Erikson's stages of psychosocial development. In *StatPearls* [Internet]. StatPearls Publishing.

Palhad, S., Onwubu, S., Singh, R., Thakur, R., Thakur, S., & Mkhize, G. (2023). The Benefits and Challenges of the Gig Economy: Perspective of Gig Workers and Small Medium and Micro Enterprises (SMMEs) in South Africa. *African Journal of Inter/Multidisciplinary Studies*, *5*(1), 1–12. DOI: 10.51415/ajims.v5i1.1051

Pande, N. (2024). WHAT ARE THE ECONOMIC IMPLICATIONS OF THE RISE OF THE GIG ECONOMY ON EMPLOYMENT STABILITY AND BENEFITS? *EPH-International Journal of Business & Management Science*, *10*(1), 53–67. DOI: 10.53555/EIJBMS.V10I1.175

Park, C. L. (2010). Making sense of the meaning literature: An integrative review of meaning-making and its effects on adjustment to stressful life events. *Psychological Bulletin*, *136*(2), 257–301. DOI: 10.1037/a0018301 PMID: 20192563

Parks, A. C., & Biswas-Diener, R. (2013). Positive interventions: Past, present, and future. In Kashdan, T. B., & Ciarrochi, J. (Eds.), *Mindfulness, acceptance, and positive psychology* (pp. 140–165). Context Press.

Parks, A. C., Schueller, S. M., & Tasimi, A. (2012). Positive psychology in digital contexts. *The American Psychologist*, *67*(6), 577–589. DOI: 10.1037/a0029121

Patel, S. S., Rogers, M. B., Amlôt, R., & Rubin, G. J. (2017). What Do We Mean by 'Community Resilience'? A Systematic Literature Review of How It Is Defined in the Literature. *PLoS currents, 9*, ecurrents.dis.db775aff25efc5ac4f0660ad9c9f7db2. DOI: 10.1371/currents.dis.db775aff25efc5ac4f0660ad9c9f7db2

Patel, V., Weiss, H. A., Chowdhary, N., Naik, S., Pednekar, S., Chatterjee, S., De Silva, M. J., Bhat, B., Araya, R., King, M., Simon, G., Verdeli, H., & Kirkwood, B. R. (2010). Effectiveness of an intervention led by lay health counsellors for depressive and anxiety disorders in primary care in Goa, India (MANAS): A cluster randomised controlled trial. *Lancet*, *376*(9758), 2086–2095. DOI: 10.1016/S0140-6736(10)61508-5 PMID: 21159375

Pennebaker, J. W., & Seagal, J. D. (1999). Forming a story: The health benefits of narrative. *Journal of Clinical Psychology*, *55*(10), 1243–1254. DOI: 10.1002/(SICI)1097-4679(199910)55:10<1243::AID-JCLP6>3.0.CO;2-N PMID: 11045774

Petitmengin, C., Van Beek, M., Bitbol, M., Nissou, J. M., & Roepstorff, A. (2019). Studying the experience of meditation through micro-phenomenology. *Current Opinion in Psychology*, *28*, 54–59. DOI: 10.1016/j.copsyc.2018.10.009 PMID: 30502663

Piaget, J. (1936/1952). *The origins of intelligence in children* (Cook, M., Trans.). International Universities Press.

Piaget, J. (1951). *Play, dreams and imitation in childhood*. Routledge & Kegan Paul.

Piaget, J. (1972). *Psychology and pedagogy*. Viking Press.

Pierce, B. S., Perrin, P. B., Dow, A. W., Dautovich, N. D., Rybarczyk, B. D., & Mishra, V. K. (2021). Changes in physician telemedicine use during COVID-19: Effects of practice setting, demographics, training, and organizational policies. *International Journal of Environmental Research and Public Health*, *18*(19), 9963. DOI: 10.3390/ijerph18199963 PMID: 34639269

Pressman, S. D., & Cohen, S. (2005). Does positive affect influence health? *Psychological Bulletin*, *131*(6), 925–971. DOI: 10.1037/0033-2909.131.6.925 PMID: 16351329

Puig, A., Lee, S. M., Goodwin, L., & Sherrard, P. (2006). The efficacy of creative arts therapies to enhance emotional expression, spirituality, and psychological well-being of newly diagnosed stage I and II breast cancer patients: A preliminary study. *The Arts in Psychotherapy*, *33*(3), 218–228. DOI: 10.1016/j.aip.2006.02.004

Ramsetty, A., & Adams, C. (2020). Impact of the digital divide in the age of COVID-19. *Journal of the American Medical Informatics Association : JAMIA*, *27*(7), 1147–1148. DOI: 10.1093/jamia/ocaa078 PMID: 32343813

Reyes-Perez, M. D., Carreño Saucedo, L., Sanchez-Levano, M. J., Cabanillas-Palomino, R., Monje-Yovera, P. F., Jaime-Rodríguez, J. P., Atoche-Silva, L. A., Alarcón-Bustíos, J. M., & Fernández-Altamirano, A. E. F. (2025). The Spirituality-Resilience-Happiness Triad: A High-Powered Model for Understanding University Student Well-Being. *European Journal of Investigation in Health, Psychology and Education*, *15*(8), 158. DOI: 10.3390/ejihpe15080158 PMID: 40863280

Rickard, N. S., & McFerran, K. (2012). Lifelong engagement with music: Benefits for mental health and wellbeing. *Arts & Health*, *4*(2), 132–142. DOI: 10.1080/17533015.2011.584884

Riva, G., Banos, R. M., Botella, C., Wiederhold, B. K., & Gaggioli, A. (2012). Positive technology: Using interactive technologies to promote positive functioning. *Cyberpsychology, Behavior, and Social Networking*, *15*(2), 69–77. DOI: 10.1089/cyber.2011.0139 PMID: 22149077

Rubin, J. A. (2016). *Approaches to art therapy: Theory and technique* (3rd ed.). Routledge. DOI: 10.4324/9781315716015

Russo, S. J., Murrough, J. W., Han, M. H., Charney, D. S., & Nestler, E. J. (2012). Neurobiology of resilience. *Nature Neuroscience*, *15*(11), 1475–1484. DOI: 10.1038/nn.3234 PMID: 23064380

Rutter, M. (2006). Implications of resilience concepts for scientific understanding. *Annals of the New York Academy of Sciences, 1094*(1), 1–12. DOI: 10.1196/annals.1376.002 PMID: 17347337

Ryan, M., & Ryznar, R. (2022). The Molecular Basis of Resilience: A Narrative Review. *Frontiers in Psychiatry, 13*, 856998. DOI: 10.3389/fpsyt.2022.856998 PMID: 35599764

Ryff, C. D. (2014). Psychological well-being revisited: Advances in the science and practice of eudaimonia. *Psychotherapy and Psychosomatics, 83*(1), 10–28. DOI: 10.1159/000353263 PMID: 24281296

Ryff, C. D., Singer, B. H., & Dienberg Love, G. (2004). Positive health: Connecting well-being with biology. *Philosophical Transactions of the Royal Society of London. Series B, Biological Sciences, 359*(1449), 1383–1394. DOI: 10.1098/rstb.2004.1521 PMID: 15347530

Saccardo, S., Clements, D., & Sarama, J. (2024). Manipulative-rich environments in early mathematics: Emotional and cognitive outcomes. *Early Childhood Research Quarterly, 65*, 1–15. DOI: 10.1016/j.ecresq.2024.102044

Sanders, E. B. N., & Stappers, P. J. (2008). Co-creation and the new landscapes of design. *CoDesign, 4*(1), 5–18. DOI: 10.1080/15710880701875068

Sani, Y., Wardany, O. F., Herlina, H., & Vernanda, G. (2021). The implementation of embodied learning: A literature review. *Edukasi, 15*(1), 1–10. DOI: 10.15294/edukasi.v15i1.30008

Sarama, J., & Clements, D. H. (2009). Building blocks and cognitive building blocks: Playing to know the world mathematically. *American Journal of Play, 1*(3), 313–337.

Sarama, J., & Clements, D. H. (2019). *Hands-on, minds-on: Learning mathematics through manipulatives*. Routledge.

Schetter, C. D., & Dolbier, C. (2011). Resilience in the Context of Chronic Stress and Health in Adults. *Social and Personality Psychology Compass, 5*(9), 634–652. DOI: 10.1111/j.1751-9004.2011.00379.x PMID: 26161137

Schueller, S. M., Tomasino, K. N., & Mohr, D. C. (2017). Integrating human support into behavioral intervention technologies: The efficiency model of support. *Clinical Psychology : a Publication of the Division of Clinical Psychology of the American Psychological Association, 24*(1), 27–45. DOI: 10.1111/cpsp.12173

Schulte, P. A., & Chun, H. K. (2009). Climate change and occupational safety and health: Establishing a preliminary framework. *Journal of Occupational and Environmental Hygiene*, *6*(9), 542–554. DOI: 10.1080/15459620903066008 PMID: 19551548

Schulz, E. K. (2002). *The meaning of spirituality in the lives and adaptation processes of individuals with disabilities*. Texas Woman's University.

Schunk, D. H., & DiBenedetto, M. K. (2020). Motivation and social-emotional learning in health psychology. *Journal of Health Psychology*, *25*(9), 1235–1247. DOI: 10.1177/1359105320913439

Seaton, C. L., Rondier, P., Rush, K. L., Li, E. P. H., Plamondon, K., Pesut, B., Oelke, N. D., Dow-Fleisner, S., Hasan, K., Currie, L. M., Kurtz, D., Jones, C., & Bottorff, J. L. (2022). Community stakeholder-driven technology solutions towards rural health equity: A concept mapping study in Western Canada. *Health Expectations*, *25*(6), 3202–3214. DOI: 10.1111/hex.13627 PMID: 36245334

Segerstrom, S. C., Carver, C. S., & Scheier, M. F. (2018). Optimism, psychosocial well-being, and adaptation to chronic illness. *Health Psychology Review*, *12*(2), 71–93.

Seligman, M. E. P. (2011). *Flourish: A visionary new understanding of happiness and well-being*. Free Press.

Seligman, M. E. P., & Csikszentmihalyi, M. (2000). Positive psychology: An introduction. *The American Psychologist*, *55*(1), 5–14. DOI: 10.1037/0003-066X.55.1.5 PMID: 11392865

Seligman, M. E. P., Steen, T. A., Park, N., & Peterson, C. (2005). Positive psychology progress: Empirical validation of interventions. *The American Psychologist*, *60*(5), 410–421. DOI: 10.1037/0003-066X.60.5.410 PMID: 16045394

Seligman, M. E., & Csikszentmihalyi, M. (2014). *Positive Psychology: An Introduction*. Springer.

Shah, A. Q., Noronha, N., Chin-See, R., Hanna, C., Kadri, Z., Marwaha, A., Rambharack, N., & Ng, J. Y. (2023). The use and effects of telemedicine on complementary, alternative, and integrative medicine practices: A scoping review. *BMC Complementary Medicine and Therapies*, *23*(1), 1–40. DOI: 10.1186/s12906-023-04100-x PMID: 37533042

Sharma, P., Sethi, M. I. S., Liem, A., Bhatti, H. B. S., Pandey, V., & Nair, A. (2023). A Review of Telemedicine Guidelines in the South-East Asia Region. In *Telemedicine Reports* (Vol. 4, Issue 1, pp. 271–278). Telemed Rep. DOI: 10.1089/tmr.2023.0040

Sharma, V., Feldman, M., & Sharma, R. (2024). Telehealth Technologies in Diabetes Self-management and Education. In *Journal of Diabetes Science and Technology* (Vol. 18, Issue 1, pp. 148–158). SAGE Publications Inc. DOI: 10.1177/19322968221093078

Sheldon, K. M., & Lyubomirsky, S. (2006). How to increase and sustain positive emotion: The effects of expressing gratitude and visualizing best possible selves. *The Journal of Positive Psychology*, *1*(2), 73–82. DOI: 10.1080/17439760500510676

Shen, Y. T., Chen, L., Yue, W. W., & Xu, H. X. (2021). Digital Technology-Based Telemedicine for the COVID-19 Pandemic. In *Frontiers in Medicine* (Vol. 8, p. 646506). DOI: 10.3389/fmed.2021.646506

Shoib, S., Hussaini, S. S., Armiya'u, A. Y., Saeed, F., Őri, D., Roza, T. H., Gürcan, A., Agrawal, A., Solerdelcoll, M., Lucero-Prisno, D. E.III, Nahidi, M., Swed, S., Ahmed, S., & Chandradasa, M. (2023). Prevention of suicides associated with global warming: Perspectives from early career psychiatrists. *Frontiers in Psychiatry*, *14*, 1251630. Advance online publication. DOI: 10.3389/fpsyt.2023.1251630 PMID: 38045615

Shukla, A. (2022). Role of art therapy in the promotion of mental health. *PubMed Central.* https://pubmed.ncbi.nlm.nih.gov/

Siegler, R. S., & Ramani, G. B. (2008). Playing linear numerical board games promotes low-income children's numerical development. *Developmental Science*, *11*(5), 655–661. DOI: 10.1111/j.1467-7687.2008.00714.x PMID: 18801120

Singh, S., & Sharma, T. (2017). Affect of adversity quotient on the occupational stress of IT managers in India. *Procedia Computer Science*, *122*, 86–93. DOI: 10.1016/j.procs.2017.11.345

Sin, N. L., & Lyubomirsky, S. (2009). Enhancing well-being and alleviating depressive symptoms with Positive Psychology Interventions: A practice-friendly meta-analysis. *Journal of Clinical Psychology*, *65*(5), 467–487. DOI: 10.1002/jclp.20593 PMID: 19301241

Slayton, S. C., D'Archer, J., & Kaplan, F. (2010). Outcome studies on the efficacy of art therapy: A review of findings. *Art Therapy: Journal of the American Art Therapy Association*, *27*(3), 108–118. DOI: 10.1080/07421656.2010.10129660

Smyth, J. M. (1998). Written emotional expression: Effect sizes, outcome types, and moderating variables. *Journal of Consulting and Clinical Psychology*, *66*(1), 174–184. DOI: 10.1037/0022-006X.66.1.174 PMID: 9489272

Sokol, J. T. (2009). Identity development throughout the lifetime: An examination of Eriksonian theory. Graduate journal of counseling psychology, 1(2), 14.

Sonke, J., Rollins, J., Brandman, R., & Graham-Pole, J. (2017). The state of the arts in healthcare in the United States. *Arts & Health*, *9*(2), 177–190. DOI: 10.1080/17533015.2016.1211283

Southwick, S. M., Bonanno, G. A., Masten, A. S., Panter-Brick, C., & Yehuda, R. (2014). Resilience definitions, theory, and challenges: interdisciplinary perspectives. European journal of psychotraumatology, 5, . DOI: 10.3402/ejpt.v5.25338

Stanberry, B. (2000). Telemedicine: Barriers and opportunities in the 21st century. In *Journal of Internal Medicine* (Vol. 247, Issue 6, pp. 615–628). DOI: 10.1046/j.1365-2796.2000.00699.x

Stańczykiewicz, B., & Senczyszyn, A. (2024). Bullying of LGBTQ+ children and adolescents in schools: Understanding the phenomenon, consequences, and international standards with a focus on the polish context. *Frontiers in Psychiatry*, *15*, 1493745. DOI: 10.3389/fpsyt.2024.1493745 PMID: 39524124

Stanford, J. (2017). The resurgence of gig work: Historical and theoretical perspectives. *Economic and Labour Relations Review*, *28*(3), 382–401. DOI: 10.1177/1035304617724303

Steptoe, A., Deaton, A., & Stone, A. A. (2015). Subjective well-being, health, and aging. *Lancet*, *385*(9968), 640–648. DOI: 10.1016/S0140-6736(13)61489-0 PMID: 25468152

Stewart, A., & Stanford, J. (2017). Regulating work in the gig economy: What are the options? *Economic and Labour Relations Review*, *28*(3), 420–437. DOI: 10.1177/1035304617722461

Stuckey, H. L., & Nobel, J. (2010). The connection between art, healing, and public health: A review of current literature. *American Journal of Public Health*, *100*(2), 254–263. DOI: 10.2105/AJPH.2008.156497 PMID: 20019311

Tan, Z. M., Aggarwal, N., Cowls, J., Morley, J., Taddeo, M., & Floridi, L. (2020). The Ethical Debate about the Gig Economy: A Review and Critical Analysis. SSRN *Electronic Journal*. DOI: 10.2139/ssrn.3669216

Taylor, S. E. (2018). *Health psychology* (10th ed.). McGraw-Hill Education.

The Trevor Project. (2022, June). *Resilience and mental health among LGBTQ youth.*

Theron, L. C., & Theron, A. M. (2014). Meaning-making and resilience: Case studies of a multifaceted process. *Journal of Psychology in Africa*, *24*(1), 24–32. DOI: 10.1080/14330237.2014.904099

Torous, J., Myrick, K. J., Rauseo-Ricupero, N., & Firth, J. (2021). Digital mental health and COVID-19: Using technology today to accelerate the curve on access and quality tomorrow. *JMIR Mental Health, 8*(3), e18848. DOI: 10.2196/18848 PMID: 32213476

UNESCO. (2006). *Road map for arts education*. UNESCO.

UNICEF. (2021). *The state of the world's children 2021: On my mind – Promoting, protecting and caring for children's mental health.* United Nations Children's Fund. https://www.unicef.org/reports/state-worlds-children-2021

Upitis, R., & Smithrim, K. (2003). *Learning through the arts: National assessment final report*. The Royal Conservatory of Music.

van Kessel, G., Milanese, S., Dizon, J., de Vries, D. H., MacGregor, H., Abramowitz, S., Enria, L., Burtscher, D., Yeoh, E. K., Thomas, B. E., Kwang, R., de Almeida, J. R., & Gobat, N. (2025). Community resilience to health emergencies: A scoping review. *BMJ Global Health, 10*(4), e016963. DOI: 10.1136/bmjgh-2024-016963 PMID: 40221140

Varela, F. J., Thompson, E., & Rosch, E. (1991). *The embodied mind: Cognitive science and human experience*. MIT Press. DOI: 10.7551/mitpress/6730.001.0001

Veinot, T. C., Mitchell, H., & Ancker, J. S. (2018). Good intentions are not enough: How informatics interventions can worsen inequality. *Journal of the American Medical Informatics Association : JAMIA, 25*(8), 1080–1088. DOI: 10.1093/jamia/ocy052 PMID: 29788380

Venugopal, V., Chinnadurai, J. S., Lucas, R. A. I., & Kjellstrom, T. (2015). Occupational heat stress profiles in selected workplaces in India. *International Journal of Environmental Research and Public Health, 13*(1), 89. Advance online publication. DOI: 10.3390/ijerph13010089 PMID: 26729144

Voth, M., Chisholm, S., Sollid, H., Jones, C., Smith-MacDonald, L., & Brémault-Phillips, S. (2022). Efficacy, effectiveness, and quality of resilience-building mobile health apps for military, veteran, and public safety personnel populations: Scoping literature review and app evaluation. *JMIR mHealth and uHealth, 10*(1), e26453. DOI: 10.2196/26453 PMID: 35044307

Vygotsky, L. S. (1978). *Mind in society: The development of higher psychological processes*. Harvard University Press.

Watts, S., Marchand, A., Bouchard, S., Gosselin, P., Langlois, F., Belleville, G., & Dugas, M. J. (2020). Telepsychotherapy for generalized anxiety disorder: A randomized controlled trial. *Cognitive Behaviour Therapy*, *49*(3), 192–205. DOI: 10.1080/16506073.2019.1699741

Wilcox, L., Larson, K., & Bartlett, R. (2021). The role of resilience in ethnic minority adolescent navigation of ecological adversity. *Journal of Child & Adolescent Trauma*, *14*(4), 507–515. DOI: 10.1007/s40653-020-00337-7 PMID: 33456643

Windle, G., Bennett, K. M., & MacLeod, C. (2020). The Influence of Life Experiences on the Development of Resilience in Older People With Co-morbid Health Problems. *Frontiers in Medicine*, *7*, 502314. DOI: 10.3389/fmed.2020.502314 PMID: 33072779

Winner, E., Goldstein, T. R., & Vincent-Lancrin, S. (2013). *Art for art's sake? The impact of arts education*. OECD Publishing. DOI: 10.1787/9789264180789-en

Wood, A., & Lehdonvirta, V. (2021). Platform Precarity: Surviving Algorithmic Insecurity in the Gig Economy. SSRN *Electronic Journal*. https://doi.org/DOI: 10.2139/SSRN.3795375

Yang, S., & Wang, W. (2022). The Role of Academic Resilience, Motivational Intensity and Their Relationship in EFL Learners' Academic Achievement. *Frontiers in Psychology*, *12*, 823537. DOI: 10.3389/fpsyg.2021.823537 PMID: 35153940

Yardley, L., Morrison, L., Bradbury, K., & Muller, I. (2015). The person-based approach to intervention development: Application to digital health-related behavior change interventions. *Journal of Medical Internet Research*, *17*(1), e30. DOI: 10.2196/jmir.4055 PMID: 25639757

Yarney, L., Mintah, N. A., Ayisi, E. K., & Adzei, F. A. (2023). Narratives of Clinicians on Telemedicine and Delivery of Quality Healthcare in Ghana. *Open Journal of Social Sciences*, *11*(08), 232–256. DOI: 10.4236/jss.2023.118017

Yassa, H. A., Hussein, A. A. R. M., Makhlouf, H. A., Makhlouf, N. A., Youssef, H. M. S., Sotohy, R. S. A., & Essa, A. A. (2022). *Pros and cons of telemedicine in diagnosis and management: A cross sectional survey*. Electronic Journal of General Medicine., DOI: 10.29333/ejgm/12236

Yoon, S., Tomlinson, C. A., Lorenzo Benavides, J., Chang, Y., Stanek, C., Wang, X., Ishiekwene, M., Susana Mariscal, E., Duron, J. F., & Howell, K. H. (2025). Resilience and Strengths Among Minoritized Racial and Ethnic Groups of Children in the United States Exposed to Trauma, Violence, and Maltreatment: A Scoping Review. *Trauma, Violence & Abuse*, *26*(2), 220–234. DOI: 10.1177/15248380241309382 PMID: 40022617

Zagorianakos, A. (2019a, February). *A phenomenological methodology based on Husserl's work in the service of mathematics education research.* Paper presented at the Eleventh Congress of the European Society for Research in Mathematics Education (CERME 11), Utrecht University, Utrecht, Netherlands. https://hal.archives-ouvertes.fr/hal-02417428

Zagorianakos, A. (2022). The capturing of Vygotskyan perezhivanie as radical Erlebnis, through the analysis of a prospective teacher's learning episode. In C. Derouet, A. Nechache, P. R. Richard, L. Vivier, I. M. Gómez-Chacón, A. Kuzniak, M. Maschietto, & E. Montoya Delgadillo (Eds.), *Actes du septième symposium d'Étude sur le Travail Mathématique* (pp. 417–430). IREM de Strasbourg.

Zagorianakos, A. (2016). The study of the intuition of essence of a prospective teacher of mathematics from a phenomenological perspective. *Mediterranean Journal for Research in Mathematics Education*, *15*, 69–94.

Zagorianakos, A. (2019b). A phenomenological approach to the mathematical lived experience: Towards a radical change of attitude to students' (mis)conceptions. In Shvarts, A. (Ed.), *Proceedings of the PME and Yandex Russian Conference: Technology and Psychology for Mathematics Education* (pp. xxx–xxx). Moscow, Russia: HSE Publishing House.

Zagorianakos, A., & Shvarts, A. (2015). The role of intuition in the process of objectification of mathematical phenomena from a Husserlian perspective: A case study. *Educational Studies in Mathematics*, *88*(1), 137–157. DOI: 10.1007/s10649-014-9576-9

Zaidel, D. W. (2013). Neuroesthetics is not just about art. *Frontiers in Human Neuroscience*, *7*, 730. https://doi.org/10

Zarghami, M. (2021). Psychiatric aspects of coronavirus (2019-nCoV) infection. *Iranian Journal of Psychiatry and Behavioral Sciences*, *14*(1), 2019–2021.

Zhang, L., Yang, J., Zhang, Y., & Xu, G. (2023). Gig worker's perceived algorithmic management, stress appraisal, and destructive deviant behavior. *PLoS ONE, 18*(11 November). DOI: 10.1371/journal.pone.0294074

Ζωγάκη, Ε. (2020). Όψεις του πραγματικού: οι εικαστικές τέχνες και η ματιά του θεατή. Οπτική αντίληψη, αισθητικές θεωρίες και καλλιτεχνικές συμβάσεις. Στο Αθανασέκου (Επιμ.) *Γιατί με αφορά η τέχνη (σελ.331-347).* Αθήνα: Ηδυέπεια.

About the Contributors

Agathi Argyriadi is a Psychologist with specialization on Cognitive – Behavioral Psychotherapy and Developmental Psychology. Her PhD thesis is entitled "The effects of "Aesthetic flow experiences" in school's environment of first graders. A psycho-educational approach". She also holds a M.Ed. on Special Education and a second Master on Counseling. She is a Lecturer in the Department of Education at Frederick University, teaching developmental and cognitive psychology. In the past she has also taught at Cyprus University of Technology (Therapeutic communication), at the East London University (Research Methods and Statistics) and at the Technological Educational Institute of Peloponnese at the department of Speech Pathology (teaching Developmental Psychology and Clinical Neuropsychology), for 3 years. She has acted as a self- employed Psychologist and for a 3-year project against violence at the Ministry of Internal Affairs of the Hellenic Republic. She has also acted for two years, as an external associate at a private school in Greece, with the aim of monitoring and supporting students with learning difficulties, psychological problems and counseling of parents. Agathi Argyriadi was also a professor at the Foundation for Youth and Lifelong Learning and specifically at the Institute for Vocational Training of the Ministry of Education. She has published articles in international journals and she has participated in numerous of training seminars. She is the writer of 10 scientific books in the field of psychology. Her research interests focus on optimizing learning environments using positive psychology and aesthetic theories, developmental psychological issues, special education field, social inclusion issues. She teaches in the Distance Learning Program of Special Education.

Alexandros Argyriadis is an Assistant Professor in mental health at the Hellenic Mediterranean University in Crete, Greece.

***

Maria Athanasekou is an Art Historian, a graduate of the School of Philosophy of the National and Kapodistrian University of Athens, with postgraduate studies in Art History at the University of London, and a PhD holder from the School of Architecture of the National Technical University of Athens (NTUA). She currently teaches at the Hellenic Open University and Frederick University, and has taught at the Department of Early Childhood Education (TEAPI) at NUA, the Faculty of Philosophy (Department of History and Archaeology) at NUA, the University of the Aegean, the University of Western Macedonia, the Alexander Technological Educational Institute of Thessaloniki, among others. She is a member of the European research team COST Action, representing Greece on the "Perinatal Mental Health and Birth-Related Trauma: Maximising Best Practice and Optimal Outcomes" (DEVoTION) CA18211, serving on its Management Committee. She regularly gives public lectures on topics related to Art History for a range of institutions. She participates actively in international conferences, and her academic work includes peer-reviewed journal articles, book chapters, and published monographs in both print and digital form. Her research interests are interdisciplinary, always oriented toward the intersection of art, therapy, and education. She has received advanced training in Art Therapy, Children's Drawing Interpretation, Intercultural Education, Digital Education, Special Education, Psychology, Neuropsychology, Folklore Studies, and more, and is a certified adult educator. Her approach to art is deeply interdisciplinary, drawing insights from related fields such as Anthropology, Psychology, Folklore, and Sociology, with the aim of fostering a meaningful connection between students and art. She is passionate about telling the stories of art, sharing them, and engaging with others through the visual image. She believes that art holds immense power and a wealth of stories—many, if not all, of which concern us or will concern us at some point in our lives, as our existential field of experience continues to expand. Her teaching invites reflection, emotional connection, and critical thinking, highlighting the transformative and therapeutic dimensions of art in education and beyond.

Shreya Ghosh is an Assistant Professor at PES University, Bangalore, and a research scholar with a strong passion for inquiry and innovation. Her interests lie in neuroscience, psychology, human relations, and sustainable development. She explores how psychological principles and neuroscientific insights support emotional regulation, cognitive balance, sustainable practices, and elder well-being, while integrating perspectives from wisdom traditions.

Antonis Zagorianakos holds a degree in Mathematics from the National and Kapodistrian University of Athens (NKUA), as well as a Master's in the Epistemology and Didactics of Mathematics from the same institution. He completed his PhD at

Manchester Metropolitan University with a full tuition scholarship, focusing on the emergence of intuition and supervision in students during mathematical activities. He currently teaches Mathematics in Secondary Education and has also taught for six years at the Department of Early Childhood Education (TEAPI, NKUA). His research has expanded to include young children in preschool and early primary school settings. His academic interests involve authoring scientific articles presented at both international and Greek conferences. In addition to his teaching and writing, Dr. Zagorianakos is actively engaged in designing educational interventions that integrate creative, tactile, and conceptual approaches to mathematics learning. His work is deeply rooted in the belief that mathematical understanding is not only cognitive but also embodied and intuitive.

Index

A

C

D

E

S

T

W

www.ingramcontent.com/pod-product-compliance
Lightning Source LLC
LaVergne TN
LVHW081521300926
849161LV00006B/1246